Nuclear Pharmacy

Nuclear Pharmacy
Concepts and Applications

Edited by
Blaine Templar Smith RPh, PhD

Saint Joseph College School of Pharmacy, West Hartford, CT, USA

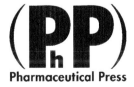

Pharmaceutical Press

This book is dedicated to Joan Templar Smith PhD, without whose
tireless and relentless editorial prowess this book would be much less
of a happy success. Many thanks and gratitude for your work.
This book is also dedicated to the authors who came together and
created what we all hope is a good teaching tool. Through all the
work, everyone kept this adventure intact despite numerous
slow-downs and speed-ups.

Published by Pharmaceutical Press
66-68 East Smithfield, London E1W 1AW, UK

© Pharmaceutical Press 2010

(**P.P**) is a trade mark of Pharmaceutical Press

Pharmaceutical Press is the publishing division of the Royal Pharmaceutical Society of
Great Britain

First published 2010

Typeset by Thomson Digital, Noida, India
Printed in Great Britain by TJ International, Padstow, Cornwall

ISBN 978 0 85369 866 1

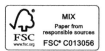

Contents

Preface

This book was written with the professional pharmacy student in mind, but also with the desire that the book would be useful to others, such as pharmacists, physicians, nuclear pharmacists, nuclear medicine technologists, and graduate students performing research in this field.

Often there is a desire to have in the pharmacy curriculum an elective or specialty track that differs from those traditionally offered in most pharmacy programs. This book is intended to provide material not only for the students but also for those instructors who may be reticent to teach an elective course in an area outside their expertise.

A synopsis of the topics covered in this book is provided in Chapter 1. The topics range from an introduction to basic nuclear physics, radioactive decay, radiopharmaceuticals, and the practice of nuclear pharmacy, to the methods for acquiring and using radiopharmaceuticals in the nuclear medicine unit.

It is hoped that teachers and students with no experience in this area can read and use this book and come away with confidence that nuclear pharmacy is not an impossible, untouchable topic. Neither teachers nor students need to become experts in the field of nuclear pharmacy in order to experience and enjoy the trip into this other world. For those wishing to pursue nuclear pharmacy further, this will provide a first step and allow them to decide if the area is of interest to them.

For teachers and instructors, it is hoped that this book will provide a practical guide to use in teaching. If you have no prior experience in nuclear pharmacy, it is hoped that by reading this book you will lose all trepidation and feel confident to teach an elective course in this area. Perhaps you will go further, and decide to begin a specialty track for your students, if none yet exists. In any case, enjoy, and best wishes.

Blaine Templar Smith
June, 2009

About the editor

Blaine Templar Smith RPh, PhD is a graduate of the University of Oklahoma College of Pharmacy and Nuclear Pharmacy programs and currently Chair of the Department of Pharmaceutical Sciences at Saint Joseph College (Connecticut) School of Pharmacy. His areas of expertise include immunology, molecular biology, and the application of radioactive and non-radioactive tracers for diagnostic and therapeutic purposes.

Dr. Smith has taught for 20 years at the university level, in the areas of pharmaceutics, immunology, molecular biology, and nuclear pharmacy. He is a member of the American Society of Health-System Pharmacists, the American Association of Colleges of Pharmacy, the Massachusetts Pharmacists Association, the Connecticut Pharmacists Association, and as a member of these organizations, has edited and published scientific and educational materials.

His primary interest has been the improvement of pedagogy and pedagogical materials for undergraduate professional pharmacy students. But his interests have also included the needs of graduate students, medical students, nuclear pharmacists, nuclear medicine technologists, pharmacists, and physicians.

Dr. Smith is an avid runner, professional cellist, and appreciator of nature and the great outdoors. He believes that, with the help of the health sciences, the world can be a healthier, happier, and safer place to live.

Contributors

Edward M. Bednarczyk   School of Pharmacy and Pharmaceutical Sciences, University at Buffalo, State University of New York, NY, USA.

William Crisp   Purdue University School of Pharmacy and Pharmaceutical Sciences, West Lafayette, IN, USA.

Wendy Galbraith   University of Oklahoma College of Pharmacy, Oklahoma City, OK, USA.

Vesper Grantham   College of Allied Health and Department of Medical Imaging and Radiation Sciences, University of Oklahoma Health Sciences Center, Oklahoma City, OK, USA.

Blaine Templar Smith   Department of Pharmaceutical Sciences, Saint Joseph College (Connecticut) School of Pharmacy, West Hartford, CT, USA.

Kara Duncan Weatherman   Purdue University School of Pharmacy and Pharmaceutical Sciences, West Lafayette, IN, USA.

Hannah Weber   Purdue University School of Pharmacy and Pharmaceutical Sciences, West Lafayette, IN, USA.

Jan M. Winn   Winn Educational Management Corporation, Edmond, OK, USA.

1

Radioactive drugs in medicine: radiopharmaceuticals

Blaine T. Smith

Learning objectives

- Describe what the field of nuclear pharmacy is
- Differentiate between a conventional and a nuclear pharmacy
- Delineate the activities and roles of a nuclear pharmacist
- Explain why radioactive drugs have usefulness
- Understand and explain the need for background knowledge in the field of nuclear pharmacy
- Define what is meant by a tracer study
- Describe the various levels of authority that regulate the practice of nuclear pharmacy
- Explain, in general, how a radioactive material can be made useful as a 'drug'
- Explain why positron-emitting radiopharmaceuticals are special
- Describe, in general, why non-radioactive drugs sometimes are used in conjunction with radioactive drugs
- Define a nuclear medicine procedure.

Nuclear pharmacy

Nuclear pharmacy, a specialty practice of pharmacy that employs the use of radioactive drugs for diagnosis and therapy, is one of the specialties recognized by the US Board of Pharmaceutical Specialties. The Board grants the nuclear pharmacist certification in nuclear pharmacy (Board Certified Nuclear Pharmacist [BCNP]).

Nuclear pharmacy regulations require the nuclear pharmacist to select the proper radioisotope and, in most cases of radiopharmaceuticals, reagent (or carrier compound) for a prescribed procedure. The joining of the reagent, or 'cold kit,' to the isotope results in a radiopharmaceutical. Before radiopharmaceuticals can be administered to patients, the pharmacist must ensure their sterility, purity, and identity, using various techniques unique to the nuclear pharmacy setting. The nuclear pharmacist is also responsible for the proper packaging, transport, and delivery of radiopharmaceuticals to the nuclear medicine facility, where the radiopharmaceutical will be used for imaging or treatment purposes.

Analogous to a traditional pharmacist, the nuclear pharmacist is responsible for providing 'radiopharmaceutical care' to patients, which includes supplying information, assessing outcomes of procedures and interventions, and assessing potential adverse effects or contraindications that may be important in some patients. Like traditional pharmacists, nuclear pharmacists evaluate and process prescriptions, but their prescriptions originate from nuclear medicine physicians or their supervised representatives.

Nuclear pharmacy is to nuclear medicine what pharmacy is to medicine. As in traditional pharmacy practice, nuclear pharmacy requires a thorough knowledge of drugs, indications, adverse effects, allergies, and contraindications. In addition, it requires the knowledge needed to become expert in the mechanisms of radioactive decay. It is necessary to understand what radiation is, how to utilize it safely, and how to protect personnel and patients from unnecessary exposure. As with traditional pharmacy, nuclear pharmacy has seen the introduction of increasing numbers of biotechnology-based drugs. And, as with traditional pharmacy, these new drugs introduce new requirements for storage, preparation, and administration.

The nuclear pharmacist

The duties of the nuclear pharmacist are, in most ways, very similar to those of a traditional pharmacist. However, since the nuclear pharmacist deals with radioactive drugs, there is an added layer of regulation, knowledge, and skill that he/she must master beyond that of the traditional pharmacist.

A nuclear pharmacist's duties are similar to those of a traditional pharmacist's in that a nuclear pharmacist procures, compounds, assures quality, dispenses, and distributes radiopharmaceuticals. The main distinguishing feature of a nuclear pharmacist's work is that most of the drugs he/she deals with are radioactive. Also, like a traditional pharmacist, the nuclear pharmacist monitors patient outcomes and provides information to, and consults with, the nuclear medicine team to ensure the highest possible quality of care.

Nuclear pharmacists are responsible for preparing or compounding radiopharmaceuticals and ensuring their safety, efficacy, and purity until administered to the patient. They work in a variety of settings. A nuclear pharmacy can stand alone in a different location from the nuclear medicine center; within a hospital, where it can be conveniently located near the nuclear medicine facility; or within an academic setting, where it serves as both pharmacy and teaching facility for students and pharmacists wishing to specialize in nuclear pharmacy. Nuclear pharmacists may also participate in industry as researchers involved in nuclear medicine 'kit' formulation and preparation (materials assembled prior to mixing radioactivity) or at government and private research institutions.

Radioactive drugs in medicine

Pharmaceuticals are dosage forms or 'drug delivery systems' that deliver a specific amount of drug to a target system. Radiopharmaceuticals are drug delivery systems that deliver radioactivity to the desired tissue(s) in the body. Among the few exceptions are diagnostic laboratory procedures that utilize human tissues outside the body, but these are encountered less frequently than those that are administered directly to the patients. Most radiopharmaceuticals are administered parenterally, though there are a few that utilize the oral route of administration. The focus of this book is on typical radiopharmaceuticals and the typical practice of nuclear pharmacy.

Radiopharmaceuticals are drugs that are radioactive. Normally, they consist of a 'cold' (non-radioactive) chemical component that will eventually be coupled with a radioisotope. This chemical component of the 'kit' is crucial to the delivery of the radiopharmaceutical to its target. Radiopharmaceuticals are useful because certain of their isotopes emit radiation that can be detected by specialized instruments, which turn the emissions into images from inside the body. These images allow actual physiological processes to be observed, rather than the static images seen with other imaging systems. Radiopharmaceuticals can also be therapeutic in nature. Some isotopes emit radioactivity that is intended to damage tissues and DNA. This can be useful when the desired outcome is to destroy aberrant or cancerous cells.

Thus, while some radiopharmaceuticals are designed to give nearly harmless emissions for imaging that can provide physiological information ('X-rays from the inside out'), other radiopharmaceuticals can be prepared that are therapeutic and intentionally harmful to targeted tissue. The importance of both types of radiopharmaceutical lies in their ability to target specific tissues and exclude others. The role of the nuclear pharmacist is to ensure the proper preparation of the chemical couplers with the correct type and amount of radioisotope.

Radioactivity and radioactive decay

To understand radiopharmaceuticals, a sound foundation knowledge of the structure of atoms, the mechanisms of radioactive decay, and the mathematics required in the preparation of radiopharmaceuticals is required. The reader must have a fundamental understanding of the effects of different radiations on the body, limits of exposure, methods of protection, and so on. These areas of study are called radiation biology and health physics.

Because this book is meant as an introduction or primer, its discussion will begin with these basic topics: (1) the components of the atom and how they act, (2) what controls the actions of the nucleus, (3) what controls radiation, (4) the different routes of radioactive decomposition and the causes, (5) the emissions that occur as a result of radioactive decay, and (6) the mathematics involved in radioactive decay. These topics will be discussed in Chapter 2.

The study of radioactivity is immersed in mathematics, at least at a college calculus level. Much of nuclear pharmacy includes mathematics derived from nuclear physics, and it therefore needs to be understood to be able to make sense of the nature and actions of radioisotopes.

Radiopharmaceuticals

Because radiopharmaceuticals show physiology, rather than anatomy, they are valuable tools for evaluating processes in the body in real time. Specialized detectors (cameras) collect the radiation emanated from the body and show spatially where the radiation originated. In this way images are made. The more radioactive emissions a specific area of the body gives off, the more 'exposed' the detector assembly is, and this correlates with what is happening and where it is happening in the body. As mentioned above, specialized equipment makes possible the creation of static pictures, and even motion pictures, of what is happening inside the body.

The amounts of radioactivity used are so small that the nuclear medicine procedures are also referred to as 'tracer procedures.' The nuclear pharmacist and nuclear medicine professionals must have a good understanding of physiological behavior in order to understand the information provided by nuclear medicine images. Like traditional drugs, radiopharmaceuticals follow the ADME sequence (absorption, distribution, metabolism, and excretion), though most bypass the absorption step, since they are parenterally administered. Cleverly designed procedures can reveal extraordinary information that is useful for diagnosing and treating patients. These topics are covered in Chapter 3.

Nuclear pharmacy operations

Radiopharmaceutical preparation and administration must follow rules set forth by the US Drug Enforcement Agency (DEA), the US *Pharmacopeia* (USP), and the Best Practices regulations. Being radioactive, radiopharmaceuticals are also subject to additional rules and oversight by the state and/or the Nuclear Regulatory Commission (NRC) and the Environmental Protection Agency.

Nuclear pharmacy practice sites can be found in many locations. Most often they are near the nuclear medicine facilities that use their products. Because positron-emitting radiopharmaceuticals have very short lifespans, they must be prepared close to the nuclear medicine facilities. Radiopharmaceuticals are prepared at a nuclear pharmacy and then transported to the various nuclear medicine departments in a timely manner.

Preparation of radiopharmaceuticals must follow state and federal regulations. Since most radiopharmaceuticals are injectible, they must also be sterile. Experience in a conventional sterile compounding facility is definitely an advantage for those intending to prepare radiopharmaceuticals. Radiopharmaceuticals, like conventional pharmaceuticals, require a valid prescription in order to be dispensed. These are usually communicated via telephone by nuclear medicine technologists in the nuclear medicine facility, acting on behalf of a nuclear medicine physician or radiologist.

Quality control is a greater consideration of the nuclear pharmacist than it is of the conventional pharmacist. Since nearly all of the radiopharmaceuticals are compounded on-site, they must be guaranteed to have sterility and accuracy of preparation.

The nuclear pharmacy also serves as a storage area for radioactive material and biohazardous materials. The radioactive material is allowed to decay in the pharmacy, or it is shipped to a location where it can be safely stored. These issues are discussed in Chapter 4.

Nuclear pharmacy practice

Nuclear pharmacy is a specialty area that requires additional training beyond that required for a standard pharmacy degree and licensure. Like other drugs, radioactive drugs have USP monographs that specify standards of purity, efficacy, and quality control.

A nuclear pharmacy uses products obtained from the decay of reactor materials and those from particle accelerators (linear accelerators and cyclotrons). Those products are purified before being used to radiolabel chemical compounds, referred to as 'kits.'

A kit contains all that is needed for the radiopharmaceutical of interest except the isotope. Proper labeling of the kit ensures a radiopharmaceutical product that localizes in a desired area of the body. A few of these products (reactor and accelerator products) are made available in large renewable bulk containers called generators.

Generators allow the nuclear pharmacy to maintain an inventory of its most essential isotopes (mainly technetium-99m [^{99m}Tc], which will be described below) without the necessity of having daily deliveries. This is because the generators create more of the isotope to replace nearly all that was taken previously. So, in essence, for ^{99m}Tc, the generator acts as a ^{99m}Tc vending machine, supplying each day's needs of that isotope, and continuing to do so for several days.

These topics are discussed in Chapter 5.

Turning radioisotopes into drugs

A nuclear pharmacist must be aware of potential chemical incompatibilities and drug interactions in patients, and take precautions to avoid these. The nuclear pharmacist must also know the indications, dosing, and so on for radiopharmaceuticals.

Ultimately, it should be of interest to the reader to find out how kits are prepared and what the various radiolabeled kits are used for. After understanding the aspects of kit compounding, applications of the radiopharmaceuticals is the next information of importance. Kits are usually used for 'tracer studies.' These are procedures that require minute amounts of radiopharmaceuticals to identify any internal abnormalities.

As with conventional pharmaceuticals, radiopharmaceuticals are studied for their pharmacology; pharmacokinetics; biodistribution; mechanisms of uptake, action, and excretion; drug interactions; and contraindications. Each radiopharmaceutical must have a drug monograph, just as conventional pharmaceuticals do.

In addition to gathering all of this information, the effects of the emitted radiation on the body also need to be studied and quantified. It is necessary for the nuclear pharmacist to be familiar with all of these data, and to be prepared to answer questions from the rest of the nuclear medicine team, especially if something wrong occurs with an administration.

These are topics that are discussed in Chapter 6.

Positron-emitting radiopharmaceuticals

A specialized category of radiopharmaceuticals includes those used for positron emission tomography (PET). These radiopharmaceuticals are often incorporated into naturally occurring biological substances or into compounds that are similar to natural substances. Positrons (β^+) offer superior imaging possibilities, when used appropriately. They require somewhat different isotope carriers and imaging equipment than standard radiopharmaceuticals. The advantage of PET is the prevalence of organic isotopes that lend themselves to imaging biochemistry-based physiological processes. The most common isotopes used for positron imaging include those of carbon, oxygen, nitrogen, and fluorine.

PET imaging requires specialized equipment, which will be described in Chapter 7. PET radiopharmaceuticals have found use in oncology, and in brain and myocardial imaging, among others. Because this is a relatively new branch of nuclear pharmacy and nuclear medicine, it is certain that more applications will be forthcoming.

Non-radioactive drugs used in nuclear medicine

Occasionally, non-radioactive drugs are used to facilitate or enhance the effects of radiopharmaceuticals. These are called interventional agents. Interventional agents are non-radioactive drugs given to patients to cause the body to react in such a way that the procedure results are optimized. The procedures using these drugs are numerous and include inducing artificial cardiac stress, causing the gall bladder to contract, and preparing the area where radiopharmaceuticals will concentrate during brain imaging.

Because interventional agents are drugs, they must be documented as to their mechanisms of action, safety, efficacy, pharmacology, pharmacokinetics, adverse effects, conditions, and contraindications. These are discussed in Chapter 8.

The nuclear medicine procedure

The nuclear pharmacist is part of a team that also includes nuclear medicine technologists, nuclear medicine physicians, and health physicists. These team members are part of a nuclear medicine unit of a hospital or imaging center. Bringing together the expertise of these team members makes possible the performance of nuclear medicine procedures.

There are many different types of procedures. Nearly every organ of the body can be targeted for imaging or therapy. The nuclear pharmacist's duties include not only preparing the radiopharmaceuticals but also providing counseling and educational insights to patients and various clinicians. It is important that the nuclear pharmacist keeps up to date on the latest information regarding the proper use of radiopharmaceuticals, the newly introduced radiopharmaceuticals, and any potential problems or benefits of radiopharmaceuticals that research reveals.

It has become increasingly important for the nuclear pharmacist to assess patient care by reviewing appropriateness of procedures, doses, and administrations. For this reason, the nuclear pharmacist must be intimately familiar not only with the instruments used in the nuclear pharmacy but also with those used for performing procedures in the nuclear medicine unit. Mastery of conventional pharmaceuticals and a solid background in physiology, anatomy, and immunology are all imperative in order to be competent in all of the functions of a nuclear pharmacist.

Nuclear medicine procedures in clinical applications are covered in Chapter 9, which is written from the unique perspective of a nuclear medicine technologist describing the procedures. This chapter will bring the entire information in this book to a sensible and practical conclusion. Instrumentation will be discussed in more detail, and each organ system will be individually analyzed in regard to the types of imaging or therapy that are currently in use in nuclear medicine units. Patient preparation, dosing of radiopharmaceuticals, imaging, treatment, patient monitoring, and scan monitoring are all discussed in this culminating chapter.

Summary

Nuclear pharmacy is a specialty practice within pharmaceutical practice, and is recognized by the Board of Pharmaceutical Specialties. With study and expertise, a pharmacist can become board certified (BCNP). Duties of the nuclear pharmacist mirror many of those of a conventional pharmacist, but there is the added layer of regulation and specialization that comes from dealing with radioactive substances.

Compounding or mixing materials (commonly known as kits) is more important in nuclear pharmacy than in most conventional settings. Mathematics, radiation physics, and radiation biology play more central roles in nuclear pharmacy than they do in conventional pharmacy. Like conventional pharmaceuticals, radiopharmaceuticals have drug monographs and all the requirements of prescription medications.

There are various types of radioactive emission from different isotopes, some requiring very different detection equipment than others. The nuclear pharmacist must be familiar with these. Of particular distinction is the category of positron-emitting radiopharmaceuticals. Though most drugs prepared by a nuclear pharmacist are radioactive, there are some that are not radioactive but still have importance in nuclear pharmacy.

The nuclear pharmacist is part of an integrated team that includes the pharmacist, nuclear medicine technologists, nuclear medicine physicians, and radiologists. When all the members work together, successful nuclear medicine procedures can be performed, leading to proper diagnosis and treatment of patients.

Self-assessment questions

1 Nuclear pharmacy is:
a a centralized pharmacy in a hospital that distributes crucial medications
b a specialty practice of pharmacy that employs the use of radioactive drugs for diagnosis and therapy
c a specialty area of pharmacy recognized by the American Association of Practicing Physicists
d an area of pharmacy that specializes in isolating subatomic particles for research purposes
e a specialty area of pharmacy that employs the use of DNA for diagnosis and therapy.

2 The difference between a conventional pharmacy and a nuclear pharmacy is that:
a a nuclear pharmacy must be located within a hospital
b a radiopharmaceutical is a hospital chart order and requires no formal prescription
c quality control is not as important in nuclear pharmacy as in conventional pharmacy
d nuclear pharmacy is responsible to the state and/or Nuclear Regulatory Commission; conventional pharmacy is not
e most radiopharmaceuticals are dispensed for therapeutic purposes.

3 The activities and roles of a nuclear pharmacist are to:
a inject radioactive drugs into patients
b prepare imaging equipment for nuclear medicine procedures
c be knowledgeable in regard to potential adverse reactions or results from studies
d perform routine inspections of nuclear medicine clinics
e prepare sterile vials containing the chemicals necessary to prepare radiopharmaceuticals.

4 Radioactive drugs are useful because:
a they decay rapidly and so are useful for diagnosis, but not for therapy
b they are the best drugs for treating congestive heart failure
c the patient is typically very compliant for fear of getting radiation poisoning
d one radiopharmaceutical can be used for all possible procedures, simplifying the job of the nuclear pharmacist
e they can show both anatomical features and also physiological features of the body.

5 Background knowledge is required for the field of nuclear pharmacy because:

   a   nuclear physics and mathematics, including calculus, are essential for the role of nuclear pharmacist

   b   injecting patients will be simplified

   c   it is the job of the nuclear pharmacist to interpret the imaging results

   d   the pharmacist must predict when each drug will be completely eliminated from each patient

   e   trigonometry is required to calculate the angle that radioactivity is coming from.

6 A 'tracer study' is:

   a   a small capsule injected into an artery and followed throughout the circulatory system

   b   reveals what the patient has eaten in the past 24 hours

   c   a procedure that require minute amounts of radiopharmaceuticals to identify any internal abnormalities

   d   reveals all of the coarse anatomy of the patient

   e   allows the patient to be found again after the administration of the radiopharmaceutical.

7 The practice of nuclear pharmacy is regulated by the following authorities:

   a   the local police department must give permission for the establishment of a nuclear pharmacy

   b   the Drug Enforcement Agency (DEA) has authority over the practice of nuclear pharmacy

   c   the National Institutes of Health must approve of each type of procedure

   d   the state boards of pharmacy must maintain copies of all radioactivity used by the nuclear pharmacy

   e   the Department of Human Services must ensure all procedures are performed without charge to the patient.

8 In general, a radioactive material can be made useful as a 'drug' by:

   a   applying it sparingly to the external area of the body so that radiation can pass through to the other side of the body and an image can be made

   b   repeated doses allows an equilibrium to be established so that the patient can be imaged

   c   preceding the radioactive drug with a traditional drug, so that the traditional drug is labeled with radioactivity and can be followed through the body

   d   attaching it to a chemical 'kit,' which enables it to localize where desired e   injecting a kit into a patient, followed by radioactivity so that it is simple to visualize details of the body.

9 Positron-emitting radiopharmaceuticals are given special treatment because:

   a   they require somewhat different isotope carriers and imaging equipment

   b   they give positive results from procedures, rather than negative results from negatrons

   c   they can be imaged from much further away from the patient than other radiopharmaceuticals

   d   they require less-complex machinery to gather an image than other types of radiopharmaceutical

   e   they are less dangerous for patients.

10 In general, non-radioactive drugs are sometimes used in conjunction with radioactive drugs:

   a   in case the radioactive drugs do not work properly

   b   to decrease life-threatening toxicity to the patient

   c   to block the radiopharmaceutical from accessing unnecessary areas of the body

   d   because they can sometimes be seen just as effectively on imaging machinery as radioactive drugs

   e   to facilitate or enhance the effects of radiopharmaceuticals.

11 The following can be called a 'nuclear medicine procedure':

   a   using radioactivity to dissolve scar tissue

   b   implanting a radioactive capsule into a patient so the patient will not get lost

   c   targeting a specific organ of the body for imaging purposes

   d   leaving a small amount of radioactivity at a surgical incision site to assist the surgeon

   e   injecting a dye into a patient before exposing the patient to an X-ray machine.

2

Introduction to radioactivity and radioactive decay

Blaine T. Smith

Learning objectives

- Name the major components of an atom
- Describe the four forces in nature and their relevance to the atom
- Calculate energy, atomic mass, and binding energy for nuclei and electrons
- Use the standard definitions and nomenclature for describing nuclides
- Understand the use and application of decay schemes for radionuclides
- Describe different radioactive emissions and how these emissions can interact with matter
- Calculate a radionuclide's decay rate, decay constant, and the amount of radionuclide remaining at different times during decay
- Discuss the units used, and the importance of the effects of radiation exposure.

The atom

The atom has at its center a positively charged nucleus. Surrounding the nucleus is a cloud of up to 100 negatively charged electrons, which rotate around the nucleus along various energy orbits. Normally, the overall nuclear charge is equal in magnitude, but opposite in sign, to the overall electron charge, leaving the atom electrically neutral. The radius of the nucleus, approximately $0.0001\,\text{Å}$ ($10^{-13}\,\text{cm}$ [NB $100\,\text{pm} = 1\,\text{Å}$]), is only a minute percentage of the volume of the entire atom. The nucleus is composed mainly of nucleons, which are protons and neutrons.

Protons

A proton is a nucleon possessing a positive charge. Its mass, $1.6726 \times 10^{-24}\,\text{g}$, is approximately 1836 times that of an orbital electron (http://hyperphysics. phy-astr.gsu.edu/hbase/Tables/funcon.html; http://periodic.lanl.gov/default. htm). The number of protons in the nucleus is referred to as the atomic number (Z).

As will be discussed below, mass can be expressed in terms of atomic mass units (AMU) or in million electronvolts (MeV). A proton has a mass of $1.00728\,\text{AMU}$ or $938.27\,\text{MeV}$.

Neutrons

A neutron is a nucleon that carries no charge. Its mass, which is similar to that of a proton, is $1.6749 \times 10^{-24}\,\text{g}$ ($1.00867\,\text{AMU}$ or $939.57\,\text{MeV}$) (http:// periodic.lanl.gov/default.htm). The total number of neutrons in the nucleus is referred to as the neutron number (N).

Neutrons and protons are held to each other by the strong interaction or nuclear binding force, one of the four fundamental forces in nature. The total number of nucleons (protons plus neutrons) in a nucleus is $Z + N$, and is given the letter A. Although the mass of a nucleus from the periodic table or chart of the nuclides is *not* an integer, it is expressed for our initial purposes as A in the equation $A = Z + N$ (MIRDTrilinear Chart of the Nuclides http://wwwndc.jaea.go.jp/CN04). This discrepancy is caused by the nuclear binding energy, which will be discussed below.

In a given element, the number of protons is equal to the number of electrons, resulting in an overall neutral charge for the atom. The electron configuration determines *chemical* properties of an element. The *nuclear structure* determines the stability and the propensity for radioactive decay of the atom's nucleus.

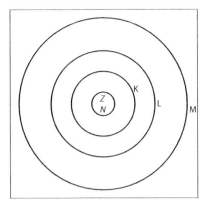

Figure 2.1 An atom with three potential orbitals levels for electrons (*K*, *L*, and *M* shells) surrounding a nucleus containing protons (*Z*) and neutrons (*N*).

Electrons

An electron, with a mass of 9.1094×10^{-28} g (0.000549 AMU, 0.511 MeV), moves in energy levels, not paths, around the nucleus (http://hyperphysics. phy-astr.gsu.edu/hbase/Tables/funcon.html). Lower orbitals (those closer to the nucleus) possess higher kinetic energy and lower potential energy. The electron cloud surrounding an atom has order, in that the electrons orbit at defined energy levels or shells (K, L, M, N, etc.). These shells increase in potential energy the farther from the nucleus they are. If an electron moves from a shell farther from the nucleus to one closer to the nucleus, energy must be released. Conversely, energy must be provided to an electron in order for it to move outward (Figure 2.1).

Again, while nuclear reactions occur in the nucleus, chemical reactions occur with the movement of electrons, and require as little as 10 eV to initiate. This will be important to remember later, when electron binding energy and radiation biology are discussed.

Atomic dimensions

An atom is approximately 10^{-8} cm (approximately 1 Å or 100 pm) in size. As mentioned above, the nucleus is approximately 10^{-13} cm or one fermi (1 F) in size. And, although it contains almost 100% of the atom's mass, its volume is approximately 1/1 000 000 000 000th of the entire volume of the atom. An analogy illustrating the extreme differences in size would be: if an entire atom were a 100 m (round) football field, the nucleus would be approximately 1 cm in size, a proton 1 mm, and an electron would be a mere dot in space.

Atoms follow the basic rules of thermodynamics and physics. Nucleons and electrons tend toward greater stability by giving off kinetic energy to lower their potential energy. Radioactive decay and the rearrangements of electrons occur in order to make more stable the lower potential energy configurations of the nuclear and electron energy levels, respectively.

Definitions: the nuclear language

- *Radioactive*. The term radioactive means the random and spontaneous disintegration(s) of atomic nuclei that are unstable because of energetically unfavorable nuclear configurations. This involves nuclei moving from higher to lower potential energy states, leading ultimately to stable (non-radioactive) nuclear arrangements. The potential energy is carried away from the nucleus or surrounding electron cloud by various particulate and photon emissions. These radiations take on the forms of α, β^- (negatron, essentially an electron), β^+ (positron), X-rays, and γ photons.
- *Nuclide*. A nuclide is any identifiable atomic species. It has a definite number of protons (Z) and a definite number of neutrons (N).
- *Radionuclide*. This is a radioactive nuclide.
- *Element*. An element is a nuclide with a defined Z (atomic number). For example, if Z is 53, the element is iodine, though the isotope (see below) is not defined.
- *Symbol identification*. A nuclide or radionuclide can be identified by labeling its symbol with three numbers that represent (1) its mass (A), the sum of the number of protons and neutrons; (2) its atomic number (Z), the number of protons; and (3) the number of neutrons (N) (Figure 2.2).
- *Isotopes*. (Derived from the Greek word for 'same place'.) These are nuclides that have the same atomic number (Z) but differ in atomic mass (A). Isotopes also have the same number of electrons and, therefore, possess the same chemical properties. (As stated above, the electron level is where chemical reactions occur.) Some isotopes are stable, others radioactive. For example, ^{14}C and ^{15}C are radioactive isotopes of carbon, while ^{12}C and ^{13}C are not. These differences reflect differing stabilities of the nuclei (Figure 2.3). Generally, elements with lower Z numbers tend to have fewer isotopes than elements with higher Z numbers.

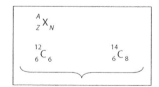

Figure 2.2 Basic nomenclature of a nuclide. A is the mass number, the sum of the number of protons and neutrons; Z is the atomic number, the number of protons; and N is the number of neutrons. The lower part of the figure shows two nuclides of carbon. Note that the number of protons remains the same in both nuclides, while the neutron numbers differ to balance.

$$^{1}_{6}C_{6} \quad ^{13}_{6}C_{7} \quad ^{14}_{6}C_{8} \quad ^{15}_{6}C_{9}$$

Figure 2.3 Isotopes. Examples here are for carbon, where the number of protons (Z) is 6 for all four isotopes of the same element.

$$^{65}_{29}Cu \quad ^{65}_{30}Zn$$

Figure 2.4 Isobars. Examples here are different elements, as it is the atomic number Z that determines the element.

- *Isobars.* These are nuclides that have the same atomic mass (A) but differ from each other in atomic number (Z) and so also in neutron number (N). An example is the pair of isobars copper-65 and zinc-65 (^{65}Cu and ^{65}Zn). These are two different elements, since it is the atomic number that determines the element (Figure 2.4).
- *Isomers.* Nuclides with the same atomic mass (A) and the same atomic number (Z) are known as isomers. The only difference is that one of the isomers is in an excited (metastable) state, and this results in two different energy levels. An example is technetium, where the isomer ^{99m}Tc 'decays' to ^{99}Tc, while emitting a gamma photon (γ) to balance the overall energy. This is written as ^{99m}Tc $\rightarrow$ ^{99}Tc $+ \gamma$. (Gamma photons will be discussed below.) An isomer is indicated by a lower case 'm' next to the atomic number. Figure 2.5 shows a general form of isomeric decay, or 'isomeric transition.' Isomeric transitions will be discussed in more detail later in the text.
- *Isotones.* Nuclides that have the same number of neutrons (N) but differ in atomic mass (A) are known as isotones; they also differ in the number of protons. An example is the two elements, hydrogen and helium. Both have one neutron, but hydrogen has one proton and helium has two (Figure 2.6).
- *Ions.* Atoms with a net electrical charge, postive or negative, are known as ions. Because ionization is an electronic state, not a nuclear state, ions can be radionuclides or simply nuclides. An ion's net charge is determined by

$$^{Am}_{Z}X_N \rightarrow ^{A}_{Z}X_N + \gamma$$

Figure 2.5 Isomers, showing a general form of isomeric decay, or isomeric transition.

$$^{2}_{1}H_1 \quad ^{3}_{2}He_1$$

Figure 2.6 Isotones: hydrogen has one proton and helium has two.

the lack, or excess, of one or more electrons from the atom's electron cloud.

Nuclear forces

There are four fundamental forces: gravitational, electromagnetic (coulombic), strong interaction (strong nuclear), and weak interaction (weak nuclear).

- *Gravitational force.* This is principally involved in interactions between large objects. It is too weak at the atomic level to be of much consequence in its effects and is, therefore, not as important at the nuclear level as other forces.
- *Electromagnetic (coulombic) force.* This force, acting mainly outside the nucleus, is exerted on electrically charged particles. An attractive force, it is responsible for holding electrons and protons together in atoms. To understand the comparative strengths of the electromagnetic and gravitational forces, consider the following. The distance between an electron and a proton is roughly 5×10^{-9} cm. The electromagnetic force between the two is approximately 9.2×10^{-3} dynes, whereas the gravitational force is only around 4×10^{-42} dynes. It is obvious that gravitational force is negligible at the atomic level.
- *Strong interaction (strong nuclear) force.* This binds the nucleons together. Although it is much stronger than the electromagnetic force, it does not act outside the nucleus. The strong interaction force is approximately 100 times stronger than the electromagnetic force, approximately 10^{13} times greater than the weak interaction force (described below), and approximately 10^{38} times greater than the gravitational force. It is involved with collisions between protons and other particles. It is strong enough to keep protons proximal in the nucleus and to overcome charge repulsion between them. The strong interaction has no direct effect on electrons since they are extremely small in mass, and at a great distance from the nucleus.
- *Weak interaction (weak nuclear) force.* This is associated with beta and other nuclear decays; it acts over a relatively small range, approximately 10^{-16} cm, which is 1000 times smaller than the diameter of a nucleus. It plays an important role, since it is involved in radioactive decay. The weak interaction force is able to transform neutrons into protons, and protons into neutrons.

So, together, these fundamental forces (mostly the last three) dictate the actions and interactions that occur in the nucleus and the atom's electron cloud. All matter moves toward the configuration that is the most stable. It forfeits kinetic energy in order to move from a point of higher potential energy to one of lower potential energy. For atoms, this is manifest as the discharge of particles and rays from within the nucleus or from the surrounding electron cloud (http://230nsc1.phy-astr.gsu.edu/hbase/forces/funfor.html; http://imagine.gsfc.nasa.gov/docs/ask_astro/answers/980127c.html). These changes, these movements toward greater stability, are the origin of radioactivity and will, therefore, be thoroughly discussed below. Harnessing these emissions is at the core of nuclear pharmacy, nuclear medicine, and nuclear physics.

Radioactivity calculations

Nuclear pharmacy and nuclear medicine use many units for quantifying such items such as mass, exposure, dose, and radioactivity.

Mass units

The atomic mass unit (AMU) was introduced above. 1 AMU is 1.66053×10^{-24} g, which is understood to be one-twelfth the mass of a ^{12}C atom (Clarke et al. 1903; Mattauch 1958; http://hyperphysics.phy-astr.gsu.edu/hbase/Tables/funcon.html). The mass of a ^{12}C atom (six protons, six neutrons, and six electrons) is 1.992×10^{-23} g. The atomic mass unit for ^{12}C is therefore its mass divided by the mass of 1 AMU:

$$\frac{1.992 \times 10^{-23} \text{ g}}{^{12}\text{C}_{\text{atom}}} \times \frac{1 \text{ AMU}}{1.660 \times 10^{-24} \text{ g}} = 12.00 \text{ AMU}$$

The periodic table mass for ^{12}C is 12.011 g. The difference between the periodic table (or chart of the nuclides) mass for an atom and its AMU mass is called the **mass defect** (http://periodic.lanl.gov/default.htm; http://wwwndc.jaea.go.jp/CN04/). This difference is where the conversion between energy and mass occurs, and it is accounted for by the energy required to hold the atom together. This energy can be converted to mass, which is the mass defect.

Energy units

Units of energy are often useful, as well. Recall from physics that force equals mass times acceleration ($F = ma$), with one available unit for expression, the dyne. So, force can be measured in **dynes**. A dyne is an unbalanced push or pull, accelerating 1 g at 1 cm/s. The unit used for the dyne is mass multiplied by distance per time squared ($g \cdot cm/s^2$).

Another useful energy unit is the **electronvolt** (eV; usually seen as MeV, one million electronvolts); 1 MeV = 23,045,000 calories/mol. The electronvolt is not an SI (International System) unit. The electronvolt can be related to another energy term, the **erg** (the amount of work done by a force of one dyne exerted for a distance of one centimeter [$g \cdot cm^2/s^2$]), by the equation

Work = force × distance = energy

One erg is equal to 1.6022×10^{-6} MeV. This can then be used to derive the energy equivalent of 1 AMU. Using $E = mc^2$ to express energy, where c (the speed of light) is 2.997925×10^{10} cm/s, the energy of a mass of 1 AMU (or 1.66053×10^{-24} g) can be calculated as

$$E = mc^2$$

$$E = 1 \text{ AMU} \times (2.997925 \times 10^{10} \text{ cm/s})^2$$

As 1 AMU=1.66053×10^{-24} g, then

$$E = [1.66053 \times 10^{-24} \text{ g}] \times (2.997925 \times 10^{10} \text{ cm/s})^2$$

$$E = 1.492 \times 10^{-3} \text{ erg}$$

As 1 erg $= 1.6022 \times 10^{-6}$ MeV, the energy equivalent of 1 AMU

$$E = \frac{1.492 \times 10^{-3} \text{ erg}}{\text{AMU}} \times \frac{1 \text{ MeV}}{1.6022 \times 10^6 \text{ erg}} = \frac{931.5 \text{ MeV}}{\text{AMU}}$$

Therefore, the mass of 1 AMU has the energy equivalence of 931.5 MeV. Substituting the value for the mass of ^{12}C into $E = mc^2$ and dividing by 12 provides the values which were described above:

$$E_{proton} = 938.27 \text{ MeV}$$

$$E_{neutron} = 939.57 \text{ MeV}$$

$$E_{electron/beta/positron} = 0.511 \text{ MeV}$$

Parenthetically, conversion of mass to million electronvolts is

$$\left(\frac{1 \text{ AMU}}{1.660 \times 10^{-24} \text{ g}} \right) \times \left(\frac{931.5 \text{ MeV}}{\text{AMU}} \right) = \frac{5.611 \times 10^{26} \text{ MeV}}{\text{g}}$$

Further application at the atomic level involves ergs and electronvolts. A volt is a unit of potential. An electronvolt is a unit of energy. One electronvolt is equal to one electron accelerated to one volt of potential energy, and is equal to 1.6×10^{-12} erg (1 eV $= 1.6 \times 10^{-12}$ erg). Radioactive emissions are usually quantified using the electronvolt: 1000 eV $= 1$ keV (thousand electronvolts) and 1000 keV $= 1$ MeV (million electronvolts). The energy or energies at which radioactive emissions occur are characteristic of certain isotopes, and this can be helpful in identifying the isotope of origin.

Units of radioactivity

Important to nuclear pharmacy and nuclear medicine are units of radioactivity. The fundamental unit of radioactivity is the curie (Ci), which is defined as 3.7×10^{10} disintegrations per second (dps). The SI unit for radioactivity is the becquerel (Bq), which is equal to 1 dps. The SI units are metric and technically are the preferred method of quantifying radioactivity. However, the older system, using curies, millicuries, and microcuries is still relatively prevalent in practice: 1 Ci $= 1000$ mCi (millicuries) and 1 mCi $= 1000\,\mu$Ci (microcuries). Originally the curie was the number of disintegrations of one gram of pure radium per second. In the 1950s, a new radium half-life was found. Now, for any atom

$$1 \text{ Ci} = 3.7 \times 10^{10} \text{ dps} = 3.7 \times 10^{10} \text{ Bq}$$

Some helpful conversions are:

$$1 \text{ mCi} = 37 \text{ MBq} = 3.7 \times 10^{7} \text{ dps} = 3.7 \times 10^{7} \text{ Bq}$$

$$1\,\mu\text{Ci} = 37 \text{ kBq} = 3.7 \times 10^{4} \text{ dps} = 3.7 \times 10^{4} \text{ Bq}$$

$$1 \text{ Bq} = 1 \text{ dps}$$

$$1 \text{ MBq} = 10^{6} \text{ Bq} = 10^{6} \text{ dps} = 2.7 \times 10^{-5} \text{ Ci} = 2.7 \times 10^{-2} \text{ mCi} = 0.027 \text{ mCi}$$
$$= 27\,\mu\text{Ci}$$

An element may be radioactive because of instability in its nucleus, and a nucleus will decay only if it is energetically favorable for it to do so, meaning that it will only do so if it leads to greater stability of the atom. Of importance to the stability (or instability) of the nucleus and electrons is the amount of potential energy required to keep nucleons or electrons in place. These energies are their respective **binding energies.**

Binding energy in the nucleus

For nucleons, the binding energy is the difference between the assigned value from the periodic table and the calculated AMU. These values do differ, and this difference represents the binding energy. The binding energy for nucleons is the energy required to keep the nucleons from dissociating.

Calculating the number of protons present in the nuclide multiplied by 1.6726×10^{-24} g/proton plus the number of neutrons present in the nuclide multiplied by 1.6749×10^{-24} g/neutron, and comparing the results with the mass appearing on the chart of the nuclides (a 'periodic table' for all nuclides) will provide a small difference in grams. This can be converted to MeV to determine the binding energy for the nucleus. Further, the total binding energy can be divided by the number of nucleons present for that isotope, thus providing the binding energy per nucleon. The binding energy for one particle can often be generalized to equal 7.1 MeV. The true range for atomic masses greater than 11 but less than 60 is 7.4–8.8 MeV. For atomic masses less than 11, the binding energy is approximately 7.1 MeV. Using the value for binding energy, the stability or instability of an element can be predicted. The prediction is based on the difference between the calculated value and the periodic table (the assigned or chart of the nuclides) value. If the nuclear binding energy is negative, the nuclide is unstable and capable of undergoing radioactive decay. If the binding energy is positive, the nuclide is stable and unlikely to undergo decay.

The binding energy for $^4\text{He} = 2m_{^1\text{H}} + 2m_n - m_{^4\text{He}}$ where $m_{^1\text{H}}$ is the mass of ^1H (a proton), m_n is the mass of a neutron, and $m_{^4\text{He}}$ is the periodic table atomic mass for helium-4 (^4He); this is equal to $2(1.0079) + 2(1.00896) - 4.00260 = 0.03054$ AMU. Since $1\ \text{AMU} = 931.5$ MeV, the binding energy for ^4He is 28.45 MeV.

So, as stated above, the binding energy for one nucleon is roughly 7.1 MeV. Figure 2.7 shows a plot of binding energy per nucleon versus mass number, and allows more precise estimates of binding energy per nucleon.

The binding energy for atomic masses less than 11 is approximately 7.1 MeV. Therefore, for elements there is a calculable nuclear binding energy. As stated above, the binding energy can be used to determine if an element is stable:

- negative binding energy: decay favorable
- if the binding energy of products is less than the binding energy of the initial nucleus ($\text{BE}_{\text{products}} - \text{BE}_{\text{initial nucleus}} = $ negative value), decay is favorable.

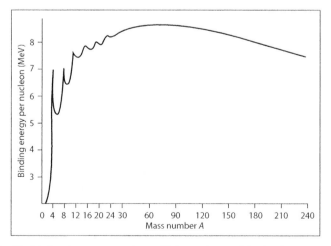

Figure 2.7 The binding energy per nucleon with increasing nuclide atomic mass number.

Because the **half-life** (the time for a radionuclide to decay to half its original value) is inversely proportional to the binding energy, the binding energy can be used to predict the stability of elements. A shorter half-life indicates greater instability.

Binding energy of orbital electrons

The binding energy of orbital electrons is also important because dislodging electrons is another mechanism by which atoms can lose potential energy to become more stable (overall). It is also a mechanism that can lead to other radiations. Like nucleons, electrons possess a binding energy, which keeps them in place in their particular orbital. However, if a collision with a particle or ray from the atom carries enough energy (i.e. energy greater than the electron binding energy), electrons can be dislodged from their orbitals. This results in rearrangements in the orbitals and radioactive emissions, which will be discussed below. The binding energy is the energy required to remove an electron from its orbit around the nucleus and is measured in electronvolts (eV).

It should be kept in mind that chemical reactions occur with electrons and require energy a minimum of only 10 eV per atom. The importance of this will also be discussed below.

Emissions from radioactive decay and their interactions with matter

The stability of an atom is dictated by the arrangement and binding energy of the nucleons. As discussed above, these have a direct bearing on whether a nuclide will be stable or prone to decay. Radionuclides decay by several mechanisms, including fission (splitting of an atom); alpha, beta, positron decay; electron capture; and isomeric transition. Various combinations are also often involved, as multiple decay steps. Of these various decays, all except fission are of consequence to nuclear pharmacy and nuclear medicine. It is often helpful to know not only the tendency of a nuclide to decay, but to be able to predict by which mechanism (or mechanisms) it will tend to decay. One way to predict the most likely decay mechanism is by noting the nuclide's **neutron to proton ratio**.

A graph of the number of neutrons in an atom versus the number of protons has a slope approximately equal to one at the beginning. The elements here, where the neutron to proton ratio is nearly one, tend to be stable. Further up the periodic table, there is a greater proportion of neutrons in nuclides and a higher preponderance of radioactivity. An abundance of neutrons implies increasing instability.

The most stable nuclides contain even numbers of protons and neutrons and, therefore, a neutron to proton ratio of one. Nuclides are less stable when either the number of protons or the number of neutrons is odd. Infrequently, nuclides have odd numbers of *both* protons and neutrons (these are all with

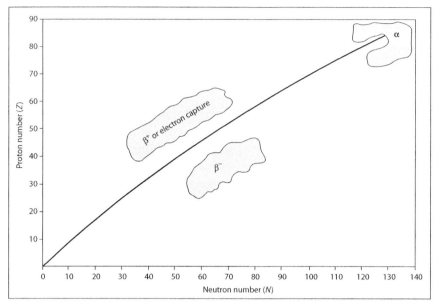

Figure 2.8 The line of stability where the neutron to proton ratio is approximately one.

mass less than 14). These too tend toward instability. Nuclides tend eventually to attain the most stable ratio possible via radioactivity, emission of particles, and/or photons.

Studying a plot of neutron to proton ratio, as it occurs in elements, illustrates, first, that a neutron to proton ratio of approximately one is stable. This line is named the 'line of stability' and has a slope of one (Figure 2.8). Nuclides 'try' to attain the highest possible stability, a position as close as possible to the line of stability. A neutron to proton ratio that is *greater than one* is above the line, indicating excess protons. The nuclides tend to correct themselves by getting rid of some positive charge. This is accomplished via positron emission or electron capture, both of which will be discussed below. A proton is converted to a neutron, and a positron (β^+, a **positively charged electron**) is discharged from the nucleus. Below the line of stability, the neutron to proton ratio is *less than one*, indicating excess neutrons. When this occurs, the nuclides tend to correct themselves by getting rid of some negative charge. This is done via beta (a fast-moving electron from within the nucleus) emission. At the same time, a neutron is converted to a proton and the beta (β^-) particle is ejected from the nucleus. All of these emissions will be discussed in more detail.

Types of radioactive decay

There are two reasons for radioactive decay in an atom. The first is a neutron to proton ratio greater than, or less than, one. The second reason for radioactive decay is an energy imbalance that creates the need for the atom to rid itself of energy in order to attain greater stability.

As mentioned above, two units are used when discussing the potential for radioactive decay and the magnitude with which it occurs. These are the AMU where one AMU is equal to 1/12th the mass of a ^{12}C nucleus. The second is the electronvolt (more conveniently, the MeV [a million electronvolts, or a mega-electronvolt] and keV [kiloelectronvolt]). Gamma emissions tend to be lower in energy than particulate emissions, so are normally expressed in kiloelectron-volts. The β^- and β^+ emissions have higher energy, so the megaelectronvolt is more commonly used as a unit for their energies. The types of radioactive decay are outlined below. Some are useful in nuclear pharmacy and nuclear medicine, while others are not. All of them need to be understood, however, since they can all impact the performance of the radiopharmaceutical, and since they are important for personal protection from radioactive emissions.

For all emissions, the end products of their interactions with matter are ionization and excitation. Ionization is the creation of positive or negative charges, and this is what we observe with equipment especially made for detecting particular types of radiation and specific energy ranges. Detection is a combination of when radiation interacts with matter and when we observe the effects through the equipment.

Alpha decay

Alpha particles are ionized helium atoms and can be a means of radioactive decay from the nucleus (Figure 2.9). Alpha decay occurs in elements with higher atomic mass, usually those with a heavy nucleus, such as radon or uranium, and those in which the neutron to proton ratio is very high (Figure 2.8).

The emission is particulate, so it carries a set amount of energy away from the nucleus. This causes the emission to be monoenergetic for the particular element in question. The helium nucleus (He^{2+}; $2n + 2p$) is a massive 4 AMU particle with a 2+ charge. The nuclear state equation shows that the atomic mass number A decreases to $A - 4$, the number of protons Z decreases to $Z - 2$, and the number of neutrons N decreases to $N - 2$ (Figure 2.10).

$$\text{Alpha}\ ^{4}_{2}\text{He}^{2+}$$

Figure 2.9   The alpha particle.

$$^{A}_{Z}\text{X}_{N} \longrightarrow\ ^{4}_{2}\text{He}^{2+}_{2} +\ ^{A-4}_{Z-2}\text{Y}_{N-2}$$

Parent isotope   Alpha particle   Daughter isotope

Figure 2.10   The nuclear equation for alpha decay.

Since alpha emission occurs in elements of high atomic number, those in which Z is greater than 82, these nuclides are rarely used in biological systems or nuclear medicine. This is because elements of high Z number are uncommon in biological systems (e.g. the human body).

Alpha particles move at a relatively slow velocity, a small fraction of the speed of light, and, being relatively massive, tend to follow a straight path through most materials. The particles carry a high kinetic energy, in the range 4–8 MeV. They lose energy by interacting with two electrons to neutralize the charge. The result is neutral helium ($He^{2+} + 2e^- \rightarrow He^0$).

The energy loss from the particle occurs because the particle, which is passing through matter, incurs elastic collisions with atomic electrons. This usually leads to ionization of the target, ultimately culminating in the alpha particle picking up the two electrons.

Because of their very biologically damaging characteristics, alpha-emitting isotopes have little use in nuclear pharmacy and nuclear medicine, other than the potential therapeutic applications. In addition, alpha particles are difficult to detect because of their short range, so they have little utility for imaging.

There are two main mechanisms by which alpha particles interact with matter: excitation and ionization. Excitation, which occurs less frequently than ionization, occurs when an alpha particle's collision with an electron raises the electron to a higher, outer shell. Then, as the electron falls back to its original shell, it emits this excess energy. Only a small portion ($< 5\%$) of the alpha particle energy is imparted, and because this is insufficient for overcoming electronic binding energy, electrons are not removed from the target atom. Therefore, there is little need to worry about personal protection when dealing with this type of interaction with matter.

The second, and more important, mechanism of alpha interaction with matter is the ionization of target atoms. Ionization occurs when the alpha particle is able to strip away an atom's orbital electron, creating a positively charged target ion. Meanwhile, the electron joins the alpha particle, leaving it with a 1+ charge. This phenomenon is called ion-pair formation. The alpha particle may continue making secondary ion-pairs until, ultimately, a chain reaction can occur, initiated by the primary and secondary ionizations that originated from the alpha particle.

The majority of ionizations caused by alpha particles do not involve direct interaction with the initiating alpha particle. Instead, they involve secondary reactions. As 34 eV is sufficient energy for ionization (ion-pair formation) to occur in an atom, a highly energetic alpha particle has more than enough energy to cause many ionizations before its energy is exhausted. As an alpha particle slows down, it has more time for interaction and, therefore, the likelihood of ion-pair formation is enhanced. The lower the alpha particle energy, the slower moving the particle is and the more ion-pairs are produced. For example, if the

Table 2.1 Linear range of 7 MeV alpha particles in various materials	
Material	Penetration (μm)
Air	59,000
Water (tissue)	74
Aluminum	34
Mica	29
Copper	14
Lead	2

emission was a 6.8 MeV alpha particle, 2×10^5 ions could be created before its energy was completely dissipated (Wang *et al.* 1975, pp. 41–42).

The **specific ionization** is the number of ion-pairs per unit length in air. For alpha particles, this is dependent on the energy with which the alpha particle is ejected from the nucleus. Being massive, alpha particles do not have excessive ranges in materials. For a 7 MeV alpha particle, penetration in general is only a few centimeters in air, 74 μm in water, and 2 μm in lead (Holloway *et al.* 1938) (Table 2.1).

Beta decay (negatron)

A beta particle is essentially an electron ejected from the nucleus at high velocity. Beta decay occurs when the neutron to proton ratio is greater than one. Inside the nucleus, a neutron is converted to a proton and β^- particle, with an antineutrino carrying away from the nucleus any excess binding energy above the energy of the β^- particle. Any excess energy may be emitted as gamma radiation, which will be discussed below. An antineutrino, a small particle with non-zero mass, has a velocity near the speed of light and has no charge (Figure 2.11).

The effects on A, Z, and N are as follows: Z increases to $Z + 1$, N decreases to $N - 1$, and the antineutrino is emitted. It should be noted that β^- particles

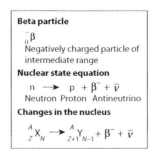

Figure 2.11 The beta particle and the nuclear equation for beta decay.

are energetic electrons in 'appearance,' but β^- particles differ from electrons in that they originate from inside the nucleus. Electrons are in orbit outside the nucleus and have no energy in their normal condition.

A beta particle is very different from an alpha particle. Weighing in at 1/7300th the mass of an alpha particle, a beta particle is considered 'very light.' Both β^- and β^+ are charged particles, but, unlike alpha particles, they have an extremely small mass and velocities that approach the speed of light. They travel in a haphazard path, caused by deflection. Because of their relatively high velocity, they have less time than alpha particles to interact with the target atoms and orbital electrons they pass. However, beta particles have higher penetrating power than alpha particles and a much longer range, a range that is as long as several meters in air. Dissipation of beta particle energy occurs when a β^- encounters a positive charge or a β^+ a negative charge, and ionization and ion-pair formation occur.

Unlike alpha particles, beta particles are not monoenergetic for a particular radionuclide but are emitted at varying energy levels over a continuous range. The antineutrino, for beta decay, and neutrino, for positron decay (below), carry some energy with them as part of their respective beta decay processes. A specific beta energy range is emitted, depending on the isotope of origin (Loevinger, 1957). Therefore, beta particles can be characterized by drawing a graph of the number of particles, or observed intensity, versus particle energy. Of interest, are the following two quantities for the same spectrum: the average energy of emission (E_{avg}) for that particular spectrum and the maximum energy emitted (E_{max}) (Franz *et al.* 1936) (Figure 2.12). The average energy of beta emission can be estimated as one-third the maximum energy of emission: $E_{avg} = \frac{1}{3}E_{max}$.

The emitting isotope can be identified by these two values. Values for E_{max} range from 0.019 MeV (19 keV) for ^{3}H up to 4.81 MeV for chlorine-38 (^{38}Cl).

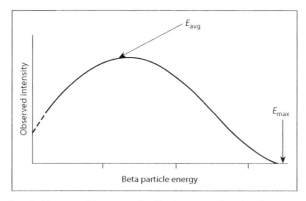

Figure 2.12 A typical beta particle energy distribution curve, showing the average energy of emission (E_{avg}) and the maximum energy emitted (E_{max}). Note that E_{avg} does not always correspond with the highest point on the curve.

For beta particles not at E_{max}, the antineutrino takes on the remaining energy. Consequently the energy emitted from the nucleus has E_{max} (i.e. E_{max} is made up of β^- emission and the antineutrino); beta decay is $n \rightarrow p + \beta^- + \bar{\nu}$ (energy $= E_{max}$); positron decay is $p \rightarrow n + \beta^+ + \nu$ (energy $= E_{max}$). A beta particle persists after dissipating all of its kinetic energy and usually becomes an atom's orbital electron.

Beta particles can be roughly categorized as 'hard' or 'soft' particles. Hard beta particles normally are those with an E_{avg} above 200–300 keV, while soft betas are under 200 keV. Because maximum ion-pair formation occurs at lower energy levels, the slower, softer beta particles make more ion-pairs than do the harder, faster beta particles. As mentioned above, ionization and ion-pair formation are means by which beta particles interact with matter and dissipate their kinetic energy.

Another mechanism by which β^- particles may interact with matter is through **Bremsstrahlung radiation**. Bremsstrahlung means 'braking radiation.' It occurs as a beta particle passes a positively charged nucleus. The beta particle is attracted and accelerated by the nuclear force field. Excess energy from acceleration is given off in the form of electromagnetic radiation (bremsstrahlung). The result is the emission of a gamma photon (Figure 2.13). This is more likely to occur near elements of high Z numbers such as lead (when approximately 10% of the beta energy is given away), because they have an abundance of protons, and have higher beta energies. These high Z materials attract the β^-, causing bremsstrahlung. For this reason, beta emitters are stored in containers of low Z numbers, such as lucite, in order to reduce exposure of personnel to the resulting electromagnetic radiation. Such exposure would occur if beta emitters were stored in *high* Z number containers such as lead.

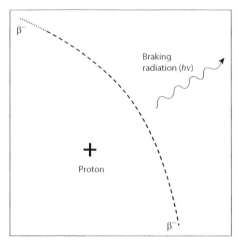

Figure 2.13   Bremsstrahlung or 'braking' radiation. As the β^- passes a proton, it is slowed (but not captured) and releases radiation.

A practical consideration is the need to measure beta particle emission. Alpha particles, having an exceptionally short range, must be measured at approximately 1 mm from the source; whereas beta particles, because they travel farther, can be measured farther from the source.

Beta particles can be used for imaging purposes, but, because of their ionization and excitation characteristics, they are more useful for their therapeutic applications.

Positron decay

Positrons are positively charged beta particles. They are emitted when the neutron to proton ratio is less than one, meaning the atom is proton rich. When a proton is converted to a neutron, a positron (β^+) and a neutrino (opposite of the antineutrino) are ejected. A neutrino is a small particle with almost no mass and no charge. It has a velocity near the speed of light, and carries away the energy difference between the atomic binding energy and the positron energy, if there is any. The nuclear state equation is a proton being converted to β^+ and a neutrino. The changes in the nucleus are a decrease in Z to $Z-1$, an increase in N to $N+1$, and emission of the neutrino (Figure 2.14).

Positrons are identical to beta particles except in charge. A positron has only a transient existence. After losing all of its kinetic energy, it interacts with an electron and is 'annihilated.'

What actually occurs is that both the mass of the positron and the mass of the electron are converted to energy during annihilation. Since each particle has the energy equivalence of 0.511 MeV, 1.022 MeV is the amount of energy that is released upon annihilation. Recall that a beta particle and an electron are basically the same with regard to charge and potential energy. Except for its charge, a positron is like a positively charged electron, in that it has characteristics of both an electron and a beta particle. From this annihilation, 0.511 MeV gamma rays are emitted at a 180° angle to each other (Figure 2.15). The predictability of 180° gamma photon release is the basis for positron emission tomography (PET) detection and the very good imaging properties of positron-emitting isotopes. One important positron decay for imaging purposes is that of ^{11}C: ^{11}C $\rightarrow$ ^{11}B $+ \beta^+$. Use of PET will be covered in detail in Chapter 7.

The energy graph for positrons differs slightly from that of beta particles, in that the E_{max} tends to be at a lower particle energy for positrons, and the positron range tends to be shorter (Figure 2.16).

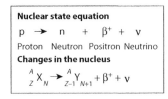

Nuclear state equation

$$p \rightarrow n + \beta^+ + \nu$$

Proton   Neutron   Positron   Neutrino

Changes in the nucleus

$$^A_Z X_N \rightarrow\ ^A_{Z-1} Y_{N+1} + \beta^+ + \nu$$

Figure 2.14   Positron emission: the nuclear state equation and changes in the nucleus.

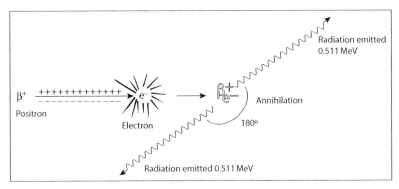

Figure 2.15 Positron annihilation. The mass of the positron and that of the electron are converted to energy during annihilation, which is released as two photons of 0.511 MeV each, at 180° to each other.

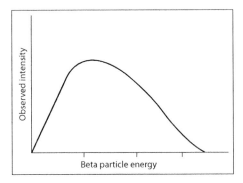

Figure 2.16 Typical energy curve for positron emission.

With positron emission, a stable nucleus is achieved. This usually occurs in elements with low Z numbers, for example $^{13}N \rightarrow {}^{13}C$ (stable).

When a proton is converted to a neutron and a β^+ particle, a mass the equivalent of two electrons is created. To maintain the conservation of energy for β^+ emission, there needs to be at least 1.022 MeV of excess nuclear energy for positron emission, which is the amount of energy required to produce the two 0.511 MeV gamma photons.

Gamma emission

The nucleus can eliminate excess excitation energy by means of photon emission. Photon emission can result from isomeric transition (discussed below), or it can occur randomly to balance the energy lost from the nucleus through a prior decay event. A gamma photon has no charge and occurs as electromagnetic radiation traveling at the speed of light. It has the longest range of any nuclear emission. Gammas have no mass, and the nucleus undergoes no atomic number change or neutron number change upon emission (Figure 2.17). Gamma emission occurs following other types of decay (β^-, β^+, electron capture, or alpha). Normally the parent and daughter are isomers, though they can be isobars, isotopes, or isotones if more than one step is involved.

Figure 2.17 The gamma photon.

The emitted photons are monoenergetic (all of the same energy or set of energies), so there is no need for an energy graph.

As with all radiation, gamma radiation is the correction of energy in the radionuclide from a higher energy state to a more stable state. The radiations occur at short wavelengths, $0.1–10\,\mu m$ (10^{-3} to $10^{-1}\,\mathring{A}$), and therefore have high energies. The energy range is $1\,keV–10\,MeV$, though most are between $10\,keV$ and $3\,MeV$ (Figure 2.18). For comparison, consider that X-rays generally have energies between $10\,eV$ and $100\,keV$.

Gamma photons have high penetrative powers, up to several meters. They penetrate matter easily, with little interaction, because, unlike alpha and beta particles, they are not ionized. This results in their range being much greater than that of either alpha or beta particles. In air, a typical alpha particle may have a range of $2–8\,cm$, a beta particle $0–10\,m$, and a gamma photon from $1\,cm$ up to $100\,m$.

Gamma photons interact with matter through direct collisions with nuclei and orbital electrons. Being monoenergetic, many gamma-emitting isotopes are extremely useful as components of imaging radiopharmaceuticals because the photons can be isolated and processed by the imaging equipment used in the nuclear medicine department.

Electron capture and X-ray emission

Electron capture (K-capture, EC), an alternative mechanism to positron emission, allows a nucleus to decrease the number of protons it contains, and achieve *nuclear* stability. Electron capture occurs when the neutron to proton ratio is less than one (excess of protons). During electron capture, an inner orbital electron is captured and drawn into the nucleus. This effectively changes a proton to a neutron, with a neutrino carrying any excess energy from the conversion: electron + proton → neutron + neutrino (ν). Similar to beta decay, the products of electron capture are isobars and therefore are different elements. The product element may also remain unstable, causing it to emit gamma photons or conversion electrons in order to discharge more energy.

Typically, a cascade reaction ensues, usually starting from the K shell. There can be an N capture or L capture, or other orbital electron capture. The end result is that electrons from outer shells move to fill vacated shells closer to the nucleus.

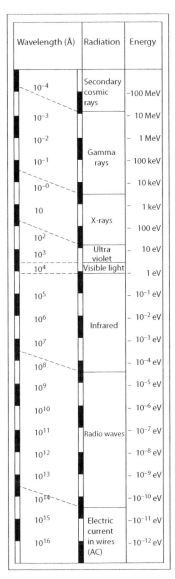

Wavelength (Å)	Radiation	Energy
10^{-4}	Secondary cosmic rays	-100 MeV
10^{-3}		$- 10$ MeV
10^{-2}		$- 1$ MeV
10^{-1}	Gamma rays	$- 100$ keV
10^{-0}		$- 10$ keV
10		$- 1$ keV
10^2	X-rays	$- 100$ eV
10^3	Ultra violet	$- 10$ eV
10^4	Visible light	1 eV
10^5		$- 10^{-1}$ eV
10^6		$- 10^{-2}$ eV
10^7	Infrared	$- 10^{-3}$ eV
10^8		$- 10^{-4}$ eV
10^9		$- 10^{-5}$ eV
10^{10}		$- 10^{-6}$ eV
10^{11}	Radio waves	$- 10^{-7}$ eV
10^{12}		$- 10^{-8}$ eV
10^{13}		$- 10^{-9}$ eV
10^{14}		-10^{-10} eV
10^{15}	Electric current in wires (AC)	-10^{-11} eV
10^{16}		-10^{-12} eV

Figure 2.18 The electromagnetic spectrum.

Electrons lose potential energy when they move inward toward lower potential energy orbits, and give off X-rays as they come closer to the nucleus. These emissions are called 'K X-rays,' or 'L X-rays,' depending on the shell of origin. It should again be emphasized that gamma rays are predominantly from inside the nucleus, and X-rays are from outside the nucleus.

For electron capture, the parent and daughter energy differences *usually* are less than 1.022 MeV, which differs from the requirements for positron emission. Another difference between electron capture and positron emission is that electron capture usually occurs in elements of high Z number, whereas positron emission occurs in elements of low Z number. Because electron shells in these elements are closer to the nucleus, the probability of electron capture being the decay modality increases along with the increasing Z number. As with positron emission, the net result of electron capture is the loss of a proton and gain of a neutron.

Isomeric transition and gamma radiation emission

Recall that isomers differ from one another because the parent nuclide is in an excited state. The *nucleus* of the parent nuclide can remain in an excited (isomeric) energy state. These isomeric nuclei decay to a ground (stable) state. The decay from an excited state to a lower energy state is called isomeric transition. Isomeric transition can accompany β^-, β^+, and electron capture decays. The energy difference between isomeric energy states may appear as gamma radiation. If the isomeric state is long lived enough to be measurable, it is called a **metastable state** and is denoted by an 'm' (e.g. ^{99m}Tc).

Internal conversion: another isomeric transition

When a gamma photon from the nucleus strikes an orbital electron (called a conversion electron), the electron is given energy. The extent of the energy transferred from the gamma photon to the electron depends on the angle at which the electron is struck. If the imparted gamma energy (conversion energy) is higher than binding energy of the electron, the orbital electron is dislodged at a high velocity from its orbit. The phenomenon is called electron conversion. This internal conversion is at a discrete energy, since the causative gamma impact has a discrete energy. As typically occurs during electron capture, the vacated orbital leads to a cascade of electrons filling subsequent orbital vacancies. The conversion *electrons* are also monoenergetic, which leads to the emission of an X-ray as a means of giving up kinetic energy to attain lower potential energy (Figure 2.19). Internal conversion is more

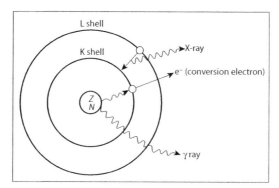

Figure 2.19 Internal conversion. The excess energy of the nucleus is initially given off as a gamma photon. This gamma photon strikes an orbital electron, ejecting it from the atom. The vacancy left by the ejected electron is then filled by electrons from the outer orbitals, which leads to secondary X-ray emission(s).

common with higher atomic number elements and transitions involving lower energy gammas.

Extranuclear events leading to X-rays and the Auger electron

These are emissions resulting from electron capture or internal conversion that cause disruption of the electron cloud. Two types of emissions can occur.

As discussed above, X-rays can be produced by the displacement of orbital electrons and the subsequent replacement of the missing electron(s). These X-rays are quantified using **fluorescence yield**, the energy difference between the orbitals of the shifting electrons. Fluorescence yield is the probability of X-ray emission caused by orbital electron displacement (Figure 2.20). Fluorescence yield is calculated via the probability of the number of X-rays emitted per number of spaces available to be filled. The probability is expressed as the inverse of the fluorescence yield (1/Fl Yld).

The second type of emission is the **Auger electron**. This method for eliminating energy occurs during isomeric transition as an alternative process to X-ray emission. When the originally displaced electron energy is transferred to another outer electron, it knocks the latter out of the atom (Figure 2.20). (This is analogous to internal conversion.) The Auger electron is a monoenergetic electron emission.

Elements with low Z numbers favor Auger electron emission, while those with high Z numbers favor X-ray emission (Figure 2.20). It follows that the probability for X-ray emission increases as Z increases. For X-ray emission to occur, its energy must be at least equal to that expended during the orbital rearrangement process: $E_{X\text{-ray}} = BE_{original} - BE_{final}$, where BE is the binding energy of the electron.

For Auger electrons to occur, the transition energy must exceed the electron binding energy. Otherwise, the emission will be an X-ray: $E_{Auger} = E_{X\text{-ray}} - E_{ejected\ electron}$, where $E_{X\text{-ray}}$ is the energy of the X-ray that would have been released had there been insufficient energy to expel the second electron.

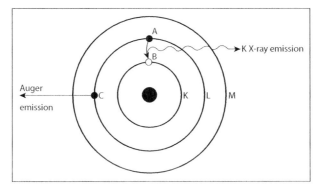

Figure 2.20   X-ray and Auger electron emission are both mechanisms to fill vacated electron orbitals.

Usually, X-rays are emitted as a result of electron capture or internal conversion, and they reflect the energy differences between the orbital electrons. The energy range is from a few electronvolts up to approximately 120 keV. The X-rays from electron capture or internal conversion are of little use in nuclear pharmacy or nuclear medicine but need to be understood for reasons of radiation protection and development of useful radioisotopes.

Photoelectric effect

This occurs when a gamma photon collides with a bound inner electron, which is usually the first K shell electron. This produces an electron with energy equal to that of the impinging gamma photon, and this, in turn, creates an ejected electron. If there is complete energy transfer, then $E_{e^-} = E_\gamma - E_{BE}$. To dislodge the orbital electron, the binding energy must equal the energy of the gamma. (All energy must be transferred for the photoelectric effect.) The loss of the orbital electron induces a cascade, and kinetic energy is lost for conservation of energy. The requirement for energy loss causes X-ray or Auger electron emission. Photoelectric electrons are in the 0–0.5 MeV range. We then detect this resultant ionization. The photoelectric effect usually occurs with elements of high Z number (e.g. there is a better chance of this happening with lead than with aluminum).

Compton effect

This is the decrease in energy (increase in wavelength) of an X-ray or gamma ray photon when it interacts with an outermost shell electron. In contrast with the photoelectric effect, only a *portion* of the gamma energy is given to the electron, leaving a lower energy gamma photon and a displaced electron; for example, there is an 80% to 20% energy distribution for the gamma photon and electron, respectively. There is a high energy spread for the resultant gamma photons and recoil electrons, since there is variability in energy transfer from the initial gamma photon. The maximum energy is imparted to the electron if the electron reflects backwards along the path: '180° back-scattering' of the photon (Figure 2.21). The resultant electron and lower energy gamma photon can then cause ionization of other atoms. The higher the energy of the gamma photon, the higher the imparted energy to the electron. The Compton effect commonly occurs with gamma photons of medium energy, in the range 0.5–1.5 MeV. It is also common in atoms of low to medium Z numbers.

Pair production from a gamma strike

This occurs when there is a direct hit by a gamma photon on a nucleus, resulting in the creation of an electron and a β^+ (Figure 2.22). The pair then undergoes annihilation, and some energy is lost to the nucleus during the interaction. This can only occur if there is enough energy available to create the pair (at least the total rest mass energy of the two particles), thus conserving both energy and momentum. For all of this to occur, the interaction must

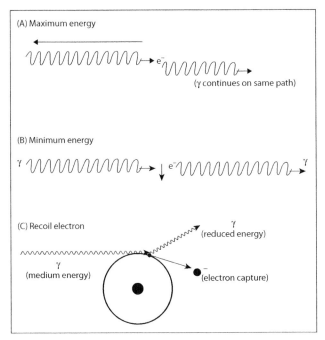

(A) Maximum energy

e⁻

(γ continues on same path)

(B) Minimum energy

γ

e⁻

γ

(C) Recoil electron

γ
(reduced energy)

γ
(medium energy)

(electron capture)

Figure 2.21 The Compton effect. (A) The maximum energy is imparted to the orbital electron by 180° backscattering. (B) The minimum energy is imparted by a 90° strike. (C) Formation of a recoil electron.

start with more energy than 1.022 MeV, the sum of the energy of two annihilation gamma photons. Although the energy is not symmetrically given to the resulting components, 1.022 MeV must be supplied to allow for the two annihilation gamma photons, and enough energy exceeding this must be given to account for the creation of the electron. Pair production occurs in elements of high Z number and with high-energy photons, those in the million electron-volt range. The electron and gamma photons can then cause ionization of other atoms.

The emission that is going to occur from these events depends on the Z number of the absorbing material and the energy of the gamma photon (Figure 2.23).

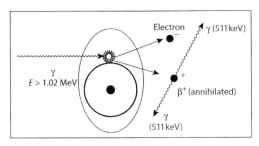

Electron

γ (511 keV)

γ
E > 1.02 MeV

β⁺ (annihilated)

γ
(511 keV)

Figure 2.22 Pair production.

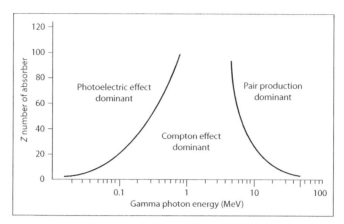

Figure 2.23 Gamma energy in the photoelectric effect, Compton effect, and pair production. The photoelectric effect dominates up to 1 MeV, the Compton effect from 1 to 10 MeV, and pair production above 10 MeV. The interaction type is dependent on the density of the matter and the gamma ray energy.

Nomenclature: decay schemes

Often it is helpful to visualize the decay of an isotope, since it can be complex and information intensive. One way to do this is to look at published **decay schemes** for isotopes. Decay schemes are simple line drawings that allow easier conceptualization of the mechanisms by which isotopes decay, their emission energies, and parent–daughter relationships (Figures 2.24–2.27).

Decay schemes are diagrams designed to help in visualization of the mechanisms by which radioisotopes decay. They use arrows and energy level lines to indicate the type(s) of decay occurring. Since some isotopes undergo more than one type of decay, the percentage 'abundance' of each type of decay and the energies of the decay emissions is also be indicated on the schematic.

Decay schemes help to reveal what is happening with an isotope of interest, including the decay energies that may be available for either imaging or therapy. The types of decay scheme illustrated below are examples of those commonly encountered in nuclear pharmacy and nuclear medicine. They are beta, positron, gamma, and isomeric transition.

The symbol, mass number, and half-life appear on the uppermost horizontal line. If there is more than one decay path, the percentage followed by each is noted in the scheme. The parent and daughter half-lives are indicated in their respective positions on the diagram. An arrow pointing down and to lower right indicates decay by β^- emission. An arrow pointing down and to lower left indicates decay by β^+, α, or electron capture. Gamma emission is represented by a line (usually wavy) moving straight down (Figure 2.26). If the daughter is not stable, multiple decays may occur (polyenergetic decay). The percentage of each type of decay is indicated on the scheme.

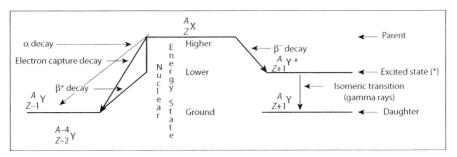

Figure 2.24   Model for general decay schemes.

Beta decay

A β^- decay is represented on a decay scheme as an arrow pointing down and to the right (Figure 2.25). Recall that $E_{\text{avg}} = \frac{1}{3}E_{\text{max}}$. An example is that of iodine-131 (^{131}I), which has a half-life of eight days:

$$^{131}_{53}\text{I} \rightarrow {}^{131}_{54}\text{Xe} + \beta^- + \tilde{\nu}$$

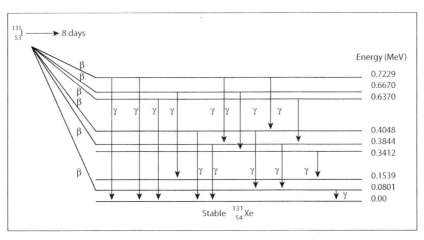

Figure 2.25   Beta decay scheme.

Gamma (isomeric transition) decay

The decay of molybdenum-99 (^{99}Mo) is initially by beta decay but is followed by isomeric transition and gamma emission, resulting in $^{99\text{m}}$Tc, ^{99}Tc, and finally by another beta decay to ruthenium (^{99}Ru) (Figure 2.26).

$$^{99}_{42}\text{Mo} \rightarrow {}^{99\text{m}}_{43}\text{Tc} + \beta^- + \tilde{\nu}$$

$$^{99}\text{Tc} \rightarrow {}^{99}\text{Ru} + \beta^- + \tilde{\nu}$$

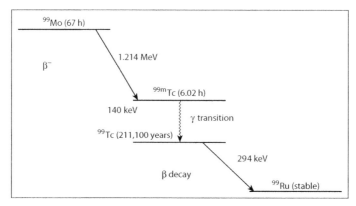

Figure 2.26 Gamma (beta and isomeric transition) decay scheme. Any excess energy left in the nucleus after β⁻ emission is emitted as gamma radiation.

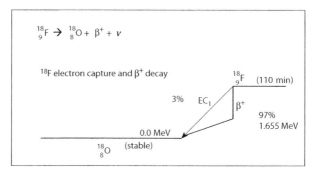

Figure 2.27 Positron decay of ¹⁸F: the nuclear state equation and the decay scheme. Any excess energy left in the nucleus after β⁺ emission is emitted as gamma radiation.

Positron decay

Figure 2.27 shows positron decay.

Mathematics involved with radioactive decay

According to the fundamental law of decay, the number of atoms that decay is exponential with respect to time, independent of physical properties (such as temperature and pressure), irreversible, and random. Radioactivity is random because it cannot be predicted which atom will decay. Only a probability that it will decay during a given time frame can be quantified. Decay is random for a given nucleus, but, for a large group of the same radionuclide, it follows a first-order decay model, with rate of decay proportional to the remaining radioactive nuclei. Because it is a geometric decay, there is no time on the graph where the number of nuclei is equal to zero.

Decay rate is specific for a particular nuclide. For calculation purposes, N represents the number of undecayed but radioactive nuclei present at time t; N is proportional to the rate of decay, where λ is the decay constant (the fraction disintegrating per unit time), expressed as inverse time for the particular isotope. The symbol λ represents the probability of disintegration for a radioactive atom. Therefore, the disintegration rate is $-dN/dt = \lambda N$. It is negative because radioactive decay is viewed as the loss of nuclei. Rearranging gives $dN/N = -\lambda dt$, and integrating gives $N_t = N_0 e^{-\lambda t}$, where N_0 is the number of atoms at the beginning of the time interval (at $t = 0$) and N_t is the number of atoms remaining after the time interval (t).

For each radionuclide there is a distinct half-life ($t_{1/2}$). The half-life is the time required for a radionuclide to decay to one half its original radioactivity, or simply, from its original 'activity.' After one half-life, N_t is reduced to $1/2N_t$, and the equation becomes $1/2N_0 = N_0 e^{-\lambda t_{1/2}}$. Solving this gives $\ln 1/2 = -\lambda t_{1/2}$. Rearranging leads to $\lambda t_{1/2} = \ln 2$, and further derivation provides $t_{1/2} = 0.693/\lambda$ and $\lambda = 0.693/t_{1/2}$.

Note that $t_{1/2}$ is in time (i.e. seconds), and λ is in reciprocal time (1/time, i.e. 1/s or s^{-1}). Since we use instruments to measure radiation indirectly, we must often consider the efficiency of the detector. Instruments do not measure 100% of all radioactive decays. However, the instrument can be presumed to have a constant error and if we know this constant, we can infer how many disintegrations are occurring per unit of time for a given sample. Decay is often described as disintegrations per minute (dpm), per second (dps), and so on. Our instruments tell us the number of 'counts' they are recording per unit of time. They report counts per minute (cpm), counts per second (cps), and so on. If, in reality, the **disintegration rate** is 1000 dps and the counter has a 70% efficiency, 700 cps will be reported by the instrument.

When describing disintegrations as counts, activity is reported as counts per minute. This can be represented by $A_t = A_0 e^{-\lambda t}$, where A is the activity detected when the same detector set-up is used for detection at both times and the efficiency of the equipment is not changing. 'Activity' means the disintegration rate for any radionuclide. Both equations (that for N_t and that for A_t) are first-order equations and can be graphed in standard Cartesian (Figure 2.28) and semi-logarithmic (Figure 2.29) fashions.

The slope of the semi-logarithmic decay curve is λ. Since $\lambda = 0.693/t_{1/2}$, the half-life can be calculated through cross-multiplication, as $0.693/\lambda$. The number of atoms of an isotope present can be determined using the equation $N = A/\lambda$, where A is activity but presumed to be converted to disintegrations per second, and λ is in units of reciprocal seconds. The mass of an isotope sample can be derived from this equation as well, since the number of atoms present is known.

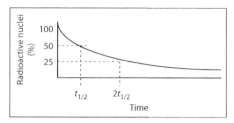

Figure 2.28 First-order decay plotted in Cartesian coordinates.

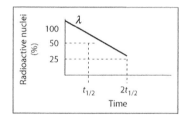

Figure 2.29 First-order decay plotted in semi-logarithmic coordinates. The slope of the line (λ) is the decay constant.

Helpful terms and equations

The number of atoms present at time t can be calculated from the number of atoms present at time 0, the decay constant for an isotope, or the elapsed time, $N_t = N_0 e^{-\lambda t}$ (N here represents the number of atoms). This equation can be arranged to solve for whichever variable is missing.

To find activity rather than number of atoms, the equation $A_t = A_0 e^{-\lambda t}$ may be used or $A_t = A_0/2^n$, where n is the number of half-lives that have occurred.

The **average life** of a group of atoms (τ) is $1/\lambda$ or $1.44 t_{1/2}$. This is also called the mean half-life. In one average life time, the activity of a group of a given type of radionuclide is reduced to 37% of its initial value. Since λ is the probability of decay per unit time, $1/\lambda$ is the mean time between decays; $1/\lambda$ has application in calculating exposure and the time required to reach the maximum amount of activity, which will be explained below.

If a radionuclide decays via multiple decay modes, a figure called the effective half-life can be calculated by finding the effective (total) decay constant, λ_e, where λ_e is the multiple of all included λ values divided by the sum of all the λ values:

$$\frac{\lambda_1 \lambda_2 \lambda_3 \dots}{\lambda_1 + \lambda_2 + \lambda_3 \dots}$$

Successive decay equations

There are a few unique aspects to calculating the decay rate of parent and daughter isotopes when their half-lives have certain relationships with each other. If they remain in contact with each other, the parent and daughter isotopes can reach a point where both have the same apparent decay rate. If a parent isotope decays to a daughter isotope that also decays, the following is true:

$$dN/dt = \lambda_p N_p - \lambda_d N_d$$

where $\lambda_p N_p$ is the growth rate of the daughter isotope from the decay of the parent and $\lambda_d N_d$ is the decay rate of the daughter. Integration gives

$$(A_d)_t = \lambda_d N_d = \frac{\lambda_d (A_p)_0}{(\lambda_d - \lambda_p)} \left(e^{-\lambda_p t} - e^{-\lambda_d t} \right)$$

If there is initial activity $(A_d)_0$, $(A_d)_0 e^{-\lambda_d t}$ is added, and $(A_d)_t$ becomes:

$$(A_d)_t = \lambda_d N_d = \frac{\lambda_d (A_p)_0}{(\lambda_d - \lambda_p)} \left(e^{-\lambda_p t} - e^{-\lambda_d t} \right) + (A_d)_0 e^{-\lambda_d t}$$

Parent–daughter relationships

Transient equilibrium occurs when the half-life of the parent nuclide is slightly longer than the daughter's half-life (Figure 2.30): $(t_{1/2})_p$ can be 10–50 times longer than $(t_{1/2})_d$. If λ_d is greater than λ_p, $(t_{1/2})_d$ is 10–50 times

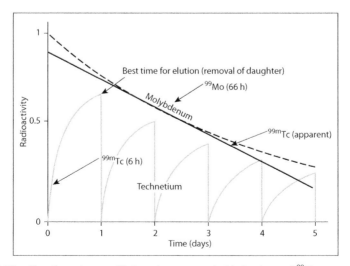

Figure 2.30 Plot of transient equilibrium, demonstrated with the decay of ^{99}Mo.

shorter than $(t_{1/2})_p$. In this case $e^{-\lambda_d t}$ is negligible compared with $e^{-\lambda_p t}$ when t is long enough.

$$(A_d)_t = \frac{\lambda_d (A_p)_0}{(\lambda_d - \lambda_p)} e^{-\lambda_p t} = \frac{\lambda_d (A_p)_t}{(\lambda_d - \lambda_p)}$$

The time to maximum activity is:

$$t_{max} = 1.44 \left[\frac{(t_{1/2})_p (t_{1/2})_d}{(t_{1/2})_p - (t_{1/2})_d} \right] \ln \left[\frac{(t_{1/2})_p}{(t_{1/2})_d} \right]$$

The value 1.44 in this equation comes from $\tau(1/\lambda)$ mentioned above, the average life of a group of atoms.

Figure 2.30 demonstrates this process for the decay of ^{99}Mo ($t_{1/2} = 66$ hours) to 86% ^{99m}Tc ($t_{1/2} = 6.0$ hours) and 14% ^{99}Tc.

If eluted (daughter isotope taken from the source) once a day, the parent regenerates the daughter to the maximum amount possible, up to the amount of parent isotope remaining.

Secular equilibrium occurs when the amount of the daughter isotope remains constant. It remains constant because the rate of decay from parent to daughter is equal to the decay rate of the daughter (Figure 2.31): $(t_{1/2})_p$ exceeds $(t_{1/2})_d$ by 100 times or more. λ_d is much greater than λ_p because the half-life of the parent is much longer than the daughter's half-life. This means that λ_p can be neglected, and $(A_d)_t = (A_p)_t$.

At the beginning, there is no daughter isotope present. Then, the parent decays and builds up the daughter. The loss of the parent isotope eventually comes to an equilibrium with the appearance of the daughter isotope.

The importance of understanding successive decay and the related equations is that many of the radiopharmaceuticals compounded and used in nuclear pharmacy rely on the decay of the parent to daughter nuclide. The daughter nuclide in these cases is the isotope that is useful for imaging or therapy. This set-up is called a **generator** and is self-contained. It is shipped to

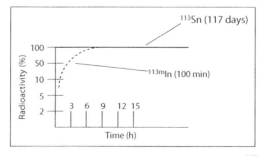

Figure 2.31 Plot of secular equilibrium, demonstrated with the decay of ^{113}Sn.

the pharmacy while the parent nuclide is decaying to the daughter. The daughter is **eluted**, or removed from the generator in its pure (no parent nuclide) form.

It is imperative to know: (1) how much daughter nuclide can be eluted at a given time, (2) the best time to remove the maximum possible amount of daughter nuclide, and (3) the amount of time required for the generator to replenish the daughter isotope after what was available has been removed. To achieve these, it is important to know the parent–daughter relationship and the half-lives of each. Then, a graph and/or computation can be made to determine the best time interval to wait before again eluting the daughter nuclide from the generator.

The terminology used includes the 'growth' of the presence of the daughter isotope and the 'growth rate' from the decay of the parent nuclide.

Effects of radiation on the body: radiation physics and radiobiology

Radiobiology is the study of the effects of radiation on biological systems and, to a great extent, this is also the study of health physics. In familiarizing themselves with these areas of study, nuclear pharmacists become aware of the limits of radiation *exposure*, the radiation *dose*, and the equivalent *dose* that are considered safe for workers and patients. Of ultimate importance is knowing how much radiation and what type of radiation a given part of the body is exposed to and for how much time.

As with other matter, radiation effects on the body include excitation (raising an electron to a higher energy level) and ionization (actual *ejection* of an electron). Radiation causing the latter is called ionizing radiation. Recall that ionization requires roughly 34 eV, which is easily sufficient to break chemical bonds (the carbon–carbon double bond is 4.9 eV). Ionizing radiation can be subcategorized as either electromagnetic or particulate ionizing radiation.

Electromagnetic radiation includes X-rays and gamma rays, all moving at the speed of light but having different wavelengths and, therefore, different energies. When X-rays or gamma rays are absorbed by the body, energy is deposited as the photon is dissipated. Electromagnetic photons are considered to be ionizing if their energy exceeds 124 eV. Particulate ionizing radiation includes alpha, beta, and positron particles plus other particles that are not of concern to nuclear pharmacy.

Radiation can be directly or indirectly ionizing. Charged particles are directly ionizing. Electromagnetic radiation is indirectly ionizing. When photons are absorbed, so is their energy, which can be converted to charged particles via mechanisms such as the Compton and photoelectric effects. Directly and indirectly, ionizing radiation can create free radicals, which, being very reactive chemically, can cause damage in the cell or in DNA. An example of initial free radical formation can occur with water:

$$H_2O \rightarrow H_2O^+ + e^-$$

$$H_2O^+ + H_2O \rightarrow H_3O^+ + OH \cdot \text{ (free radical)}$$

The smaller the area of focus of exposure to radiation, the higher the probability of interactions between radiation and the targets, such as DNA, water molecules, and other molecules.

Damage to DNA can cause cell death, mutations, or carcinogenesis. Usually, a single-stranded break is easily repaired by the cell using the opposite strand as a template. If a double-stranded break occurs, especially in slightly offset portions of DNA, the DNA can misrepair (improperly rejoin), leading to cell death or cancerous growth. Therefore, radiation exposure and absorption must be measured. The measurement involves various units.

The units most important to nuclear pharmacy and nuclear medicine are described below. There are actually duplications within these units. Some of the older ones are still in use, and are called 'common units,' while equivalent measurements, such as SI units, are now considered more official. State and federal regulatory agencies set limits for workers, patients, and the general public, but at this point simply the units and their definitions will be introduced (http://www.physics.isu.edu/radinf/terms.htm; http://web.princeton.edu/sites/ehs/radsafeguide/rsg_app_e.htm).

Common terms and units

- *Exposure*. Assessment of exposure has utility in that it is an indicator of how much energy is being emitted into a space, such as a work environment, so it is useful for a quick assessment of electromagnetic radiation workers are, or have been, near.
- *Roentgen (R)*. The roentgen is a measure of exposure, applicable only to gamma and X-rays, and only in air: 1 R is the deposition, in dry air, of enough energy to cause an electric charge of 2.58×10^{-4} coulombs/kg. One roentgen is the amount of radiation required to liberate one unit of positive or negative charge in 1 cm^3 of dry air at standard temperature and pressure. Its main utility is its ease of use in the pharmacy or laboratory for quickly identifying how much exposure one has had to X-rays or gamma radiation.
- *Absorbed dose*. The common unit is the rad (radiation absorbed dose); the SI unit is the gray. It is often useful to assess what has likely been absorbed by tissues in workers or patients from *any* type of radiation in the nuclear pharmacy or nuclear medicine departments. In addition, there is a need to account for the resulting effects that the different types of radiation will

inevitably have on tissues, since particulate and electromagnetic radiations differ in their abilities to inflict damage (see the discussion regarding excitation and ionization above). The equivalent dose can be used to account for these differences.

- *Radiation absorbed dose (rad).* The radiation absorbed dose (rad) is used to measure absorbed dose and is equal to 10^{-2} J/kg. 1 rad is the absorption of 100 erg/g material. This is the energy given from either particulate or electromagnetic radiation to some material at a specific point.
- *Gray (Gy).* The gray is the SI unit of absorbed radiation dose from ionizing radiation: 1 Gy is equal to the deposition of one joule of energy per kilogram of a material by any type of radiation. A smaller unit used is 1/100th of a gray, a centigray (cGy). The conversion between gray and rad is 1 Gy = 100 rad.
- *The equivalent dose.* The equivalent dose allows weighting for different types of radiation in order to reflect more accurately differences in their interactions with matter (and tissues). The common unit is the rem (roentgen-equivalent man); the SI unit is the sievert. The weighting is achieved using a *quality factor* (see below), which has been derived from research and is standardized for all radiation workers and patients. It is important to avoid any risk of confusion between the absorbed dose and the equivalent dose by using the corresponding special units, since both are measured in joules per kilogram.
- *Rem (roentgen-equivalent man).* The rem is a unit quantifying equivalent or effective dose. It relates the dose absorbed in human tissue to the effective biological damage of the radiation. Particulate and electromagnetic radiations have differing effects on tissue, even if the absorbed dose is the same. A smaller unit used is the millirem (mrem), which is 1/1000th of a rem. To calculate the equivalent dose, the absorbed dose (rad) is multiplied by a quality factor (QF) that is unique to the type of radiation. Values for these are shown in Table 2.2.
- *Sievert (Sv).* The SI unit of equivalent dose is the sievert. A smaller unit used is one-millionth of a sievert, or the microsievert (µSv). To calculate the equivalent dose the absorbed dose (Gy) is multiplied by a quality factor (QF) that is unique to the type of radiation (Table 2.2). The conversion between Sieverts and Rems is 1 Sv = 100 Rem.

Table 2.2 Quality factor assignments for radiation

Types of radiation	Quality factor
X- or gamma-rays	1
Beta particles	1
Alpha particles	20

- *Quality factor (QF)*. The quality factor values Table 2.2 are from the International Commission on Radiological Protection (ICRP) publication 26 in 1978 and revised publication 60 in 1990. These values are based on the type of radiation and the tissue mass in which the energy is distributed (Lawson, 1999), and allow authorities and employers to monitor the potential amount of radiation damage occurring in a person's body. Armed with these numbers, they can intervene if exposure, dose, or equivalent dose exceeds periodic limits. For the nuclear pharmacist, monitoring the pharmacy and personal exposure enables completion of procedures with nominal risk. It is helpful to understand the types of emission occurring in materials being handled so that adequate protection can be used.

Penetration potential

As described above, various emissions have different characteristics, depending on their energies, and whether they are particulate or electromagnetic in nature (Figures 2.32 and 2.33).

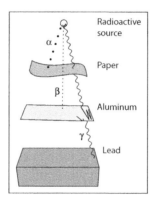

Figure 2.32   Penetration potential in materials for different radiation types.

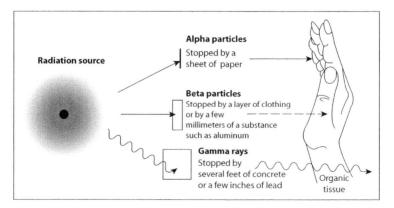

Figure 2.33   Penetration potential in tissue for different radiation types.

Alpha particles

Alpha particles have the shortest range of all the emissions, so only a small distance is required to avoid exposure. Alpha particles can be stopped with paper. They cause effective cell death when in close contact and, therefore, are sometimes used in cancer treatment. If ingested, alpha particles can cause extensive damage in a concentrated area, and, because of their typically long half-lives, provide prolonged exposure.

Skin is thick enough to protect from alpha radiation. One simply needs to wash the hands and avoid breathing it. So, exposure is not normally an issue with alpha emitters, especially since the alpha emitters are rarely used in a nuclear pharmacy. However, being difficult to monitor, exposure can be very insidious.

Beta particles

Ionization and excitation of atoms occur when beta particles interact with matter, similar to the manner in which alpha particles interact with matter. One way beta particle energy is lost is via bremsstrahlung radiation (see above). Beta particles can be stopped by plastic, aluminum, or other materials of low Z number. Therefore, lucite, plastic, glass, or aluminum are used for shielding and protection.

Ingestion of beta-emitting isotopes can have severe consequences, especially radioisotopes of carbon, hydrogen, sulfur, and phosphorus, since these can be incorporated into biochemical materials in the body. They can be deposited in tissues or DNA and cause extensive damage. In addition, many of these isotopes have long half-lives, so they can stay in the body for long periods of time, leading to genetic problems and molecular destruction for many years. Fortunately, beta emission is easy to monitor, so workers can be aware of shielding needs and deficiencies.

Gamma photons

Gamma photon energies usually are larger than chemical bond energies, and can therefore cause chemical reactions or destroy structures in biological (and non-biological) systems. Recall that gamma photons can cause ionization and excitation, though not as effectively as alpha and beta particles.

Shielding requirements for gamma-emitting isotopes depend on the energy of the gamma rays. Low-energy gamma rays require only plastic containers, while high-energy gamma rays require the use of lead or materials of high Z number.

Gamma photons penetrate skin and tissue easily. The photoelectric effect occurs mostly in tissue. There is no 'safe' level of exposure to gamma radiation. However, of the typical emissions encountered in nuclear pharmacy, gamma radiation is the least worrisome regarding tissue damage.

Summary

Atoms consist of three main components: neutrons, protons, and electrons. Atoms are defined by numbers representing the numbers of neutrons, protons, and the sum of the numbers of neutrons and protons. These numbers can be represented schematically by the three letters N, Z, and A, respectively.

Two atoms that differ only in their number of neutrons are called isotopes, while those differing in the number of protons are either isobars or isotones. By virtue of possessing differing numbers of protons, isotones and isobars are actually different elements.

Energy and mass are interchangeable, and the units most pertinent to expressing these are the AMU, erg, and electronvolt.

Atoms may be either stable nuclides or unstable *radionuclides*. If an atom is radioactive, meaning it emits either particulate or electromagnetic radiation, its degree of radioactivity can be expressed in either curies or becquerels.

An element is radioactive because of an energy instability within the nucleus. By emitting various forms of radioactivity, the nucleus is eventually able to attain energy stability. The mechanisms by which atoms rid themselves of energy include beta, positron, and gamma radiations. These emissions interact with matter in either a destructive or medically useful manner. Beta particles can be used therapeutically. Positron and gamma emissions can be used diagnostically.

It is wise for the practitioner to be aware of direct and ancillary radiations that can interact with tissues, sometimes from unsuspected origins.

Decay schemes are often used in order to gain understanding of how radionuclides decay, and by which radioactive emission type.

Radioactive decay follows a first-order mathematical process. By understanding a radioisotope's half-life and decay mechanisms, its use can be optimized. This is true for the preparation and use of radiopharmaceuticals and understanding source materials such as radionuclide generators.

Having an awareness of the effects of radioactivity on the body allows the nuclear pharmacist to safely handle, monitor, and prepare doses of radiopharmaceuticals for patients. Monitoring radiation in the work environment and evaluating radiation exposure to personnel and patients is quantified by using the units of roentgens, rads, grays, rems, and sieverts. Some of these units express the exposure of air to radioactivity, while others express the amount of radiation absorbed by tissues. By using knowledge of the type of radiation encountered, the nuclear pharmacist is better able to assess risks and benefits of radiation exposure to personnel and patients. This knowledge is based on a sound understanding of radioactivity and radioactive decay.

Self-assessment questions

1 What are the three major components of atoms?
2 What are nucleons?
3 What are the differences among isotopes, isobars, isomers, isotones, and ions?
4 What are the four fundamental forces?
5 Rank the four forces, from most important to least important, in regard to their effects on the nucleus.
6 The mass of ^{32}P is 31.9739 (http://wwwndc.jaea.go.jp/CN04/). (a) Calculate the mass defect in MeV. (b) Calculate the average binding energy for each nucleon.
7 How does the neutron to proton ratio for radionuclides predict whether they will decay by beta, positron emission, or electron capture?
8 Write the nuclear state equations for alpha, beta, and positron decay.
9 Which of the decays mentioned in question 8 has the most energy?
10 Which of the decays mentioned in question 8 has/have use in nuclear pharmacy and nuclear medicine?
11 What are the main mechanisms of interaction with matter for each of the decays mentioned in question 8?
12 Which emission can have bremsstrahlung associated with it?
13 What type of decay is indicated by (a) an arrow pointing down and to the right; (b) down and to the left; (c) straight down?
14 The half-life of ^{32}P is 14.262 days. Calculate its decay constant.
15 Calculate the half-life, in seconds, of an isotope for which $\lambda = 0.0825$/h.
16 A ^{99m}Tc-sodium pertechnitate injection has a labeled activity of $550\,\mu$Ci. Express this activity in terms of MBq.
17 A ^{201}Tl-thallous chloride (^{201}TlCl) injection has a labeled activity of 132 MBq. Express this activity in terms of mCi.
18 Express the radioactivity in MBq for a substance with 5.15×10^7 dps.
19 How many dps are represented by a material whose activity is 13.25 mCi?
20 At 10:00 am ^{99m}Tc radioactivity was measured as 19 mCi (703 MBq) on a certain day. What was the activity at (a) 8:00 am and (b) 5:00 pm on the same day (half-life for ^{99m}Tc is 6.02 h)?
21 The original quantity of an isotope is measured as $750\,\mu$Ci/mL (27.8 MBq/mL). If the quantity remaining after 16 days is

187.5 µCi/mL (6.9 MBq/mL), calculate (a) the decay constant and (b) the half-life.
22 Calculate (a) the total number of atoms and (b) the total mass of ^{99m}Tc present in 8 mCi (296 MBq) ^{99m}Tc (half-life 6.02 h).
23 Define the terms roentgen, rad, rem, gray, and sievert.
24 What is the most damaging type of radiation?
25 What radiation has the longest range?

References

Clarke FW *et al.* (1903). Report of the International Commission on Atomic Weights. *J Am Chem Soc* 25.

Franz N *et al.* (1936). The radiations emitted from artificially produced radioactive substances. I. The upper limits and shapes of the β-ray spectra from several elements. *Phys Rev* 49: 368–381.

Holloway MG, Livingston Stanley M (1938). Range and specific ionization of alpha-particles. *Phys Rev* 54: 18–37.

International Commission on Radiological Protection (1978). *Publication* 26. New York: Pergamon.

International Commission on Radiological Protection (1990). *Publication 60: Recommendations of the International Commission on Radiological Protection* [*Annals of the International Commission on Radiological Protection*, Vol 21/1-3]. New York: Elsevier.

Lawson RS (1999). *Introduction to Radioactivity* http://www.e-radiography.net/articles/Introduction%20to%20Radioactivity.pdf.

Loevinger R (Apr 1957). "Average energy of allowed beta-particle spectra". *Phys Med Biol* 1(4): 330–339.

Mattauch J (1958). The rational choice of a unified scale for atomic weights and nuclidic masses. Supplement to E. Wichers *Report on Atomic Weights for 1956-57*. *J Am Chem Soc* 80: 4121.

Wang C *et al.* (1975). *Radiotracer Methodology in the Biological Environmental, and Physical Sciences*. Englewood Cliffs, NJ: Prentice-Hall.

Further reading and web sources

Georgia State University (2008). *Fundamental Physical Constants* http://hyperphysics.phy-astr.gsu.edu/hbase/Tables/funcon.html (accessed March 7, 2009).

Georgia State University (2008). *Fundamental Forces* http://230nsc1.phy-astr.gsu.edu/hbase/forces/funfor.html (accessed March 7, 2009).

Hall E (2000). *Radiobiology for the Radiobiologist*. Philadelphia, PA: Lippincott Williams & Wilkins.

Idaho State University *Radiation Related Terms* http://www.physics.isu.edu/radinf/terms.htm.

Java Applet depicting Radioactive Decay http://lectureonline.cl.msu.edu/~mmp/applist/decay/decay.htm.

Kowalsky R, Falen S (2004). *Radiopharmaceuticals in Nuclear Pharmacy and Nuclear Medicine*, 2nd edn. Washington, DC: American Pharmacists Association.

Los Alamos Laboratory *Periodic Table of the Elements* http://periodic.lanl.gov/default.htm (accessed July 2, 2009).

MIRD *Radionuclide Data and Decay Schemes and Trilinear Chart of the Nuclides* http://wwwndc.jaea.go.jp/CN04/.

Nuclear Chain Reaction http://lectureonline.cl.msu.edu/~mmp/applist/chain/chain.htm.

Nuclear Isotopes Half Life http://lectureonline.cl.msu.edu/~mmp/kap30/Nuclear/nuc.htm.
Periodic Table http://periodic.lanl.gov/default.htm.
Princeton University http://web.princeton.edu/sites/ehs/radsafeguide/rsg_app_e.htm.
Saha G (2004). *Fundamentals of Nuclear Pharmacy*. New York: Springer.
Silvis J, Kowitt M, Goddard Space Flight Center *Ask an Astrophysicist* http://imagine.gsfc.nasa.gov/docs/ask_astro/answers/980127c.html.

3

The physiological basis of radiopharmaceuticals

Kara Duncan Weatherman, William Crisp,

and Hannah Weber

Learning objectives

- Understand the tracer principle and how it relates to nuclear medicine imaging
- Recognize the physiological mechanisms that are mapped when performing nuclear medicine imaging
- Identify how select radiopharmaceuticals map a particular physiological process.

Introduction

Nuclear medicine is an area of medical practice that uses radioactive materials for both diagnostic and therapeutic purposes. Nuclear medicine is primarily a diagnostic imaging specialty, combining the biological behavior of a radioactive pharmaceutical with the ability to image the resulting radioactive emissions, giving both anatomical and functional information about the tissues or organs being studied. Nuclear medicine also can be used for therapeutic delivery of radioisotopes for the treatment of disease and as an *in vitro* tracer to evaluate binding processes or concentration determinations. Understanding the physiological behavior that the radioactive tracer exhibits once administered is essential in understanding the role that the nuclear medicine study plays in the diagnosis or treatment of disease. This chapter covers most of the major physiological mechanisms that are mapped by various radiopharmaceuticals to assist in the understanding of how specific nuclear medicine studies can provide essential information to support diagnosis and treatment of various diseases. Each physiological mechanism will be discussed, with examples of the imaging procedures that use that mechanism as well as the type of information that can be obtained when each study is performed. The scope of this chapter is not to discuss every radiopharmaceutical product, just give representative examples of imaging studies that follow the physiological process in question. Further discussion of the radiopharmaceuticals in subsequent chapters should provide greater discussion of the specific physiological mechanisms for each product.

Tracer principle

Before discussing any physiological process in the body, it is imperative to understand the concept of the tracer principle. The tracer principle helps to explain the ability of nuclear medicine studies to show organ function. In nuclear medicine, a radioactive isotope is associated with a compound that is known to behave in a specific manner in the body. This molecule is referred to as a tracer because of the quantity of the molecule that is administered. In most cases, the mass amount of the tracer is in the microgram or milligram range. The tracer principle is important because the imaging process attempts to map the physiological process being studied accurately without imparting any change in the process caused by the physiological effect of the tracer molecule. In the very small amounts of tracer used for nuclear medicine studies, the tracer can 'map' the physiological process as it exists in the patient receiving the radiopharmaceutical. The administration of the radiopharmaceutical will not change (either improve or further degrade) the physiological process being studied.

During imaging, the path of the radiotracer outlines mechanisms of chemical or biological processes occurring in the body. A quality radiotracer will be subjected to the same mechanisms of absorption, distribution, metabolism, and elimination (ADME) as the material it is designed to mimic. Since most radiopharmaceuticals are administered by intravenous injection, the absorption step is generally not necessary. Function of organs and organ systems is determined based upon how the body treats the imported radiotracer relative to the normal process or expected mechanism(s). Ideally, the radiotracer is highly specific for its targeted process, such that other biochemical processes in the body are not affected. Some tracers will remain in the cavity in which the tracer was injected, whereas other radiotracers will leave the site of injection and migrate elsewhere in the body. Radiotracers can also be used to obtain a more quantitative analysis based upon the redistribution of the radiotracer in the body.

Isotope dilution

Isotope dilution is a technique to obtain quantitative biochemical data including plasma volume and red blood cell (RBC) volume. These *in vivo* nuclear medicine blood studies utilize isotope dilution techniques by injecting a radiotracer, of a known volume and concentration, into a cavity of unknown volume. By withdrawing samples of the patient's blood at various time points after equilibration has occurred, the change in concentration of the injected radiotracer is then observed and is used to calculate the unknown volume of the cavity. The magnitude of the unknown volume is inversely related to the concentration of the radiotracer in the unknown volume by the relationship $C_1 V_1 = C_2 V_2$, where C_1 is the measured concentration of the radiotracer in some initial, known volume (V_1). After administration of the radiotracer, a sample can be removed from the patient and its concentration (C_2) can be determined. From these three variables, the unknown volume (V_2) can be determined. The value of using radioactive tracers for studies such as these is that it allows quantification of the concentration of the radioactive component in the sample using commonly available detection methods (Kowalsky & Falen 2004, pp. 753–761).

An example of the isotope dilution concept is seen when performing various hematological blood volume studies to determine such variables as whole blood volume, RBC volume, or plasma volume. While these studies are performed fairly infrequently today in light of advances in hematological testing methods, they may still be utilized when traditional testing does not provide sufficient diagnostic information. Red blood cells can be radiolabeled with chromium-51 (^{51}Cr). Plasma volume studies use human serum albumin (HSA) labeled with iodine-125 (^{125}I). As described above, a standardized sample containing a known activity of radiolabeled RBC or HSA prepared in known volume, is injected into a patient. Following adequate time for equilibration, a blood sample is drawn and the amount of radioactivity in the specimen can be determined. Using the formula above, plasma volume and red cell volume can be determined. Other types of data that can be obtained using the isotope dilution concept include total blood volume (calculated with a known hematocrit) and RBC survival (Lewis *et al.* 2006).

Simple (passive) diffusion

Simple diffusion is one of the most basic ways that substances can get into and out of cells. Radiopharmaceuticals use simple diffusion as a mechanism of localization in target organs for several different nuclear medicine studies. Simple diffusion is the movement of a molecule from a region of high concentration to one of low concentration. In this method of transport, the molecule does not require a protein to aid its movement to another region. In order for a molecule to pass through the lipid bilayer of a cell membrane using simple diffusion, the molecule must be non-polar and lipophilic (hydrophobic). If a hydrophilic molecule attempted to participate in simple diffusion, it would be rejected as it moved into the hydrophobic region of the membrane. The rate of diffusion is directly proportional to the concentration of the molecule; the greater the concentration of the radiotracer, the greater the transport of the molecule. The rate of diffusion is also affected by the lipid solubility of the substance. Using simple diffusion, a highly lipophilic radiotracer will diffuse across a membrane and either bind to a cellular component or redistribute to another location. Charged molecules can also participate in passive diffusion, with movement driven by the electrochemical potential that exists across a membrane.

Xenon-133 is an example of a radiotracer that undergoes the process of simple diffusion. It is administered as a gas and is inhaled during pulmonary ventilation imaging. In the lungs, the lipophilic ^{133}Xe gas moves through the airways, and with time, will be able to diffuse into obstructed areas of the lungs. A small proportion of the lipophilic molecules diffuse across the alveolar membrane in the lungs into the bloodstream where they circulate throughout the vasculature. The gas molecules eventually return to the lungs where they diffuse again over the alveolar membrane and will be excreted when the patient exhales. While most of the tracer ends up back in the lungs to be exhaled, if the tracer encounters another highly lipophilic barrier within the body, it can diffuse into these areas and be retained. ^{133}Xe uptake may sometimes be seen in the liver due to the high fatty content of this organ (Kowalsky & Falen 2004, pp. 569–571).

Facilitated diffusion

Facilitated diffusion, like passive diffusion, functions to move substrates down a concentration gradient. However, in facilitated diffusion, the use of transport proteins is required to move substrates across the cell membrane. Generally, substances that are not lipid soluble but are still required for cellular viability must cross the cell membrane using facilitated diffusion (Ganong 1997, p. 29). While there is no energy requirement for facilitated diffusion, the rate of transport of substrates across cell membranes by this method can be affected by several factors. The rate of facilitated diffusion is dependent upon the extent of the concentration gradient and the availability of the transport protein to transport substrate across the membrane. The transport process is generally specific for a particular substance and the transport mechanism can be saturated.

The PET imaging agent ^{18}F-fluorodeoxyglucose (^{18}F-FDG) is a hydrophilic glucose analog. It is transported into cells, as is glucose, using facilitated diffusion. Glucose moves across cell membranes with the assistance of transport proteins (Ganong 1997, pp. 315–316). There are 13 known facilitative glucose transporters (GLUTs) that move glucose, ^{18}F-FDG and other sugars down a concentration gradient. The most commonly expressed transport protein, GLUT-1, is overexpressed in certain tumor types (Avril 2004). This leads to an increase in the uptake of the ^{18}F-FDG in these tissues compared with surrounding tissues.

Active transport

Active transport across a cell membrane is the energy-dependent transport of a substance against its concentration gradient. This direction of cellular transport is sometimes referred to as an uphill movement, as the substance is moved from an area of lower concentration to an area of higher concentration. In addition, if the substance is an electrolyte, the movement occurs from a lower to a higher electrochemical potential. In active transport, the substance must be combined with a carrier protein or an enzyme at the outer membrane of the cell. The material then is passed through the membrane, cleaved from the carrier, and released into the cytoplasm. Generally, the energy required for this process comes from adenosine triphosphate (ATP). In primary active transport, the energy source used to carry out transport of a substance comes directly from ATP (Kowalsky & Falen 2004, p. 453). In secondary active transport, the energy used to drive transport of a substance comes from the gradient potential created by a primary transport mechanism. More specifically, the gradient created by a primary active transport mechanism contains stored energy that can be used to drive transport with a secondary transport protein. Co-transport is referred to as moving two substances across a membrane in the same direction. The contrary, secondary active transport involving the movement of two substances across a membrane in opposite directions, is referred to as antiport (Ganong 1997, p. 29).

In nuclear medicine imaging, one of the most common approaches utilizing active transport is the movement of radioactive iodine compounds into the thyroid tissue, by way of the Na^+/I^- symporter. This process is used to evaluate the functional capacity of the thyroid gland by measuring the uptake of radioactivity into the gland after the administration of a known amount of radioactive iodine. This process can also be used if radioactive iodine is administered for therapeutic purposes. The iodine molecules that are taken up in the thyroid tissue are incorporated into thyroid hormones, effectively trapping the radioactive material in the thyroid gland and allowing the therapeutic effect. Another use of active transport occurs when using thallium-201 (^{201}Tl) as a marker of myocardial perfusion. ^{201}Tl is a potassium analog that must be transported across the myocardial membrane using the Na^+/K^+-ATPase pump in order to get into cells. The Na^+/K^+-ATPase carrier is present in all tissues of the body and moves two potassium ions (or in nuclear imaging, ^{201}Tl) into the cell while moving three sodium ions out of the cell (Ganong 1997, p. 29). In myocardial perfusion imaging, the viability of myocardial cells can be assessed by determining the movement of ^{201}Tl into the cell. If the tissue is non-viable, the Na^+/K^+-ATPase pump is no longer functional, and there will be no movement of ^{201}Tl into or out of the myocardial cells.

Capillary blockade

Capillary blockade is most commonly used in nuclear medicine to visualize and determine the perfusion to organs such as the heart, lung, and brain. Capillary blockade is the intentional obstruction of blood flow through a capillary bed. The diameter of a human capillary averages 8 µm (with a range between 6 and 10 µm). When performing capillary blockade, small particles of appropriate size (usually 10 µm) are radiolabeled with an isotope and then injected into the vascular space (Kowalsky & Falen 2004, pp. 561–562). Depending on the site of injection, the particles will travel through the system until they reach the first capillary bed. At the capillary level, the particles will become trapped in the capillary vasculature through a process termed microembolization. The blockage of blood flow at the capillary level should be maintained for a sufficient period of time to allow imaging, but it is important that the particles are fragile enough to be degraded and removed from the capillary bed as a result of the normal hemodynamic pressure in the pulmonary vasculature. When imaging, the relative distribution or trapping of the radiolabeled particles provides insight into the regional blood perfusion that occurs in the tissues being studied. There will be increased particle accumulation in areas of increased perfusion and an absence of particles in area where there is no perfusion.

One tracer used for this capillary blockage technique is ^{99m}Tc-macroaggregated albumin (^{99m}Tc-MAA), which is a radiopharmaceutical used to determine the perfusion of the lungs. The pulmonary artery branches into arteries that are 60–100 µm in diameter; these then branch into arterioles of 25–30 µm diameter and end in capillaries. The average diameter of the pulmonary capillaries ranges from 7 to 10 µm, which is large enough to allow the passage of a single RBC (Saha 2004, p. 261). The ^{99m}Tc-MAA particles, which have a slightly larger diameter (approximately 10–50 µm), mechanically lodge in or near the pulmonary capillary bed and temporarily block the blood flow through the capillaries. Imaging of particle distribution provides insight into the distribution of blood flow throughout the lungs.

Compartmental localization

Compartmental localization involves the placement of a radiotracer into a fluid-filled space in the body. The radiotracer must be retained in the space long enough to obtain an image of the space. Once administered, the tracer can remain localized at the site of administration or can move with fluid movement within the space. Radiopharmaceutical imaging using compartmental localization can be used to assess normal fluid migration, to evaluate for potential blockages that inhibit normal migration of fluid, and to evaluate the compartmental space to identify the presence of fluid leakage from the space. Examples of fluid-filled compartments in the human body are the cerebrospinal cavity (encompassing the brain and spinal cord) and the vascular system.

In nuclear medicine, radionuclide cisternography can be used to study the migration and flow of cerebrospinal fluid (CSF). CSF is produced in the choroid plexus at a rate of 30–35 mL/h. At any time, the total volume of CSF in the cerebrospinal cavity is approximately 150 mL, 30 mL of which is found surrounding the spinal cord (Ganong 1997, p. 568; Kowalsky & Falen 2004, p. 473). Cisternography involves the administration diethylenetriaminepentaacetic acid (DTPA) labeled with indium-111 (^{111}In-DTPA), as a lumbar injection. The DTPA component of the radiopharmaceutical is hydrophilic and will not diffuse across the membrane surrounding the spinal column, effectively trapping the tracer in the cerebrospinal canal. The molecule is also resistant to degradation by enzymes found in the CSF (Kowalsky & Falen 2004, p. 476). The radiotracer moves slowly from the site of injection toward the head. Whole-body imaging of the patient allows visualization of any areas where CSF movement is blocked or where CSF fluid is leaking out of the cerebrospinal space. Another example of compartmental localization is blood pool imaging using ^{99m}Tc-labeled RBCs. In this process, a patient's own RBCs are removed and radiolabeled, then reinjected into the vascular space and allowed to circulate. Since the vascular space is closed, the RBCs should circulate and remain contained within the vasculature. For nuclear medicine applications, labeled RBC movement through the cardiac chambers can be used to measure the cardiac ejection fraction (amount of blood being pumped with each heartbeat). Labeled RBCs can also be used to evaluate sites of abnormal bleeding within the body, most commonly in the gastrointestinal tract. If a site of bleeding occurs within the tract, the labeled RBCs will leak out of the vascular space and into the tract lumen. Visualization of radioactivity in the gastrointestinal tract is indicative of gastrointestinal bleeding.

Chemisorption

Chemisorption, also known as physicochemical adsorption, is the binding of a radiopharmaceutical to the surface of a solid structure. This mechanism of localization is commonly used in radionuclide bone imaging. Bone comprises inorganic and organic constituents. The organic matrix includes collagen fibers and cartilage, which gives bone flexibility. The inorganic matrix includes the hydroxyapatite structure of the bone. This is formed from the crystallization of amorphous calcium phosphorus salts and gives the bone its strength and rigidity. New bone formation requires the delivery of various minerals to the bone through increased blood flow to the area. Areas of new bone formation are referred to as reactive bone (Ganong 1997, p. 361).

In nuclear medicine bone imaging, many of the bone imaging agents include a phosphonate or phosphate group, which has high affinity for the calcium of the inorganic mineral structure. This allows the radiotracer to localize in the mineral component of the bone and be absorbed into the inorganic matrix of the bone (Kowalsky & Falen 2004, p. 697). Increased uptake of the radiotracer is seen in areas of reactive bone. Blood flow is increased to this area and this adds to the increased presentation of the radioactive tracer to the site, which further enhances uptake. Today, the most common bone imaging agents that use this mechanism of localization include ^{99m}Tc-labeled methylene diphosphonate (bisphosphonate; ^{99m}Tc-MDP) and ^{99m}Tc hydroxymethylene diphosphonate (bisphosphonate; ^{99m}Tc-HDP). These agents are used to evaluate arthritis, Paget's disease, osteomyelitis, and the metastatic spread of cancer to the bone.

Phagocytosis

Phagocytosis is a cellular process in which immune cells within the body engulf particulate material such as bacteria. When particulate material comes in contact with the outer surface of the phagocytic cell, the cellular membrane invaginates to encircle the foreign material and engulf it into a vacuole or tiny cavity. This process can be both receptor and non-receptor mediated (Ganong 1997, p. 26). In the body, much of the phagocytic activity occurs in the organs of the reticuloendothelial system, which is made up of the liver, spleen, and bone marrow. Specialized cells called monocytes and macrophages are produced in the bone marrow and released into the circulation, where they eventually move into tissues in various places throughout the body and remain as fixed macrophages. Monocytes will mature to different types of macrophage depending on their anatomical location (Naito *et al.* 1997). In the reticuloendothelial system, the mature macrophage is termed a Kupffer cell.

Nuclear medicine imaging can be performed to identify the functional capacity of the Kupffer cells. In patients with diffuse and focal liver disease, ^{99m}Tc-labeled sulfur colloid imaging assesses the functional capacity of the liver; it can also identify disorders of the spleen, such as trauma, infarcts, and tumors. The radiopharmaceutical ^{99m}Tc-sulfur colloid is a suspension made up of small ($< 1\,\mu m$) colloidal particles and created by heating ^{99m}Tc and sodium thiosulfate in the presence of acid. Once the particles have been injected into the body, they circulate until they reach the reticuloendothelial system. Kupffer cells of the liver remove 80–85% of the colloidal particles injected, while the spleen (5–10%) and the bone marrow ($\sim 5\%$) take up the remainder (Saha 2004, p. 271).

Antigen–antibody binding

Radioactively labeled monoclonal antibodies with high affinities for tumor antigens can be used to localize radiopharmaceuticals at any site of tumor development. Antibodies, also called immunoglobulins, are large Y-shaped proteins that are produced by plasma cells in response to exposure to foreign substances (antigens). Antibodies identify the shapes of specific binding sites on the surface of the antigen. The location that each antibody binds to on the antigen is called the epitope. A monoclonal antibody binds to one specific epitope. Targeting human tumors requires the identification of tumor-associated or tumor-specific antigens that are expressed on tumor cell surfaces. There are several monoclonal antibodies that have been developed against tumor-specific antigens for both diagnostic and therapeutic use. The uptake of a radiopharmaceutical in this case is a result of specific binding of a radiolabeled antibody to a surface antigen on a specific tumor.

Radiolabeled monoclonal antibodies that are highly specific for a particular antigen are injected intravenously then imaged at a later time, once the monoclonal antibody has been given time to localize at the antigenic site. The injected antibody binds to a specific cell marker and allows imaging of the affected area, which can include both the primary tumor and any metastases. While radiolabeled antibodies have had moderate success in diagnostic applications in nuclear medicine, their use for therapy of certain types of cancer has become more prevalent in recent years. Currently, two monoclonal antibodies, yttrium-90 (^{90}Y)-ibritumomab tiuxetan (Y-90 Zevalin) and ^{131}I-tositumomab (I-131 Bexxar) are used for the treatment of non-Hodgkin's lymphoma in patients who have failed traditional therapy. The non-radioactive monoclonal antibody component of these agents produces a cytotoxic effect on tumor cells by stimulating the body's immune responses through a variety of mechanisms. The addition of a radioactive label to a monoclonal antibody allows a dual approach to killing cancer cells. The monoclonal antibody continues to promote immune responses, while the radioactive label adds cellular damage from the interaction of radioactive emissions with the tumor cell. The addition of the radioactive component also promotes cellular damage across several cell widths because of the path of travel of the radioactive emission. This phenomenon, called the 'crossfire effect,' enhances the destructive potential of the therapeutic agent (Kowalsky & Falen 2004, p. 768).

Receptor binding

Radiopharmaceuticals can localize within the body by binding to a specific receptor found on various tissues in the body. The receptor in most cases is simply a binding site on a membrane or surface protein that has the ability to form a complex with a biomolecule that matches the configuration of the binding site. Once the desired comound has bound to the receptor, the receptor protein has the ability to change conformation and activate specific signaling mechanisms within a cell, leading to a physiological effect.

In humans, the somatostatin receptor system is an example of this type of binding and has been used as the basis for the development of a radiopharmaceutical used for both diagnostic and therapeutic purposes. Somatostatin is a peptide that is secreted by a broad range of tissues in the body. Somatostatin is well known to have an inhibitory action on the secretion of many other hormones in the body, including growth hormone from the pituitary gland and insulin and glucagon from the pancreas. In nuclear medicine, somatostatin analogs have been developed that have similar binding affinities to somatostatin for its receptors. In many disease states, there is upregulation of somatostatin receptors, creating cells with a high density of somatostatin receptors compared with normal tissues. The radiopharmaceutical ^{111}In-pentetreotide (In-111 OctreoScan) has an amino acid sequence that is very similar to that of endogenous somatostatin and so has a very high affinity for the receptor. The radiolabeled product will accumulate in higher concentrations in tumor cells, both primary and metastatic, than in normal cells because of the increased number of somatostatin receptors, providing a tool for accurate localization of the affected tissues (Kowalsky & Falen 2004, p. 706).

Summary

Nuclear medicine is a diagnostic imaging modality that is used to provide functional information about various organs and organ systems within the body. This is done by using a small quantity of material, called a tracer, to follow the physiological interaction that occurs within a specific patient. The small mass of material used allows the tracer to map the physiological process without imparting any pharmacological effect. This provides a view of the functional capacity of the system being studied. This chapter provided a brief view of some of the common physiological processes that are studied using nuclear medicine imaging. While it was not intended to provide a complete picture of the processes being studied, it should provide the foundation for understanding the mechanisms by which radiopharmaceuticals provide both diagnostic and therapeutic information regarding the functional capacity of the system being studied.

Self-assessment questions

1 Nuclear medicine provides both anatomical and physiological information about the tissues or organs being studied: true or false?

2 Which of the following is *true* regarding the tracer principle?
 a the tracer is present in large quantities to provide sufficient information about the process being studied
 b the administration of the tracer will impart a change in the physiological process being studied
 c the tracer is able to map the physiological process as it exists in the patient
 d none of the above is true.

3 Isotope dilution is used to assist in the determination of the unknown volume of a cavity: true or false?

4 Which of the following is *not true* regarding simple or passive diffusion?
 a movement occurs from high concentration to low concentration
 b there is no need for a carrier molecule (like a protein) to assist in the movement
 c movement requires input of energy, usually from ATP
 d charged molecules can undergo passive diffusion.

5 Facilitated diffusion:
 a moves substrates down a concentration gradient
 b requires a transport protein to move substances across the cellular membrane
 c does not require energy to occur
 d all of a–c
 e none of a–c.

6 The most common energy source used to drive molecules moving through a membrane using active transport is

a adenosine triphosphate (ATP)

b cyclic adenosine monophosphate (cAMP)

c electrochemical potential

d methylene diphosphonate (MDP).

7 In capillary blockade, the blockage of blood flow that occurs at the capillary level is permanent: true or false?

8 Which of the following is an example of a 'compartment' in the human body that could be studied using compartmental localization?

a spinal column

b gastrointestinal tract

c vasculature

d all of a–c

e none of a–c.

9 Which part of the body would be imaged to view the physiological process of chemisorption?

a bone

b heart

c liver

d kidneys.

10 Which of the following require specific binding of a molecule to a specific binding site in the body?

a antigen–antibody interactions

b chemisorption

c compartmental localization

d passive diffusion.

References

Avril N (2004). GLUT1 expression in tissue and F-18-FDG uptake. *J Nucl Med* 45: 930–932.

Ganong W (1997). *Review of Medical Physiology*. Stamford, CT: Appleton & Lange.

Kowalsky R, Falen S (2004). *Radiopharmaceuticals in Nuclear Pharmacy and Nuclear Medicine*, 2nd edn. Washington, DC: American Pharmacists Association.

Lewis SM *et al.* (2006). *Dacie and Lewis Practical Haematology*. Edinburgh: Churchill Livingstone, pp. 361–366.

Naito M *et al.* (1997). Development, differentiation, and maturation of Kupffer cells. *Microsc Res Technol* 39: 350–364.

Saha G. (2004). *Fundamentals of Nuclear Pharmacy*. New York: Springer.

4

Nuclear pharmacy operations

Kara Duncan Weatherman

Learning objectives

- Understand the basic aspects of nuclear pharmacy practice
- Recognize the similarities and differences between traditional pharmacy practice and nuclear pharmacy practice
- Identify the various areas of regulatory oversight required in nuclear pharmacy practice.

Introduction

Nuclear pharmacy is an area of pharmacy practice focusing on the preparation and dispensing of radiopharmaceuticals used in both the diagnosis and the treatment of various diseases. The practice of nuclear pharmacy shares some commonalities with traditional types of pharmacy practice, but the use of radioactivity in the compounding and dispensing functions provides a number of challenges and issues that truly make this area of practice unique. This chapter will cover the basic operational and regulatory aspects of nuclear pharmacy practice.

The nuclear pharmacy laboratory

Location

Nuclear pharmacy practice sites can be found in both hospital settings and as centralized laboratories in communities throughout the world. In most countries outside of the USA, nuclear pharmacy laboratories are located in a hospital, in close proximity to the nuclear medicine department. These laboratories can range in size and function, depending on the size of the department being serviced. In some instances, these nuclear pharmacy laboratories are staffed with a dedicated radiopharmacist, while in a smaller institution, the preparation and dispensing duties are carried out by a physicist or a nuclear medicine technologist under the supervision of the nuclear medicine physician of record. In the USA, there are limited numbers of dedicated nuclear pharmacy practice sites found in institutional practice locations. Most of these sites are found primarily in academic, tertiary care medical centers where patient care and research applications can both be serviced by an in-house pharmacy (Ponto & Hung 2000). In the late 1970s and early 1980s, the face of nuclear pharmacy practice in the USA began to change, as several centralized nuclear pharmacy companies were established. These nuclear pharmacy 'laboratories' were opened at various locations throughout the USA, first in large metropolitan areas and, in recent years, spreading to smaller cities and towns in geographic proximity to hospitals, clinics, and physician offices where nuclear medicine procedures are performed. The centralized nuclear pharmacy concept has been attempted with varying levels of success in several countries worldwide, but has not attained the level of use that is seen in the USA.

Centralized nuclear pharmacies are not located on every street corner in every city or town, as might be the case with traditional community pharmacy practice. The key placement issue for a nuclear pharmacy is a large collection of hospitals, clinics, and specialty physician offices in a fairly close geographic area. Since the main component of this specialty is handling radioactive material, which has a limited period of useful activity, most pharmacies are set up to deliver materials to end users within a two or three hour travel distance. Centralized nuclear pharmacy operations may be located in a unit found within a strip mall, in a medical office complex, and occasionally, in a free-standing building. Usually, there are very few indications that the occupant is classified as a pharmacy. Since there are significant rules and regulations that are imposed on nuclear pharmacies for the safe use and control of radioactive materials, it is desirable to limit movement of people into and out of the facility; consequently the pharmacies are generally designed so that it would be highly unlikely that someone would be able to walk in from the street unless they had a need to be there. Since nuclear pharmacies must deliver their products to the end user, the pharmacy must be located somewhere that allows an ample fleet of delivery vehicles to be maintained, and where the delivery staff will have quick and easy access to interstate and highway transportation routes.

As with most commercial pharmacy operations, the development of 'chain' nuclear pharmacies has come about over the years. Currently, there are three major chain nuclear pharmacy companies: Cardinal Health Nuclear Pharmacy Services, Covidien/Mallinckrodt Imaging, and GE Healthcare. These three chain companies combined have over 200 sites throughout the USA, along with a handful of sites in various cites across the world. Unlike traditional commercial pharmacies, however, there is also still a very strong presence of independent nuclear pharmacies throughout the USA. Currently, there are more than 100 independently owned nuclear pharmacies throughout the USA (United Pharmacy Partners 2008). In addition, some nuclear pharmacists chose to specialize in the production and dispensing of radiopharmaceuticals for PET imaging. This modality uses extremely short-lived radionuclides and is increasing in popularity (Callahan & Dragotakes 1999). This growth of PET imaging has influenced the development of institutional and centralized facilities dedicated to the production and dispensing of the radiopharmaceuticals used in this specialized imaging area.

Areas of the pharmacy

As stated earlier, nuclear pharmacy laboratories are generally centralized facilities with limited access for the general public. This is probably the most striking difference between community pharmacy practice and nuclear pharmacy practice. In a nuclear pharmacy, the most common interactions occur between the pharmacy staff and the nuclear medicine technologists and physicians working at the hospitals and clinics that are serviced. In general, there is no contact between the nuclear pharmacy staff and the patients themselves. Nuclear pharmacists that practice in an institutional setting may have some limited interaction with the patients, but again, they are more closely in contact with the physician and technologist staff who are carrying out the imaging procedure.

The nuclear pharmacy is generally divided into two general spaces: the non-restricted area and the restricted area. The non-restricted area includes all of the general areas of the pharmacy where staff and visitors should have no opportunity for contact with radioactive materials. These areas include the kitchen, eating areas, office areas, restrooms, storage areas, and the general reception areas. The restricted area includes any area of the pharmacy where radioactive materials are stored, handled, and dispensed. Since these areas have the potential for someone to come into contact with radioactive materials, the restricted area is closely controlled and monitored to ensure that there is minimal risk for inadvertent exposure to radioactive materials.

While each radiopharmacy will have a specific layout based on the size and structure of the building in which it is located, all radiopharmacy operations have similar areas located in the restricted area and that correlate with the usual tasks being performed on a day-to-day basis. These areas are described below.

Compounding area

Given that the prescription products that are dispensed from a nuclear pharmacy comprise radioactive material with a discrete and limited duration of use, the major function of the nuclear pharmacist is the continual preparation of radiopharmaceuticals to meet the needs of their customer base. The daily tasks of the nuclear pharmacist include the procurement of radioactive materials to be used in the preparation of a radiopharmaceutical and the physical manipulations necessary to combine the radioactive material and the material to be labeled to form the final radiopharmaceutical product. Since most radiopharmaceuticals will be administered to patients by intravenous injection, it is essential that all manipulations are carried out under strict sterile product compounding guidelines. The compounding area of a radiopharmacy will be found in a fairly segregated area of the pharmacy, away from major traffic areas yet close to the areas where the radioactive material is stored until needed. Most compounding is performed in a vertical laminar flow hood to avoid unnecessary exposure to radioactive materials for the compounding personnel. The hoods used in a nuclear pharmacy will be very similar to those used when compounding hazardous materials (e.g. for chemotherapy) in a hospital setting. The release of the recent USP revised general chapter <797> *Pharmaceutical Compounding – Sterile Preparations* has required most nuclear pharmacy operations to evaluate critically their sterile compounding procedures and possibly to increase the level of compliance. While discussions of USP <797> are out of the scope of this particular chapter, the interpretation of these requirements has varied among nuclear pharmacy practitioners, with some pharmacies outfitting the compounding area as a separate, dedicated 'cleanroom' located within the restricted area. The release of USP <797> has made substantial changes and improvements in the daily compounding operations of nuclear pharmacies (US Pharmacopeia 2008).

Dispensing area

After the nuclear pharmacist has prepared the radiopharmaceutical product, it must be subdivided into individual unit doses for each patient. Each unit dose is based on a prescription order that is communicated to the pharmacy by a staff member from the nuclear medicine department at a hospital or clinic. The order must indicate the desired product to be dispensed, as well as the desired amount of radioactive material needed at the specified time of day when the dose will be administered to the patient. Dispensing of the unit doses is usually done in a separate laminar flow hood found in close proximity to the hood used for compounding the radiopharmaceutical. In this area, pharmacy technicians are primarily responsible for the actual dispensing of the radio-pharmaceutical, drawing the correct amount of the compounded material into a unit dose syringe, checking the amount of radioactivity present in the syringe, and verifying that it matches the desired activity that will be dispensed to the patient. It must be kept in mind that this is somewhat more challenging since the dose will be administered to the patient at some point in time later than the time that the dose is dispensed from the pharmacy. It is the job of the nuclear pharmacy technician, working under the supervision of the nuclear pharmacist, to assure that the amount of material in the syringe at the time of dispensing will be sufficiently high to ensure that the amount of radioactive decay that occurs between the time of dispensing and the time of administration to the patient results in the desired amount of radioactivity for the patient. Again, because of the new USP <797> regulations, in most pharmacies, the compounding and dispensing hoods will be found in close proximity to each other. In addition, in fairly large pharmacies, there may be several dedicated dispensing hoods to allow the pharmacy staff to dispense the number of ordered doses in a timely fashion.

Blood labeling area

A common procedure performed in a nuclear pharmacy involves the isolation and separation of white blood cells from a sample of whole blood from a patient in the hospital nuclear medicine department. The blood is sent to the nuclear pharmacy, where the nuclear pharmacist or nuclear pharmacy technician separates the white blood cells from the sample, isolates the white cells from other cellular components, and then radiolabels the cells with a radioactive isotope. The labeled cells are then prepared for return to the hospital where they will be reinjected into the patient with the goal of identifying sites of infection in the body. The blood labeling area is segregated from the other areas of the pharmacy because of the inherent biohazard risk of handling blood products. However, since the blood will be labeled with radioactive materials, this area must still be found within the restricted area of the pharmacy.

Quality control area

Since the radiopharmaceuticals prepared in the radiopharmacy are compounded products, it is important that the compounding radiopharmacist is able to verify that the labeling reaction has occurred as expected, and the final product is, in fact, the desired radiopharmaceutical product. Small samples of each product compounded will be tested to confirm that the end product is acceptable for administration to the patient. The quality control procedures used in nuclear pharmacy utilize thin-layer chromatography, allowing the desired compound to be separated from any impurities and quantified. Generally, quality control testing is performed before or during the time that the nuclear pharmacy technician is dispensing the unit doses, so that any kits and doses that do not meet the required standards can be removed and replaced with new materials. Luckily, this process is fairly rapid and can easily be done before any doses are ready to be released from the pharmacy for delivery to the end user. In addition, the products that are used in nuclear pharmacy today are very stable and the chance of a radiopharmaceutical kit failure is very minimal.

Packaging and transport area

Every dose dispensed from a centralized nuclear pharmacy must be delivered to the end user at an outside facility, so a large component of the restricted area will be dedicated to the packaging and shipping of the final unit dose products. Each nuclear pharmacy will have driver/courier staff who will be responsible for securely closing and sealing each unit dose container, ensuring that the containers are not inadvertently contaminated with radioactive materials, placing the correct unit doses in the correct shipping containers for the end user, completing an inventory of each container, and following the appropriate regulatory requirements for shipping radioactive materials. Nuclear pharmacy technicians, and even the nuclear pharmacist, may be involved in this process to expedite the shipping process. The packaging and shipping process occurs throughout the day as doses are needed by the end users. Nuclear pharmacy facilities located within a hospital setting generally do not have significant package and transport needs since the doses are utilized within the department where they are prepared. There are some hospital-based nuclear pharmacies that do supply a limited number of doses to other nuclear medicine departments, generally in fairly close proximity to their facility. Regardless of the distance traveled, if materials are delivered outside the hospital, all shipments must comply with the regulations for packaging and transporting radioactive materials.

Order entry area

All radiopharmaceutical unit doses are dispensed pursuant to an order from a nuclear medicine physician or radiologist. A nuclear medicine technologist, working under the supervision of the physician, generally telephones in the orders to the pharmacy each afternoon, providing the dose requirements for the next day's imaging procedures. Orders are transcribed as they are called in, either by the nuclear pharmacist or by the nuclear pharmacy technician if state regulations allow technicians to take orders, and will be entered into the pharmacy computer system, which will generate legally valid prescription labels to accompany the patient dose to the hospital.

Radioactive material storage areas

Given that each nuclear pharmacy handles several different radioactive materials in the course of daily preparation and dispensing, each pharmacy will have one or more dedicated areas for the storage of radioactive materials. The storage area will generally be found in a secure area to prevent unintentional release of radioactive materials or unauthorized removal of radioactive materials from the restricted area. Unlike the inventory in most pharmacy facilities, radioactive material brings added storage requirements to prevent members of the pharmacy staff from having excessive exposure to radioactivity. Consequently, most storage areas in the pharmacy are heavily shielded with a dense material such as lead or tungsten to prevent excessive radioactive exposure during the normal movements of the pharmacy staff within the restricted area.

Radioactive waste areas

Unlike most other types of pharmacy practice, one of the major benefits of the centralized nuclear pharmacy services is the handling of waste products. The unit dose syringe after the patient has been injected is still a biohazard and it most likely still contains small but detectable amounts of radioactive materials. Federal and state regulations require that these syringes must be treated as biohazardous waste, but the presence of even small amounts of radioactive materials prohibits normal biohazard handling procedures (incineration of the waste materials). Any material for disposal must no longer be radioactive before sending to the biohazard incineration facility. The easiest way to eliminate the radioactive component is to hold the waste until the material naturally decays away. Depending on the isotope, this could be as short as a few hours, or as long as several years. Since most nuclear medicine departments have limited space for waste storage, one of the added benefits that a centralized nuclear pharmacy provides to its customers is the ability for the end user to return radioactive waste to the pharmacy for storage and disposal. After administration, the unit dose syringes are returned to the nuclear pharmacy in the original storage containers. Once in the pharmacy, members of the pharmacy staff are responsible for removing all waste from the shipping containers, segregating the waste based on the time needed for acceptable decay, then ensuring that all containers are cleaned and disinfected before they are used again. The radioactive waste is held in appropriately shielded containers until ready for disposal with a commercial waste service.

The size of most commercial nuclear pharmacies varies depending on the number of doses dispensed from the facility, the amount of equipment needed, and the number of staff members necessary to complete the daily tasks of the pharmacy. The number of doses that are dispensed from a centralized nuclear pharmacy will differ depending on the geographic location and the number of hospitals and clinics that are serviced by the pharmacy. Generally, smaller nuclear pharmacies may dispense between 100 and 300 doses each day, while medium-sized pharmacies may dispense between 300 and 800 doses each day, and some very large pharmacies that service very large populations may dispense between 1000 and 1500 doses each day. More than 75% of the doses dispensed from a nuclear pharmacy are dispensed within a four to six hour period each morning, with the remaining doses dispensed as needed throughout the day.

Staffing needs

To understand the staffing needs of a nuclear pharmacy, one must understand the normal operation schedule of the pharmacy. Nuclear pharmacy is a 24-hour a day service which is offered 365 days a year. Some nuclear pharmacies are open 24 hours a day, while other pharmacies close at 5 pm and cover the needs of their customers as an 'on-call' service. Generally, the operating hours of the pharmacy are dictated by the needs of their customers.

In nuclear pharmacies, there are standard 'shifts' that must be covered at all times. The busiest part of the day is the shift referred to as the 'early,' the 'opening,' or the 'night' shift. Since radiopharmaceuticals must be compounded daily because of the short duration of the radioactivity, and most nuclear medicine departments start seeing patients as early as 7 or 8 am, the nuclear pharmacy must prepare, dispense, and deliver the radiopharmaceutical doses before the first patient is ready to be imaged. This early shift is the one in which most of the doses dispensed from the pharmacy are prepared and delivered to the end users. Nuclear pharmacies that are open 24 hours will generally start preparing for this shift between 10 pm and midnight. In pharmacies that are not 24-hour operations, the first shift generally begins between midnight and 2 am, depending on the number of doses that must be prepared. The morning shift will generally be covered by one or two nuclear pharmacists, one or more nuclear pharmacy technicians, and several driver/couriers. The organizational flow of the pharmacy during this time is hectic but well organized. As the nuclear pharmacist prepares products, one member of the staff begins quality control testing while a nuclear pharmacy technician begins dispensing unit dose prescriptions. The driver/couriers package the materials into approved transport containers and prepare these containers for delivery to the end user. Delivery runs are arranged so that a single driver/courier will make deliveries to several hospitals along the route. Often, some members of the delivery staff will leave the pharmacy as early as 3 am to reach the all of the hospitals, some of which may be two or three hours away from the pharmacy. The early shift usually concludes by 6 am, with a majority of the daily doses dispensed from the pharmacy on the road for delivery. At this time, the morning nuclear pharmacist and nuclear pharmacy technician complete paperwork, carry out several required regulatory tests, and prepare for the second shift.

The second shift generally begins as members of the nuclear medicine department arrive for work between 6 and 7 am. In most departments, there will be additional orders that were scheduled after the department closed the evening before and called in to the pharmacy at this time. In addition, doses that were scheduled for later in the morning or early afternoon are generally held in the pharmacy and not dispensed on the earliest delivery run because of the potential problems with product stability at extended time points or limitations in the amount of radioactive material available during the early morning preparation. Usually, the early morning pharmacy staff are responsible for coordinating the second shift as well, as they are most aware of the daily workflow and how the delivery schedule was determined. In busy pharmacies, however, a second pharmacist and technician may be scheduled to assist in the second run preparation. There will be several driver/couriers present, including those who are just starting their work day as well as those early morning staff returning from their deliveries. The second shift is also a fairly busy time in the pharmacy, but it generally is complete by 9 or 10 am.

Staffing for the remainder of the daily operation schedule will depend on the logistics of the pharmacy. Generally, there will be one or two pharmacists available at any time, one or more pharmacy technicians, and several driver/couriers. Most of the day shift in a nuclear pharmacy involves filling additional 'add-on' doses called in by customers, performing white blood cell labeling, and completing various daily regulatory tasks. As the afternoon begins, customers generally start phoning in orders for studies that will be performed the next day, and so the nuclear pharmacist and technician will be busy taking orders, entering them into the computer system, and generally setting up the pharmacy to prepare as much as possible to alleviate some of the workload of the early shift the next morning. If the pharmacy is open 24 hours, this task may be carried out during the early evening hours. Nuclear pharmacies that are not open 24 hours generally close between 4 and 5 pm each day. Once the last nuclear pharmacist leaves the facility, the 'on-call' pharmacist begins coverage. All nuclear pharmacies have a dedicated emergency number that is given to customers to call if emergency doses are needed. When the last pharmacist leaves the facility, the emergency number is forwarded to the on-call cell phone. If called, the nuclear pharmacist speaks directly with the nuclear medicine technologist, then must return to the pharmacy and prepare the desired dose for the customer. Most pharmacies also have a driver/courier on call who will meet the pharmacist at the pharmacy to package and deliver the dose to the customer. The on-call coverage generally lasts until the early-shift pharmacist arrives in the pharmacy.

A nuclear pharmacy must also be available for service on weekends and holidays. Usually, a single nuclear pharmacist, a nuclear pharmacy technician, and several driver/couriers will cover an entire weekend or holiday. Most weekend hours in a nuclear pharmacy involve a few early morning hours in the pharmacy as well as on-call coverage. Some nuclear medicine departments operate on Saturdays, so doses must be prepared and dispensed for delivery to the hospital before 7 am. Most of the doses dispensed during a weekend shift are termed 'backup' doses, and are sent to some hospitals in anticipation of potential studies being ordered. Many facilities request only backup doses on Saturdays, Sundays, or holidays, so most dispensing and regulatory work is complete before noon.

Patient care issues

For some pharmacists, working in a nuclear pharmacy is an ideal practice location because it lacks the level of patient contact seen in community pharmacy practice. Since the nuclear pharmacy is a free-standing laboratory that services several medical institutions, patients do not present to the nuclear pharmacy to pick up their doses. All doses are ordered by members of the hospital's or clinic's nuclear medicine staff and are delivered by a member of the pharmacy's driver/courier staff directly to the facility where the actual dose will be administered to the patient by a nuclear medicine technologist. Most nuclear pharmacists develop relationships with the nuclear medicine technologist staff over the phone but may not ever get the chance to meet these people in person. While the possibility for disagreements or conflict can occur when dealing with the nuclear medicine staff at the hospital, most issues are resolved fairly quickly as a result of long-standing relationships between the department and the nuclear pharmacy. Occasionally, the nuclear pharmacist may have the opportunity to consult with the technologist or even the nuclear medicine physician or radiologist on staff when issues related to potential abnormal distribution of a radiopharmaceutical occur. Generally, nuclear pharmacists have the opportunity to play an important role in continuing education and training of members of the nuclear medicine community through involvement in local nuclear medicine societies. There are several initiatives relating to hospital Joint Commission requirements that have the potential for greater involvement of nuclear pharmacists in the provision of patient care. The provision of medication therapy management services for patients presenting for nuclear medicine imaging procedures is an area where nuclear pharmacists traditionally have not been active participants. While it is difficult for a nuclear pharmacist in a centralized nuclear pharmacy to obtain access to patient-specific information, this is an area of nuclear pharmacy practice that could allow greater involvement by nuclear pharmacy practitioners who would like to increase their level of direct patient care.

Regulations

Pharmacy regulations

Radiopharmaceuticals are regulated as a prescription drug through the US Food and Drug Administration (FDA). The FDA is involved in regulating all aspects of drug production to ensure that the drugs are safe and effective. The FDA has legislative authority via the US Food, Drug and Cosmetic Act. Since radiopharmaceuticals are considered legend drugs, they fall under the global jurisdiction of the FDA. The FDA also requires drug manufacturers to register as a drug establishment and they must operate under Current Good Manufacturing Practices (cGMP) guidelines. These guidelines are quite stringent and require significant quality assurance and quality assessment programs to assure the safety of the products being produced.

Nuclear pharmacies do not need to register as a drug establishment if they operate in conformance with applicable local laws regulating the practice of pharmacy; are regularly engaged in dispensing legend drugs pursuant to a prescription from a practitioner licensed to administer prescription drugs to patients; and do not manufacture, propagate, compound, or process drugs or devices for sale other than in the regular course of business of dispensing or selling at retail. In simplest terms, a nuclear pharmacy operates under the laws of the state board of pharmacy as a licensed pharmacy.

In most states, a nuclear pharmacy is not specifically recognized as anything other than a pharmacy entity, and all state board of pharmacy rules that pertain to the operation of any other type of pharmacy also apply to the daily operation of a nuclear pharmacy. Establishing a nuclear pharmacy in any state requires following specific state requirements for establishing a pharmacy entity, including the application to establish a pharmacy, the pharmacist staffing requirements, the role of pharmacy technicians, electronic processing of prescriptions, contents of a prescription label, preparation of sterile pharmaceuticals, and many others. The state board of pharmacy inspects nuclear pharmacies; however, an interesting issue in most states is that there are so few nuclear pharmacies that few if any of the board inspectors are well versed in the daily operation of such a pharmacy. Many inspectors are unsure or uncomfortable with the prospect of inspecting a facility that houses radioactive materials. It is imperative that the staff members of the nuclear pharmacy are aware of the state pharmacy requirements and that they are comfortable relating the daily operations of the nuclear pharmacy to the state requirements for the operation of a pharmacy. It is not uncommon for members of the nuclear pharmacy staff to engage in discussions with board of pharmacy inspectors about the activities that go on within the pharmacy during the inspection process, with the state inspectors learning more about this area of practice during each inspection.

Radioactivity regulations

Regulatory oversight of nuclear pharmacy operations with respect to the use of radioactive materials is provided by both federal and state regulatory agencies. The primary oversight for the handling of radioactive materials comes from the Nuclear Regulatory Commission (NRC). The NRC was first created in 1946 as the Atomic Energy Commission (AEC) and in subsequent years was split into two entities, the NRC and the Department of Energy. The NRC has the authority at the federal level to regulate the use of by-product material (radioactivity made in a nuclear reactor as well as fission by-products, both of which are discussed in more depth in Chapter 5). Until 2007, the NRC had no oversight over accelerator-produced materials; this oversight was provided by state regulatory agencies. In 2007, revision of the regulatory landscape removed the oversight of cyclotron-produced materials from the states and placed it under NRC jurisdiction. Even with this regulatory change, the NRC does not solely inspect all facilities in every state. The Atomic Energy Act of 1954 provided a statutory basis allowing the NRC to relinquish oversight to individual states that wished to establish a state program to assume NRC regulatory authority. This gives the states the authority to license and regulate radioisotopes, source materials, and certain quantities of special nuclear materials. A state must request this transfer of the NRC authority, and the transfer will occur in agreement form signed by the governor of the state and the chairman of the NRC. The first state to achieve agreement status was Kentucky in 1962. As of June 1, 2009, there are 36 states currently participating in agreement with the NRC, 13 states (including the District of Columbia) that continue to maintain NRC status, and two states in discussions to assume state oversight of the nuclear regulatory requirements (Nuclear Regulatory Commission 2009). It is important to note that the state must maintain at the minimum the NRC requirements as put forth in the *Code of Federal Regulations*; however, they are able to put forth state-specific regulatory requirements provided they are equally or more stringent than similar regulations set out by the NRC. For a practitioner in an agreement state, knowledge of the NRC regulations is the minimum requirement for compliance. If the agreement state's regulatory body has instituted a regulatory requirement that differs from the NRC requirement and is more stringent than these regulations, it will be the state version that will be enforced when inspections occur.

Rules pertaining to the safe handling and use of radioactive materials are published in the *Federal Register* as the *Code of Federal Regulations Title 10* (Nuclear Regulatory Commission 2006). The first publication was in 2004 and the rules are updated regularly. This document is extensive and not specific to nuclear pharmacy so the regulations specific to nuclear pharmacy practice are not neatly packaged in a single area of the regulations, but spread out over several sections. The most significant areas pertaining to nuclear pharmacy practice and nuclear medicine applications are discussed below.

PART 19: Notices, Instructions and Reports to Workers; Inspections and Investigations

Part 19 focuses on the rights of the workers who will be working in an environment where they have the potential of occupational exposure to radioactive materials. It is the responsibility of the employer to maintain a safe workplace. Areas covered in this section include the following.

- *Posting of notices to workers.* A licensee must post or make available current copies of the regulations, the facility license, any documents or amendments, operating procedures and notices of violations. This ensures that all employees are informed of any issues related to the operation of the facility.
- *Instructions to workers.* This section requires licensees to provide 'full disclosure' to any employee who has the potential to come in contact with radioactive materials in the course of their employment. This means that the employer may not attempt to withhold information about potential exposure to radioactive materials. This section also covers storage, transfer, and use of radioactive materials in the facility, education of employees about the health risks of exposure, and precautions to prevent or minimize exposure including protective devices used. This section also emphasizes the worker's rights to report conditions that may violate NRC regulations.
- *Notifications and reports to individuals.* This section requires employers to advise each worker of their annual dose, both annually and at termination of employment, as well as giving the worker the right to request a report of exposure after termination.
- *Inspections.* A licensee must make available to the NRC at any time any materials requested during the course of an inspection. This also requires employers to allow inspectors to consult privately with individual workers during the course of an inspection. This section also emphasizes the rights of a worker to request an inspection if they believe that there are violations of NRC regulations occurring at the workplace.

PART 20: Standards for Protection Against Radiation

Part 20 contains information pertaining to radiation protection. This section covers a significant number of points, from maximum permissible doses that an employee is allowed to accumulate in the course of their work practice to record-keeping and posting requirements for the pharmacy. Part 20 is a document that any employee in a nuclear pharmacy should review and be familiar with to help in understanding the basic tenets of radiation protection and why some tasks are performed as part of the daily operation of the pharmacy. The following is a very basic overview of the types of material covered in the subsections of Part 20.

- *Radiation dose issues.* The underlying requirement for various tasks and procedures performed in a nuclear pharmacy is ALARA: as low as reasonably achievable. The goal of the limits set forth in this chapter are designed to control occupational exposure for workers and exposure to the general public in the course of carrying out the tasks required in the course of nuclear pharmacy practice. Occupational and public dose limits have been established to prevent occurrence of clinically significant radiation-induced effects. The dose limits have been determined so that the average annual risk to an individual of developing a fatal cancer from exposure to radiation is comparable to or less than the risk of fatal accidents in 'safe' industries (approximately 10^{-4} per year), while exposure at the annual dose limit should result in a maximum risk comparable to more hazardous jobs (approximately 4×10^{-4} per year).
- *Dose monitoring.* Employers are required to supply monitoring devices for both external and internal occupational dosage based on the projected dose an employee is likely to receive in the course of employment. In most nuclear pharmacy operations, personnel monitoring is performed by having all employees wear a radiation dosimeter on their collar, a small device that records the amount of radiation dose that the employee has been exposed to in the course of the monitoring period, as well as ring badges on one finger of each hand to monitor hand (extremity) exposure.
- *Survey requirements.* Part 20 requires that each licensee should develop a system designed to monitor the extent of radiation levels, the concentration or quantities of radioactive materials, and the potential radiological hazards that could be present. The licensee is required to maintain sufficient equipment to measure these variables.
- *Posting requirements.* Nuclear pharmacies, and any other area where radioactive materials are stored or used, must visually post signage that indicates to the employees and other potential visitors to the facility the level of radiation present in the area they are entering. These levels vary depending on the type of radioactivity being used in the facility. These signs are to be posted unless the facility meets one of the listed exemptions for posting requirements, also listed in Part 20.
- *Labeling containers.* All containers which contain radioactive materials must bear the radioactive symbol and the words 'CAUTION: RADIOACTIVE MATERIAL' along with sufficient information to permit anyone handling the containers or working near the containers to recognize the presence of radioactive material and to take precautions to

minimize or avoid exposure. Again, there are cases that are exempt from labeling, which are also clearly stated in Part 20.

- *Procedures receiving and opening packages*. All radioactive material coming into and going out of the nuclear pharmacy must meet certain requirements set forth in the regulatory guidance. Part 20 specifies requirements for incoming packages to ensure that there has been no damage during the shipping process that may have inadvertently created a situation in which someone could receive an increased amount of radiation exposure when handling the package. These requirements include external monitoring of the surface, visual inspection of the package for damage, time limits for opening a package received in the facility, and requirements for notification if set limits are exceeded. In addition, each facility must develop written procedures for safely opening packages containing radioactive materials, maintain records of packages received, and ensure that staff follow the procedures as written.

- *Waste disposal*. Since nuclear pharmacies are heavily involved with handling waste materials, Subpart K discusses requirements for how waste should be disposed, the limits for certain types of disposal, and requirements for disposal of materials into sanitary sewage (disposal down sinks, waste water used to clean up spills, etc).

- *Records*. Provisions for keeping records pertaining to radiation safety programs are discussed in Subpart L of Part 20. While too detailed to cover here, this section discusses what records need to be kept, the length of time that the record must be kept, and the acceptable forms and requirements for maintaining the records.

- *Reports of loss or theft of licensed materials*. Subpart M reviews procedures as to how a licensee should report any theft or loss of materials, both by phone and as a written report. Depending on the quantity of material lost, this must be done immediately to the NRC (by telephone) or within 30 days if smaller quantities are lost and still missing at that time. All telephone reports must be followed by a written report within 30 days of making a telephone report.

- *Notification of incidents*. Guidance is given in this section of when the NRC must be notified if certain events pertaining to radioactive materials occur. These include exposures to an individual above normal levels or the release of radioactive materials outside of the restricted area that could have resulted in increased exposure to an individual. Depending on the severity, some reports would be required to be made immediately by telephone, others require a written report within 30 days of the incident.

PART 30: Rules of General Applicability to Domestic Licensing

Part 30 is specifically focused on licensing; in the case of a nuclear pharmacy, this section gives guidance on what type of license is required, how to apply for a license, records required to be kept, and exemptions. This section has considerable detail, not only for nuclear pharmacy operations but also for the licensing of hospitals, clinics, and other areas where radioactive materials will be used (Nuclear Regulatory Commission 2006).

PART 32: Specific Domestic Licenses to Manufacture or Transfer Certain Items Containing Radioactive Material

Part 32 is probably the most important section for nuclear pharmacy operations, as this covers most of the daily tasks of a nuclear pharmacy in the preparation of radioactive materials for medical use. For a nuclear pharmacy, this section is applicable as long as in the application process the applicant can show proof of license as a pharmacy by a state board of pharmacy. This part of the regulatory document identifies several areas that must be addressed when submitting an application for a nuclear pharmacy license. These include many of the basic requirements for operation of the pharmacy, including the types of radioactive material that will be used/dispensed, the maximum amount of activity of each type of radioactive material that will be used or stored in the facility, the types of packaging to be used, examples of the labeling that will be used, types of equipment used, testing requirements for ensuring that the equipment is working correctly, other specific issues related to the daily manipulation of radioactive materials, and the movement of that material to an end user. In addition, this section discusses the requirements that must be met for a pharmacist to be qualified as an Authorized Nuclear Pharmacist (ANP). This section states that radiopharmaceuticals may be prepared for medical use either by an authorized nuclear pharmacist or by an individual under the supervision of an authorized nuclear pharmacist (Nuclear Regulatory Commission 2006).

PART 35: Medical Use of Radioactive Material

Part 35 is primarily aimed at the end user of radioactive materials: the hospitals, clinics, and physicians who administer radioactive materials to the patient. However, since nuclear pharmacy is so closely related to the medical use of radioactive materials, most nuclear pharmacies follow the rules set out in Part 35 since these are the rules that their customers will be required to follow. Part 35 is an extensive section that covers virtually every aspect of practice and is far too complex to discuss in detail here. The following bullet points should give an idea of the scope of this section:

- *technical requirements*: instrumentation to be used, instrumentation quality control tests (type and frequency)
- *measurement of dosages for medical use*: requirements for measurement, records to be kept (name, dose, date and time of measurement, person measuring)

- *use of syringe shields and labels*: all syringes must be labeled adequately and users must utilize a syringe shield for radiation safety purposes when preparing a kit
- *vial shields and labels*: radiopharmaceutical kits being prepared and dispensed should be kept in a vial shield of some type, which should be adequately labeled with the contents
- *surveys for contamination*: how and when surveys should be performed, type of equipment to be used, and records to be kept
- *decay in storage*: types of radioactive material that can be held for decay before disposal; how materials that have been held for decay should be disposed of; the disposal of non-biohazardous waste in ordinary trash; record-keeping for waste disposal
- *imaging and localization*: issues related to the administration of radioactive materials to a patient, including issues pertaining to minimizing radiation exposure for the patient while maximizing the diagnostic or therapeutic benefit of using radioactive materials.

While this text does not attempt to provide a full review of the regulatory aspects related to nuclear pharmacy practice, it should be obvious that almost every action that is performed in a nuclear pharmacy as part of the scope of practice is dictated by some regulatory requirement listed in the *Code of Federal Regulations*. The regulatory coverage of nuclear pharmacy practice is extensive and for further reading and greater detail, readers should refer to the NRC web site (http://www.nrc.gov) where the regulations are given in full. These regulations should be reviewed by all personnel practicing in nuclear pharmacy.

Other regulations

While the state board of pharmacy and the NRC have the most obvious regulatory oversight of nuclear pharmacy practice, there are other agencies that may have some involvement in the daily operation of the nuclear pharmacy, and, consequently, some of the daily tasks performed in a nuclear pharmacy are in response to the requirements of these other federal agencies. While this is not designed to be an exhaustive list, a few of the more common regulatory agencies and their jurisdiction are listed below:

Department of Transportation

Since the radioactive materials received and shipped from a nuclear pharmacy must travel by way of common transportation routes (air, roads, etc.), the Department of Transportation is intimately involved in the regulatory oversight of the transportation process used by a nuclear pharmacy. While many regulations relating to transportation are included in the *Code of Federal*

Regulations Title 10, the Department of Transportation has separate regulations (found in *Code of Federal Regulations Title 49*; Department of Transportation 2008), relating to the transport of radioactive materials. In many places, the regulations listed in one document reference regulations found in the other, so to become well versed in the regulations pertaining to the transport of radioactive materials, one must review both the transportation segments in *Title 10* and those in *Title 49* for full understanding.

Occupational Safety and Health Administration

The Occupational Safety and Health Administration produces regulations that are designed to maintain acceptable personnel working environments, so the use of radioactivity (which is considered a hazardous material) as well as the handling of biohazardous materials (in the form of blood products during white blood cell labeling and in the waste materials returned to the pharmacy) requires some level of oversight by this agency. Many of these regulations are built into the daily tasks performed in a nuclear pharmacy.

Environmental Protection Agency

There are some aspects of nuclear pharmacy practice that raise the interest of the Environmental Protection Agency, which is responsible for protection from toxic materials. In most cases, the regulatory guidance set forth by the NRC regulations incorporates issues of concern to the Environmental Protection Agency; however, the latter also regulates issues such as effluent release and release of materials into sewage as areas where members of the general public may be exposed to toxic substances unknowingly.

Local agencies

In most areas, the opening of a nuclear pharmacy brings a unique set of issues to local enforcement agencies, such as the local police or fire departments. In a situation where a nuclear pharmacy is broken into and alarms are sent to local police enforcement, or if the building containing a nuclear pharmacy catches fire and prompts involvement of the fire department, it is essential that the responders are aware of the potential risk of radioactive contamination. This includes risks to the actual responders themselves as well as the potential risk to others in the area. Most nuclear pharmacies have contacts in both the local police and local fire departments and have plans of action in place in case of unexpected issues that would require immediate action by the first responder teams.

Summary

Nuclear pharmacy is one of the first recognized areas of specialty pharmacy practice, providing practitioners with elements of traditional pharmacy practice along with the unique opportunity to incorporate radioactive materials into the compounding and dispensing process. Since the development of centralized nuclear pharmacy services, nuclear pharmacy practice involves aspects of preparation, dispensing, quality control, shipping, and receiving of radioactive pharmaceuticals for use in diagnostic imaging and therapeutic treatment of different diseases. Practitioners interested in entering this area of pharmacy practice must also be familiar with increased levels of regulatory oversight required because of the use of radioactive materials in the final products.

Self-assessment questions

1   Nuclear pharmacists work in which of the following practice settings?
   a   centralized radiopharmacy laboratories
   b   hospital radiopharmacy/nuclear medicine departments
   c   PET radiopharmacies
   d   all of the above.
2   The 'non-radioactive' areas of a nuclear pharmacy include all of the following *except*:
   a   radioactive storage areas
   b   restroom facilities
   c   lunchroom/kitchen area
   d   pharmacist desk/office area.
3   The compounding area of the pharmacy is part of the non-restricted area of the pharmacy: true or false?
4   Nuclear pharmacy compounding should follow guidelines set forth in USP <797>: *Pharmaceutical Compounding – Sterile Preparations*: true or false?
5   Which of the following is *not true* about staffing a nuclear pharmacy?
   a   there is an on-call component to most nuclear pharmacist positions
   b   nuclear pharmacy uses pharmacy technicians to assist in the dispensing of radiopharmaceuticals
   c   some nuclear pharmacies are open 24 hours a day
   d   nuclear pharmacists are not required to work weekends.
6   Nuclear pharmacists have ample opportunity to have direct patient contact with people receiving radiopharmaceuticals: true or false?
7   Which of the following regulatory agencies have some authority over nuclear pharmacy operations?
   a   Nuclear Regulatory Commission
   b   Department of Transportation
   c   Occupational Safety and Health Administration

> d Nuclear Regulatory Commission and Department of Transportation only
> e Nuclear Regulatory Commission and Occupational Safety and Health Administration only
> f All of a–c.

References

Callahan RJ, Dragotakes SC (1999). The role of the practice of nuclear pharmacy in positron emission tomography. *Clin Positron Imaging* 2: 211–216.

Department of Transportation (2009). *Code of Federal Regulations, Title 49*. Washington DC: Department of Transportation; http://www.access.gpo.gov/cgi-bin/cfrassemble.cgi?title=200649 (accessed February 18, 2009).

Nuclear Regulatory Commission (2006). *Code of Federal Regulations, Title 10*, Parts 19, 20, 30, 32, 35. Washington, DC: Nuclear Regulatory Commission; http://www.nrc.gov/reading-rm/doc-collections/cfr/ (accessed February 13, 2009).

Nuclear Regulatory Commission (2009). *Agreement State Program*. Washington, DC: Nuclear Regulatory Commission; http://www.nrc.gov/about-nrc/state-tribal/agreement-states.html (accessed February 13, 2009).

Ponto JA, Hung JC (2000). Nuclear pharmacy, Part II. Nuclear pharmacy practice today. *J Nucl Med Technol* 28: 76–81.

United Pharmacy Partners (2008). *Pharmacy Locations*. Suwanee, GA: United Pharmacy Partners; http://www.uppi.org (accessed January 23, 2009).

US Pharmacopeia (2008). *National Formulary: USP<797> Guidebook to Pharmaceutical Compounding – Sterile Preparations*. Washington DC: US Pharmacopeia.

Further reading and web sources

Callahan RJ (1996). The role of commercial nuclear pharmacy in the future practice of nuclear medicine. *Semin Nucl Med* 26: 85–90.

US Nuclear Regulatory Commission http://www.nrc.gov.

5

Nuclear pharmacy practice

Kara Duncan Weatherman

Learning objectives

- Understand the common methods of radionuclide production
- Recognize the fundamental components of a radionuclide generator system
- Identify the key components of a radiopharmaceutical kit
- Recognize the differences between manufacturing and compounding.

Introduction

While there are well over 3000 different radioactive isotopes, the number with potential for use in nuclear pharmacy and nuclear medicine application is somewhat limited (approximately 200; http://www.Radiochemistry.org). Some forms of radioactivity are present as naturally occurring isotopes, originating from the decay of thorium-232, actinium-235 or uranium-238. The decay of these three starting materials leads to a decay chain or series of several radioactive isotopes with varying half-lives and decay spectra. The medical application for radioactivity involves radioactive materials that have been produced by artificial means in which a stable nuclide is transformed into a radioactive one.

In 1907, the physicist Ernest Rutherford developed the Rutherford model of the atom, in which he put proposed that atoms contain a small, charged nucleus surrounded by electrons. In 1919, Rutherford became the first person to transmute or change the character of an atom by bombarding the nucleus of stable nitrogen with alpha particles and producing a completely different stable element – an oxygen atom. By 1934, Frederick Joliot and Irene Curie Joliot (the daughter of Pierre and Marie Curie) developed the first artificially produced radioactive isotopes when they bombarded a piece of aluminum foil with an alpha-emitting radioactive source. Today, artificial forms of radio-activity are produced for medical applications using either nuclear reactors or through a particle accelerator (cyclotron or a linear accelerator).

Production methods for radionuclides

Reactor production

To understand reactor production of radionuclides, it is imperative to understand the concept of a nuclear reactor. A nuclear reactor comprises fuel rods containing an enriched form of uranium, uranium-235 (^{235}U). Since ^{235}U is a very small component (0.7%) of naturally occurring uranium-238, the naturally occurring uranium must be enriched to yield sufficient quantities of ^{235}U for use in the reactor. Nuclear fission involves splitting the heavy ^{235}U atom by bombarding the atom with a slow moving (thermal) neutron. The heavy ^{235}U nucleus will capture the thermal neutron, which causes the ^{235}U atom to split. The splitting of the heavy nucleus yields two new elements, along with two or three new neutrons moving at high speed. The neutrons produced will be slowed using a moderator to the appropriate thermal energy, making them available for fission of another heavy ^{235}U atom. This creates a constant, sustainable chain reaction (World Nuclear Association 2009).

The primary use of nuclear reactors is for the generation of power in the form of electricity. At the end of 2008, there were 104 operating nuclear power reactors in the USA and 443 commercial nuclear-generating units worldwide (http://www.eia.doe.gov). Nuclear reactors have the capacity to generate huge amounts of power by harnessing the energy that is given off during a nuclear reaction. In the fission process, heat is produced that is removed from the reactor core by water or some other coolant material. The heated water is cooled to create steam, which is routed to a turbine generator and the generated energy is converted into electricity. It is estimated that a nuclear power reactor creates 2.5 million times as much energy per pound of starting material than can be obtained from coal.

An isotope production reactor also generates significant amounts of energy during the fission reaction, but this energy is not used for power purposes. In an isotope production reactor, isotopes can be produced both by nuclear fission and nuclear activation. In nuclear fission, when a ^{235}U atom takes up a neutron, the instability of the nucleus causes it to split and form two new atoms. The fission fragments that are formed generally split unevenly, with a segment of atoms with approximately one-third the mass of ^{235}U and a segment of atoms with approximately two-thirds the mass of the starting material. The fission fragments can be removed from the reactor and chemically separated to isolate the particular radioactive material. In a nuclear activation reaction, a specific target material can be introduced into the field of neutrons produced during the fission process. The stable target atom will take up a neutron. Depending on the speed of the neutron and the energy imparted, a new isotope will be created. In some instances, an intermediate product with a short half-life is formed by the initial transformation and this then decays to a longer-lived and useful radionuclide.

There are several medically useful isotopes that are produced in a nuclear reactor. The most useful, ^{99}Mo, is used in the manufacture of a radionuclide generator since its decay product, ^{99m}Tc, is the most common isotope for medical use. Other isotopes produced in a reactor include ^{131}I (thyroid diagnosis and therapy), phosphorus-32 (various therapeutic applications), and ^{133}Xe (pulmonary ventilation studies). Most radionuclides produced in a nuclear reactor give off beta particles when they decay.

Accelerator production

The production of radionuclides can also be accomplished using a particle accelerator, a device that accelerates a charged particle to a sufficient energy to overcome the repulsive charge surrounding a positively charged nucleus when the particle is directed towards that target nucleus. This allows the charged particle to bombard and be taken up in the nucleus of the target atom. There are two main types of particle accelerators: a cyclotron and a linear accelerator. The concepts of these two machines are similar, but the type of machine used will depend on the type of nuclear reaction desired and the final yield of material desired.

A cyclotron consists of two semicircular chambers called 'Dees.' The Dees are placed in a magnetic field with a gap between them; they are then coupled to an electrical system that is used to change the electrical potential on each Dee, changing the charge from positive to negative as needed during the operation of the cyclotron. When a charged particle is introduced in the gap between the two Dees, it will move to the Dee that holds the opposite charge. This causes the particle to be accelerated into the Dee in a semicircular direction. When the particle traverses through the first Dee, the charges on the Dees are switched. At this point, the first Dee now carries the same charge as the particle, causing it to be repelled, while the opposite Dee is now charged with the opposite charge, pulling the particle across the gap and accelerating it as it moves. This process is repeated, with the charged particle gaining significant amounts of energy in the process. When the charged particle reaches a point where it carries enough energy to penetrate the electrical field around the nucleus of the target atom, the charged particle is deflected out of the magnetic field on to a target containing the desired target material and the particle is taken up in the nucleus of the target atom (Kowalsky & Falen 2004).

A linear accelerator follows the same procedure, although the charged particle will be moving in a linear not a circular pattern. A linear accelerator consists of a series of cylindrical drift tubes that have electromagnetic waves passing through. When a charged particle is introduced into a drift tube, it will be carried forward by the electromagnetic wave; it then passes through subsequent drift tubes until it has obtained the desired amount of energy. A major difference between the cyclotron and the linear accelerator is the amount of energy that can be imparted to the charged particle. A cyclotron has the ability to accelerate a charged particle up to approximately 30 MeV, while the linear accelerator has the capability of producing a charged particle with energies in the 200 MeV range. The type of accelerator used will depend on the amount of energy needed to overcome the repulsive forces of the target atom. Most medically used isotopes can be produced in a cyclotron.

Particle accelerators can accelerate both positively and negatively charged particles. A positive ion cyclotron accelerates protons, while negative ion cyclotrons utilize a proton that is associated with two electrons, giving it a net negative charge. This negatively charged particle is called a **positronium**. In a negative ion cyclotron, the actual bombardment of the positively charged target nucleus still requires a positive particle, so as the negatively charged particle is passed out of the cyclotron toward the target material, it passes through a carbon foil that strips away the two electrons, leaving a free proton with a positive charge available to bombard the target material. Most current cyclotrons are actually negative ion cyclotrons because the acceleration of a positively charge particle creates issues with activation of the internal components of the cyclotron itself. By moving a negatively charged particle through the system, there is less loss of particles through interaction with the materials used to build the cyclotron itself, while the carbon foil step at the end still allows bombardment of the target material with a positively charged particle.

Many of the radionuclides used in nuclear pharmacy and nuclear medicine are produced in a cyclotron. One group of isotopes (^{201}Tl, iodine-123 [^{123}I], gallium-67 [^{67}Ga] and ^{111}In) tends to decay by electron capture after bombardment. These isotopes are 'proton rich,' but they do not have enough excess energy to emit a positron. In decay by electron capture, proton-rich nuclei will capture an inner orbital electron, leading to the conversion of the excess proton to a neutron. An outer shell electron will drop down into the vacancy left by the captured electron, leading to the emission of a characteristic X-ray. This group of cyclotron-produced isotopes has sufficiently long half-lives to allow production in a commercial manufacturing facility and distribution to the end facility. However, there are several cyclotron-produced isotopes that decay by positron emission (oxygen-15, nitrogen-13, carbon-11, and ^{18}F). These nuclei, which are also proton rich after bombardment, also carry enough excess energy to cause the excess proton to be converted to a neutron in the decay process. Along with the formation of a new neutron, the nuclei will also emit a positron (a positively charged beta particle) and a neutrino. These isotopes have such short half-lives that production must be carried out at or near the site of use, requiring the presence of an on-site cyclotron.

Generator production

Radionuclide generators are truly the workhorses of the nuclear pharmacy. The advent of the radionuclide generator system was one of the technological advances that allowed centralized nuclear pharmacy operations to become a viable means for providing radiopharmaceutical services. The ability to have on-site production and acquisition of radioactive material is probably the single most important reason that commercial nuclear pharmacies exist today.

The most common generator system used in practice is the ^{99}Mo/^{99m}Tc generator. Following World War II, on December 8, 1953, President Dwight D. Eisenhower delivered the *Atoms For Peace* address to the United Nations, encouraging all world leaders to increase focus on the peaceful use of radioactive materials in medicine, agriculture, and other humanitarian purposes (http://www.iaea.org/About/history_speech.html). This historic call led to a significant increase in research and development initiatives designed to apply nuclear materials for civilian use (http://www.iaea.org). In the late 1950s and early 1960s, scientists at the US Department of Energy's Brookhaven National Laboratories were focusing on the development of suitable parent/daughter combinations that could be used to create a ready to use source of radioactive materials. The ^{99}Mo/^{99m}Tc pair was not the only parent/daughter pair to be evaluated, but it proved to be the most useful for medical diagnostic purposes. The scientists from Brookhaven first presented the use of ^{99m}Tc at the *7th International Electronic and Nuclear Symposium* in June of 1960. Within a year, the first medical use of ^{99m}Tc for blood flow measurements was carried out at the University of Chicago Hospital. By

1966, Brookhaven National Laboratories were unable to meet the demand for ^{99}Mo/^{99m}Tc generators, and they withdrew from production and distribution, making the generator system available for commercial production and distribution. While the ^{99}Mo/^{99m}Tc generator system is the most prevalent, there are several other generator systems that have been approved for human use and are available commercially, as well as several systems being studied for clinical use. Each system will be discussed further a little later in this chapter after discussion of general concepts related to a radionuclide generator system.

To understand fully a radionuclide generator system, the relationship between 'parent' and 'daughter' should be understood. A parent isotope is a radioactive nuclide that serves as the starting material in the nuclear decay reaction to obtain a new radionuclide. The new radionuclide being produced from the decay of the parent isotope is called the daughter. This daughter should also be radioactive, and it should be suitable for use in medical applications. The daughter will continue to decay, either to a stable isotope or to another radioactive component that will itself continue to decay until a stable isotope is reached. An ideal generator system will have the following characteristics.

- *Parent that is easy to obtain.* The creation of a generator system is only feasible if the parent isotope can be obtained and manipulated in such a way that the generator can be created. If the acquisition of the parent itself is difficult or if the parent isotope is limited in supply, it would not be useful to develop a generator system.
- *Parent half-life.* Ideally, a generator system will utilize a parent isotope with a half-life that is significantly longer than the half-life of the desired daughter isotope. The parent half-life should be sufficiently long to allow the generator system to be obtained and used over an extended period of time, allowing continuous production and acquisition of the daughter radionuclide over the useful life of the generator system.
- *Effective separation technique.* The key to a generator system is finding a method of removing the daughter isotope formed when the parent decays, while leaving the parent isotope behind so that additional radioactive decay can be allowed to occur. Ideally, this separation process can be carried out quickly and easily with limited need for manipulations, which increase the radiation exposure to the user who is obtaining the daughter isotope.
- *Reasonable cost of generation.* In today's environment, cost of materials can often be the single factor that limits the usefulness of a medical product.
- *Reasonable generator size.* The system must be designed to be fairly portable and easy to ship from production site to the end user. The

generator itself should also be small enough to fit into areas or departments with limited space.

The daughter isotope in the decay scheme should be one with character-istics that make its use in medical applications feasible. Ideally, for diagnostic imaging, the daughter should have the following features.

- *Short half-life.* The half-life of the isotope should be long enough to allow it to be obtained from the generator, prepared in the desired radiopharmaceutical dose, delivered and administered in the desired dose to the patient, and localized in the desired site for imaging, yet short enough to minimize radiation exposure to the patient by decaying to a non-radioactive component in a timely fashion.
- *No particulate radiation.* The daughter should not emit alpha or beta radiation, which would increase radiation exposure to the patient.
- *Gamma photon production.* This should be within the ideal energy range (100–300 keV) for optimal image acquisition using today's gamma cameras. Production should also be of sufficient abundance to allow an image to be obtained. Isotopes with low abundance require that larger amounts of material must be administered to obtain images of sufficient quality, and this greatly increases the patient's radiation exposure.
- *Chemically reactivity.* The distribution of a daughter isotope administered alone would be fairly limited within the body. Biodistribution can be maximized by attaching the daughter isotope to another molecule that behaves in a specific way when administered to the patient. It is essential that the daughter isotope be chemically reactive enough to carry out the chemical reactions required for this radiolabeling to occur. The more reactive the daughter, the greater the number of products that can be developed for use.

Generator equilibrium

In a radionuclide generator, both the parent and the daughter are radioactive. The parent will follow first-order decay with a particular set of characteristics to create the daughter isotope, which also follows first-order decay with a distinctly different set of characteristics. Since the daughter is formed from the decay of the parent, the parent and daughter isotopes are present together in the generator until the daughter is physically removed from the generator, leaving the parent available for further decay to form more daughters. The kinetics of a radionuclide generator relating to the formation of the desired daughter is fairly cumbersome because the daughter also will decay with time. At some point in the system, there will be an equilibrium established between

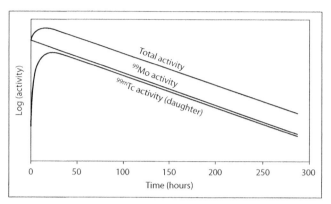

Figure 5.1 Transient equilibrium of decay as demonstrated by the semi-log plot of the ^{99}Mo/^{99m}Tc generator system.

parent decay, daughter formation, and daughter decay. Radionuclide generators can be described by the type of equilibrium that exists.

- *Transient equilibrium.* For generators with a parent isotope that has a half-life that is significantly longer than the daughter (assume up to 100 times as long), a condition of transient equilibrium will be established if the daughter is allowed to remain on the column. In transient equilibrium, the rate of daughter formation is rapid initially, because the rate of formation greatly exceeds the rate of decay. Over time, the rate of daughter atom formation appears to slow as the rate of decay becomes more significant. After this, the ratio between the activity of the parent and the activity of the daughter becomes constant and the activity of the daughter appears to decay with the same rate of decay as the parent. The ^{99}Mo/^{99m}Tc system is an example of a generator that will undergo transient equilibrium. At some point (between 48 and 72 hours), the rate of daughter formation and decay mimics the rate of parent decay, as is evidenced in the graph shown in Figure 5.1.
- *Secular equilibrium.* Generators with a parent isotope that has a half-life that is 1000 or more times longer than that of the daughter isotope are described as having secular equilibrium. As with any generator system, the rate of daughter formation will initially be rapid, and at some point, the rate of formation will equal the rate of decay. However, since the half-life of the parent isotope is so long, there will be very little appreciable decay of the parent in this time frame, and it appears that the daughter will decay with the same half-life as the parent. In this condition, the activity is essentially 'saturated' and will remain constant regardless of the amount of time elapsed. Figure 5.2 shows an example of a generator that achieves secular equilibrium.

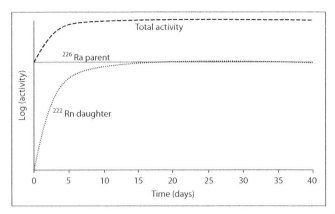

Figure 5.2 Secular equilibrium of decay as demonstrated by the semi-log plot of the ^{226}Ra/^{222}Rn generator system.

Radionuclide generator systems

The molybdenum-99/technetium-99m generator

As stated above, the ^{99}Mo/$^{99\mathrm{m}}$Tc generator is the most common generator used in nuclear pharmacy and nuclear medicine applications today. The parent isotope, ^{99}Mo, is a reactor-produced radioisotope with a half-life of 66.7 hours that decays by both beta and gamma decay (Figure 5.3). The parent decays 86% of the time to $^{99\mathrm{m}}$Tc, the daughter isotope of interest, which itself has a half-life of 6.02 hours and decays by isomeric transition with the emission of a 140 keV gamma photon. $^{99\mathrm{m}}$Tc has several of the ideal characteristics for a diagnostic imaging tool, and it accounts for between 80 and 85% of all nuclear medicine procedures performed today. The parent isotope, ^{99}Mo, also decays 14% of the time to ^{99}Tc, a daughter isotope with a half-life of 2.1×10^{5} years. This extremely long half-life is not acceptable for

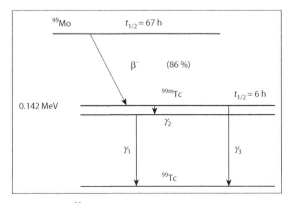

Figure 5.3 Decay scheme for ^{99}Mo.

imaging, and is so long that ^{99}Tc appears to be non-radioactive. The desired daughter in this system, ^{99m}Tc, will also decay to ^{99}Tc.

The ^{99}Mo/^{99m}Tc generators are produced by acidifying ^{99}Mo to form the anionic species molybdate (MoO_4^{2-}) and paramolybdate ($Mo_7O_{24}^{6-}$). The ^{99}Mo anions are loaded on to a generator column packed with alumina (Al_2O_3) that has been washed with a solution of saline with a pH of 5 and carries a positive charge. The anionic ^{99}Mo species is firmly adsorbed to the alumina within the column. The column is sterilized and assembled into final form under strict aseptic conditions. The column is attached to tubing and needle assemblies that are required for removal of the formed ^{99m}Tc daughter during elution of the generator. The generator system undergoes a series of quality control tests to ensure efficiency of elution, purity of the final product, sterility, and apyrogenicity (Kowalsky & Falen 2004).

Currently, the ^{99}Mo/^{99m}Tc generator is available in two basic conformations, a dry column generator and a wet column generator. The dry column generator assembly is shown in Figure 5.4. In this conformation, a source of saline is introduced through the saline port located on the top of the generator system and connected to one side of the alumina column containing ^{99}Mo and the ^{99m}Tc formed from ^{99}Mo decay. A shielded evacuated vial is connected to a separated 'collection' port at the opposite end of the alumina column. The evacuated vial pulls the saline over the column assembly from the saline vial. As the saline passes over the column, ^{99m}Tc (present as pertechnetate [TcO_4^-]) is displaced by chloride ions (Cl^-) of the saline solution and and removed from the column. The ^{99}Mo is insoluble in saline and firmly adsorbed to the alumina in the column, so it is retained on the column. The saline solution containing ^{99m}Tc is pulled into the evacuated vial. This process

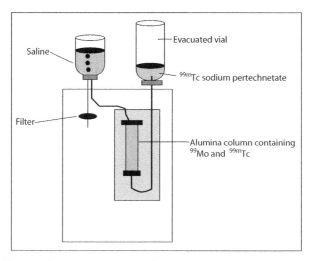

Figure 5.4 The dry column generator assembly.

is termed eluting the generator, and the final solution of ^{99m}Tc obtained is called the eluate. In the dry column generator, the volume for evacuation inside the evacuated collection vial should be greater than the volume of saline used to wash the column, so once all the saline is pulled over the column, the evacuated vial will pull air over the column. This process 'dries' the column between uses, giving this type of generator system its name. When it is time to elute the generator again, a new saline source and new evacuated vial must be utilized and the process is repeated.

In a wet column generator, the manufacturer provides a saline source of sufficient volume to meet the elution needs for the duration of the generator's useful life (two weeks). When a wet column generator arrives on site for use, the saline is placed on the appropriate saline port. When eluting, a shielded evacuated vial is placed on the collection port and the evacuation of the vial will pull saline from the saline source over the column, removing soluble ^{99m}Tc in the process. The major difference between this system and the dry system is that the evacuation space in the collection vial will eventually run out, leaving saline in the tubing and bathing the column at all times.

Yields of ^{99m}Tc

The formation of ^{99m}Tc in a ^{99}Mo/^{99m}Tc generator can be described graphically (Figure 5.5). The decay of the parent isotope is constant and is shown by the straight line at the top of the graph. The buildup and removal of ^{99m}Tc is shown in the curves under the ^{99}Mo decay line. When the generator is eluted, the daughter materials are removed from the column and the amount of ^{99m}Tc on the column approaches zero. The buildup of ^{99m}Tc occurs fairly rapidly immediately after elution and reaches a maximum at approximately 23 hours after elution. The benefit of the generator system is that elution can occur at any time and the amount of ^{99m}Tc obtained will be described by the position

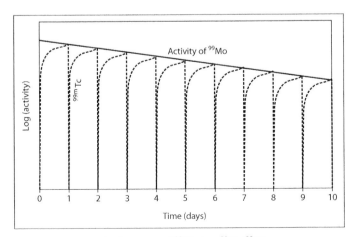

Figure 5.5 Generator curves for formation of ^{99m}Tc in a ^{99}Mo/^{99m}Tc generator.

on the graph at that point in time. Once the generator is eluted, the process begins again from zero. Since the parent isotope is decaying as well (although at a much slower rate), the amount of ^{99m}Tc obtained will decrease daily, as the amount formed is directly related to the amount of the parent ^{99}Mo present on the column. A ^{99}Mo/^{99m}Tc generator has a useful life of two weeks, but in practice, most generators will only provide sufficiently large quantities of ^{99m}Tc to be useful in a nuclear pharmacy setting for about one week. Usually, new generators are obtained once or twice each week, depending on the needs of the pharmacy.

Knowing and understanding generator kinetics allows prediction of the yield of ^{99m}Tc that can be removed from a radionuclide generator at any given time, using the equation:

$$(A_0)_{daughter} = \left[(A_0)_{parent}\left\{\frac{\lambda_{daughter}}{\lambda_{daughter} - \lambda_{parent}}\right\}e^{-\lambda_{parent(t)}} - e^{-\lambda_{daughter(t)}}\right]0.86 \quad (5.1)$$

This equation, while cumbersome in appearance, is simply a combination of the decay equation for the parent isotope (^{99}Mo) and the decay equation of the daughter isotope (^{99m}Tc). To predict the amount of ^{99m}Tc that can be obtained from a radionuclide generator at any time, there are two variables that must be identified:

- the amount of ^{99}Mo present on the column when the buildup process started (generally, at the time of the last elution of the generator when the daughter was removed from the column); in the equation, this is the variable $(A_0)_{parent}$
- the time elapsed between the start of the buildup process (the time of the last elution) and the time the generator will be eluted again; in the equation, this is the variable t.

In practice, this equation is able to approximate the amount of ^{99m}Tc on the column at any given time fairly closely; however, there are some limitations of the generator system itself that slightly skew the actual amount obtained compared with the amount calculated. In general, the amount of ^{99m}Tc removed from the column during elution ranges between 70 and 90% of the material that is actually on the column. This leaves a small amount of material on the column that will continue to decay and would possibly be available at the time of the next elution. In practice, knowing the exact amount of ^{99m}Tc that will be obtained from the column is not essential. Generally, most radiopharmacies receive the same size generator each week and elute the generator at approximately the same time each day. By reviewing the amount of activity obtained from the generators in previous weeks, it is fairly easy to predict the approximate amount of ^{99m}Tc that should be obtained when a specific generator is eluted.

Quality control testing

One of the requirements when eluting the ^{99}Mo/^{99m}Tc radionuclide generator is ensuring that the ^{99m}Tc eluate that is obtained is acceptable for use in humans. This can be done by performing simple quality control testing on the eluate that was obtained during the elution process. The quality control tests should be done prior to using the eluate in the kit preparation process to prevent unnecessary wastage of the radiopharmaceutical kits. There are three tests that must be performed on a generator eluate: radionuclidic impurity testing, radiochemical impurity testing, and chemical impurity testing. Each will be discussed in detail.

Radionuclidic impurity testing

A radionuclidic impurity is the presence of an isotope that differs than the desired species. In a ^{99m}Tc elution, the most obvious radionuclidic impurity would be ^{99}Mo. A radionuclidic impurity can be identified if the isotope is a different element (in this case, molybdenum not technetium) or if the isotope has a different atomic number (e.g. ^{200}Tl in a solution of ^{201}Tl). The presence of ^{99}Mo in a ^{99m}Tc elution is concerning because ^{99}Mo has significantly different radioactive characteristics: the 66.7 hour half-life and the emission of beta particles makes ^{99}Mo less than ideal for administration to a patient. At normal pH, ^{99}Mo is insoluble, and so if it is injected into a patient it will form an insoluble precipitate and will be removed from the bloodstream by the reticuloendothelial system. This leads to the potential for a substantially higher than expected radiation dose to the liver, spleen, and bone marrow and should be avoided.

A generator eluate is tested for the presence of ^{99}Mo in addition to ^{99m}Tc by utilizing the difference in their gamma spectra: ^{99}Mo produces photons of very high energy (740 and 780 keV), while ^{99m}Tc produces photons at 140 keV. To identify the amount of ^{99}Mo present in a generator elution, the eluate is placed in a radionuclide dose calibrator; however, because the dose calibrator does not have the capability to differentiate between the high- and low-energy photons, the ^{99m}Tc photons must be 'removed' before the reading can be taken. To do this, the generator eluate is placed in a special lead shield. The shield is thick enough that all of the 140 keV gamma photons from ^{99m}Tc will be absorbed and will not penetrate through the shielding, effectively removing them from the reading when placed in the dose calibrator. Approximately 50% of the high-energy ^{99}Mo photons will penetrate the lead shield and can be detected. The dose calibrators currently in use automatically adjust the reading obtained to compensate for this loss and display the 'true' amount of ^{99}Mo present in the elution. To determine ^{99}Mo breakthrough, the amount of ^{99}Mo (in microcuries) will be divided by the total amount of ^{99m}Tc present in the eluate. To determine the latter, the eluate is removed from the lead shield and placed in the dose calibrator. Again, many new dose calibrators have automated testing tools in place that step the user through the acquisition of all the necessary parameters needed to calculate the amount of ^{99}Mo breakthrough in a generator eluate, and even perform all the calculations necessary to determine if the eluate is acceptable for use. The NRC has set the limit for ^{99}Mo contamination in a ^{99m}Tc eluate to be no greater than 0.15 µCi ^{99}Mo per millicurie ^{99m}Tc at the time of administration to the patient. This creates some confusion because the ^{99}Mo breakthrough test is performed at the time the generator is eluted, not at the time the dose is administered. It is the responsibility of the nuclear pharmacist eluting the generator to ensure that the ^{99}Mo concentration will not be exceeded at any time point that a patient could potentially receive a dose prepared with a given ^{99m}Tc eluate. Since the manufacturers' recommended expiration for a generator eluate is 12 hours after elution, the maximum acceptable ^{99}Mo breakthrough at the time of elution would be 0.425 µCi/mCi ^{99m}Tc.

Radiochemical impurity testing

Radiochemical impurity testing tries to evaluate the percentage of radioactivity present in forms other than the desired radiochemical form. When a generator is eluted, the ^{99m}Tc is removed from the column as sodium pertechnetate (NaTcO$_4$). In the generator eluate, the primary radiochemical impurity of interest would be hydrolyzed-reduced (HR) ^{99m}Tc species that were formed on the generator column and removed during the elution process. These HR-^{99m}Tc species are insoluble precipitates that are formed in the column. When the generator is eluted, these insoluble species carry a ^{99m}Tc molecule and so contribute to the overall activity of the generator eluate. However, when they are given to a patient, the insoluble precipitate will be taken up in the reticuloendothelial system of the patient as described for insoluble ^{99}Mo above. Since the isotope emits the same 140 keV gamma photon as the desired radiopharmaceutical, the presence of HR-^{99m}Tc can lead to difficulty in evaluating the final image. The limit for HR-^{99m}Tc in a generator eluate is 5%, requiring more than 95% of the activity in the eluate to be in sodium pertechnetate. To evaluate the radiochemical purity of the generator eluate, a small sample of the solution is spotted on chromatography paper and placed in a small amount of solvent. The solvent moves up the paper, pulling the soluble sodium pertechnetate up the strip and leaving the insoluble HR-^{99m}Tc at the origin. The paper strip can be cut into two sections and each section counted using a scintillation detector. The number of counts in the bottom section of the strip divided by the number of counts in the top and bottom strips combined, and multiplied by 100, will give the percentage of activity present in the HR-^{99m}Tc form. In practice, because the radionuclide generators are eluted so frequently, there is limited time for HR-^{99m}Tc to form and so most generators have minimal if any HR-^{99m}Tc when tested immediately after elution. In many pharmacies, each individual generator eluate is used to prepare radiopharmaceutical kits, and then the radiopharmaceutical kit itself undergoes quality control testing. One component evaluated when testing radiopharmaceutical kits is the presence of insoluble precipitates, and so if any HR-^{99m}Tc was present in the generator eluate used to make the kit, it should show up when evaluating the kit itself. While this is not the most ideal method, historically, the amount of HR-^{99m}Tc in a generator eluate has been so low that the pharmacist preparing the kit assumes it is well below the 5% level and verifies this after the kit has been prepared.

Chemical impurity testing

The major potential chemical impurity that can be found in a ^{99m}Tc elution is the aluminum ions that may leach off the generator column itself. In some radiopharmaceutical kits, the presence of excess aluminum ions could interfere with the radiolabeling reaction, and so testing prior to using the generator eluate to prepare radiopharmaceutical kits is standard practice in many pharmacies. Since the aluminum ion is not radioactive, traditional radiation detection equipment cannot be used to identify the presence of this impurity. The most common test for evaluating aluminum in a generator eluate is a colorimetric spot test. Commercially available aluminum testing kits contain a paper strip impregnated with the ammonium salt of aurintricarboxylic acid, an aluminum-specific indicator. A small spot of the generator eluate is placed on the strip of paper, along with a spot of an aluminum ion solution with a known concentration of aluminum ions (10 µg/mL). The aluminum ions react with the indicator to produce a pink color with intensity proportional to the amount of aluminum ion present. The limit for aluminum concentration is 10 µg/mL, so the color intensity of the aluminum ion solution is the basis for comparison. If the color of the spot from the generator elution is less intense than the comparison spot, the amount of aluminum ion in the generator eluate is acceptable for use.

Other generator systems

While the ^{99}Mo/^{99m}Tc generator system is by far the most commonly encountered generator system in nuclear medicine, there are several others that have been made available for commercial use and which are currently being studied. This section will discuss briefly some of the other generator systems, although in considerably less detail than the ^{99}Mo/^{99m}Tc generator system.

The rubidium-81//krypton-81m generator

The rubidium-81/krypton-81m (^{81}Rb/^{81m}Kr) generator system was a commercially available generator system that allowed production of ^{81m}Kr. This generator system, with a parent half-life of 4.5 hours decayed to ^{81m}Kr with a

13 second half-life and a 191 keV gamma photon. The generator system was available in strengths between 2 and 10 mCi of ^{81}Rb and could be eluted with distilled water to obtain the daughter isotope, which was used in pulmonary ventilation imaging and for measurement of tissue blood flow. However, the generator expired 12 hours after calibration, which greatly limited its usefulness. Pulmonary ventilation studies are commonly carried out today using ^{133}Xe gas (five day half-life) or an aerosolized form of the ^{99m}Tc-labeled diethylenetriaminepentaacetic acid (^{99m}Tc-DTPA), which are more readily available and more cost effective.

The strontium-82/rubidium-82 generator

Rubidium-82 (^{82}Rb) is a positron-emitting isotope and the strontium-82/rubidium-82 ^{82}Sr/^{82}Rb generator was the first generator system commercially available for the production of a positron-emitting isotope. As ^{82}Rb has a half-life of 75 seconds, on-site production is necessary for its use, making a generator system an ideal mechanism for production to allow use in an expanded number of clinical sites. The value of ^{82}Rb is that it is a potassium analog and can be used to assess regional myocardial perfusion. The parent isotope, ^{82}Sr, has a 25 day half-life, allowing the generator to have a 28 day useful life. Because of the extremely short half-life of the daughter isotope, this generator must be eluted and the elution infused directly into the patient. Upon receipt, the commercial generator is placed in a special infusion system that is self-contained in a lead-lined mobile cart. When the patient is ready for the study, the cart is rolled to the bedside, connected to intravenous tubing, and the eluate is directly administered to the patient.

The ^{82}Sr/^{82}Rb generator does have specific quality control tests that must be performed, but unlike the ^{99m}Tc eluate from a ^{99}Mo/^{99m}Tc generator, the ^{82}Rb eluate decays too quickly to perform quality control tests on each eluate. Quality control testing of the ^{82}Sr/^{82}Rb generator is done daily, before the generator is used. Quality control tests on this generator system include ^{82}Sr (25 day half-life) and ^{85}Sr (84.8 day half-life) breakthrough testing. To perform quality control testing, the generator is eluted and the eluate is discarded to eliminate the materials that have built up within the generator since the time of last elution. Because of the kinetics of this parent/daughter system, the generator requires only 10 minutes between elutions to regenerate and produce a sufficient amount of ^{82}Rb. A second elution is performed and the time at the end of the elution is noted. The vial is placed in the dose calibrator and the amount of ^{82}Rb is recorded, and then back-calculated to determine the amount of ^{82}Rb present at the end of elution. The sample is allowed to decay for 1 hour to allow complete decay of ^{82}Rb. The sample is then placed in a dose calibrator, and the amount of ^{82}Sr recorded. The ratio of ^{85}Sr/^{82}Sr can be determined using charts provided in the package insert and the ratio of ^{85}Sr/^{82}Sr on the day of calibration, which is provided on the generator label.

From this ratio, the amount of ^{82}Sr in the sample (^{82}Sr breakthrough) can be determined using an equation provided in the package insert; this is then divided by the activity of ^{82}Rb at the end of elution. The limit for ^{82}Sr breakthrough is 2×10^{-2} μCi/mCi ^{82}Rb at the end of elution. To determine ^{85}Sr breakthrough, the result from the ^{82}Sr breakthrough is multiplied by the ratio of ^{85}Sr to ^{82}Sr that was determined earlier. The limit for ^{85}Sr breakthrough is no more than 0.2 μCi/mCi ^{82}Rb at end of elution. Most nuclear pharmacists, unless they work on-site in a facility that uses ^{82}Rb, will most likely never see a ^{82}Rb generator, much less be required to perform these quality control tests. All manipulations of this generator system must be performed on-site because of the short half-life of the agent (CardioGen-82 package insert 2000).

The germanium-68/gallium-68 generator

The germanium-68/gallium-68 (^{68}Ge/^{68}Ga) generator is designed for production of the positron emitter ^{68}Ga. The parent ^{68}Ge has a half-life of 275 days, and the daughter ^{68}Ga has a half-life of 68 minutes. It is most commonly being studied as a replacement for ^{111}In since the chemistries of gallium and indium are so similar.

Radiopharmaceutical kits

The preparation of radiolabeled pharmaceuticals in the nuclear pharmacy is possible because of the development of radiopharmaceutical kit formulations that allow pharmacists to radiolabel a desired ligand to create a specific radiopharmaceutical product without the need for extensive chemistry skills. The development of these kits is an extensive process of which most nuclear pharmacists have limited knowledge or understanding in spite of the fact that the development of radiopharmaceutical kit formulations was an essential step that lead to the development of nuclear pharmacy as a profession.

Components

A radiopharmaceutical kit consists of a sterile reaction vial and all of the non-radioactive chemicals required for the chemical reaction that will occur when a specific radioisotope is added. Most radiopharmaceutical kits are designed to utilize ^{99m}Tc as the radiolabel; however, other isotopes can be used in kit formulations. The development of radiopharmaceutical kit formulations truly begins in the most basic chemistry laboratories. Before a radiopharmaceutical kit can be designed, the basic chemistry must be determined to identify the steps necessary to get the radioactive molecule attached to the specific component to be labeled. Once this is achieved, the chemical reaction must be clarified and refined to the point where a non-chemist user can carry it out seamlessly in a small reaction vessel. The primary components of most radio-pharmaceutical kits include the following.

Ligand. The ligand is molecule or compound that will be radiolabeled with the radioactive isotope. The properties of the ligand are primarily responsible for dictating how the product will behave in the body, although there are some instances when the binding of the radioactive material causes enough of a conformational change in the ligand that a different biodistribution pattern can be seen.

Reducing agent. This is most commonly the stannous ion. The reducing agent is required to reduce the ^{99m}Tc molecule obtained from the generator at valence 7+ to some lower valence state that will allow binding to the ligand.

Other agents. Depending on the physical characteristics of the ligand and the requirements for the chemical reaction that need to occur, several other compounds may be found in a radiopharmaceutical kit. These include stabilizers, transfer ligands, buffers, and solubilizing agents.

The production of radiopharmaceutical kits can be greatly simplified for better understanding, although there are kit-specific issues with each product. On the simplest level, the formulation of a radiopharmaceutical kit involves combining the ligand to be labeled with a stannous ion solution and other miscellaneous agents needed for the radiolabeling process. The mixture is divided into presterilized vials, then frozen and lyophilized in a vacuum. The vials are sealed under nitrogen or argon gas.

Legend drug status

Since the late 1960s and early 1970s, radiopharmaceutical kits have been under the jurisdiction of the FDA. At this time, the FDA required that diagnostic products could not be sold commercially until approved as a legend drug as defined by the US Food Drug and Cosmetic Act. With this, the development of new radiopharmaceuticals must follow the same regulatory process as is seen with any other prescription drug. New radiopharmaceuticals must be approved under a New Drug Application (NDA), which is backed up by extensive clinical trial and safety data. As a result of this requirement, all radiopharmaceuticals also must be labeled in the same manner as any prescription product, including the inclusion of package inserts. A package insert for a radiopharmaceutical product is similar to any other package insert with the exception that radiopharmaceutical package inserts carry both the FDA required labeling information and the NRC radiation safety standards. In addition, each radiopharmaceutical is listed as a monograph in the USP, which provides a description of the product, product packaging, storage and labeling information, as well as identification and quality control standards.

Manufacturing versus compounding

Nuclear pharmacy activities are traditionally considered to be compounding functions as opposed to manufacturing; however, it is important to understand the differences between these two activities to clarify why we consider our activities to be compounding. Compounding of medications has existed for centuries, long before the development of large-scale drug manufacturers that produce drug products in final form. Today, the need for compounding still exists to allow physicians and pharmacists the latitude to prescribe and compound drugs in forms that may not be commercially available. The FDA has oversight of all areas of drug development, manufacture, and use, and the right to compound has long been an issue of discussion between the FDA and practitioners. Section 510(g) of the Food, Drug and Cosmetic Act (FDCA) discusses the pharmacist's right to compound and differentiates between the physical acts of compounding and manufacturing. Pharmacies are exempt from registering as a drug manufacturer if they 'do not manufacture, prepare, propagate, compound or process drugs or devices for sale other than in the regular course of their business of dispensing or selling drugs or devices at retail.' This exception in the FDCA allows pharmacy to practice the art of compounding without the need for registering with the FDA as a drug establishment, which would introduce significantly more regulatory compliance issues since the pharmacy would need to follow current good manufacturing processes. This mandate also maintains the regulatory oversight of the pharmacy at the state level (Abood 2005, pp. 112–113).

Unfortunately, in the late 1980s, there were several publicized incidents calling into question the safety of compounded medications and the role of pharmacists and the process of compounding in the errors that occurred. In 1990, the FDA published an alert letter for all compounding pharmacies that highlighted incorrect procedures and controls that could negatively impact the quality of compounded sterile products. Several of the reported issues were related to large-batch compounding, and the FDA emphasized the need for pharmacists to utilize good manufacturing practices to maintain a sterile product for use in humans. The FDA's position at this time was not to limit or discourage compounding but to serve as a reminder to pharmacy of the seriousness of compounding sterile drugs. Unfortunately, these issues enhanced the FDA's scrutiny of compounding pharmacies, with the growing concern that the FDA intended to eliminate the rights of pharmacists to compound medications.

In March of 1992, after meetings with key state and national pharmacy organizations, the FDA published *Compliance Policy Guide 7132.16*. This document reiterated that the FDA did not intend to regulate pharmacists' rights to compound drugs. It also gave some insight into the FDA's interpretation of the compounding process. Under the policy guide, pharmacists had the right to compound drugs pursuant to a legal prescription, but the guide also stated that a pharmacist has the right to prepare 'very limited quantities' of drugs before receiving valid prescriptions, assuming that the anticipated quantities can be documented by showing historic prescribing patterns for the pharmacy. However, the compliance guide also indicated that the FDA believed that some compounding pharmacies were, in fact, engaging in manufacturing outside the scope of traditional pharmacy practice and, as such, they were violating the FDCA. This final statement created significant concern in the compounding community that the FDA had intentions of increasing enforcement of compounding activities (Abood 2005, pp. 113–114).

The FDA Modernization Act of 1997 (FDAMA) amended the FDCA, adding Section 503A, which rescinded the 1992 *Compliance Policy Guide* (US Food and Drug Administration 1997). Under the provisions of this section, compounded drug products prepared by a physician or a pharmacist for an individual patient were exempt from several provisions of the FDCA, one of which inherently gave the right to consider a compounded product a 'new drug,' which would allow the agency the right to regulate the product at its discretion. To qualify for the exemptions, the compounded drug had to be compounded for an individual patient. Pharmacies could continue to produce limited quantities of a drug in anticipation of the receipt of a prescription, again based on historic prescribing patterns in the pharmacy. Section 503A also added that pharmacies could not compound 'essentially copies of a commercially available product' in order to stop compounding pharmacies that were abusing the exemption by 'compounding' a commercially available product. Compounded drugs also were required to be compounded from approved ingredients (FDAMA). Two additional provisions of Section 503A created significant controversy and were challenged at the Supreme Court level. Section 503A stated that prescriptions for compounded products could not be solicited and that physicians and pharmacists could not promote the compounding of any particular drug, drug class, or type of drug. In 2002, the Supreme Court ruled that these requirements were unconstitutional in that they violated the First Amendment. This decision invalidated Section 503A in its entirety (Thompson *et al.* v. Western States Medical Center *et al.* 2002). The FDA released a new *Compliance Policy Guide* on May 29, 2002, stating that pharmacists have the right to compound drugs extemporaneously in reasonable quantities, but again noted that it believes that increasing numbers of pharmacies are engaging in manufacturing processes. The agency deferred to the state regulatory agencies for less significant actions of the FDCA but would consider becoming involved in enforcement actions for significant violations (US Food and Drug Administration 2002).

In traditional nuclear pharmacy practice, the tenets of pharmaceutical compounding are met by the general activities carried out when preparing radiopharmaceutical products. Radiopharmaceutical kits are compounded pursuant to a prescription order. However, since there are often instances where 'add-on' doses are phoned in, most products are compounded with a specific amount of radioactivity, and the number of doses withdrawn is dependent on the time for which the doses are calibrated. While compounding standards vary from pharmacy to pharmacy, there are several 'general' guides to compounding. If the product being compounded is expensive or a product that is routinely ordered throughout the day, most pharmacies will compound using the maximum amount of radioactivity allowed for that particular kit, regardless of the number of doses needed. Generally, this will leave some amount of material in excess of what is needed, but this allows for easy dispensing of additional doses that may be phoned in throughout the day. If historical patterns in the pharmacy indicate that the product is something that is dispensed fairly infrequently, the amount of activity added during the compounding process will probably be just slightly more than what is needed to dispense the ordered doses. Since 'add on' doses are rare, it is unlikely that additional material will be needed, so there is no need to waste radioactivity to compound excess material. If an additional dose is needed, most likely an additional kit will need to be compounded. The physical act of compounding requires that the pharmacist makes the decision about how much radioactivity needs to be used. Given that most kits will have an identified maximum amount of activity that can be added to the kit, it is fairly difficult to compound 'excessive quantities' of product. In addition, the short half-life of the radioactive component limits the duration of use to several hours; consequently, in most cases, even if 'excessive quantities' of material were compounded, it would be impossible to use them in the time frame dictated by the decay of the radioactive materials. In short, the activities related to radiopharmaceutical preparation are considered to be compounding and not manufacturing in this setting.

Summary

Nuclear pharmacy practice is based on the use of radioactive materials that most commonly are artificially produced in either a nuclear reactor or a particle accelerator. This allows selection of isotopes that have ideal characteristics for imaging, while maintaining patient safety and diagnostic or therapeutic efficacy. The production of ^{99}Mo, a reactor-produced isotope that can be incorporated into a radionuclide generator system is the fundamental backbone of nuclear pharmacy practice, without which this field of practice would most likely not exist. A practicing nuclear pharmacist should have a clear understanding of both radionuclide generators and radiopharmaceutical kit preparation when compounding radiopharmaceutical kits.

Self-assessment questions

1 Molybdenum-99 is a radionuclide that is produced by a:
a   nuclear reactor
b   particle accelerator
c   radionuclide generator
d   all of the above.

2 The following accelerator-produced radionuclides decays by electron capture:
a ^{11}C
b ^{18}F
c ^{15}O
d ^{201}Tl.

3 The most commonly used radionuclide generator system is:
a $^{69}Ge/^{68}Ga$
b $^{99}Mo/^{99m}Tc$
c $^{81}Rb/^{81m}Kr$
d $^{82}Sr/^{82}Rb$.

4 The following is *not* an ideal characteristic for a radionuclide generator system:
a   sufficiently long parent half-life
b   gamma photon emission with sufficient abundance
c   chemically reactive to form other products
d   emission of alpha or beta particulate radiation.

5 The $^{99}Mo/^{99m}Tc$ generator system is an example of:
a   transient equilibrium
b   secular equilibrium.

6 Molybdenum-99 atoms will decay 100% to ^{99m}Tc: true or false?

7 The $^{99}Mo/^{99m}Tc$ radionuclide generator systems must pass which type of quality control tests before the eluate can be used in humans:
a   chemical purity testing
b   radiochemical purity testing
c   radionuclidic purity testing
d   all of the above
e   quality control tests are not required before use in humans.

8 A radiopharmaceutical kit is a ligand drug that falls under FDA approval: true or false?

9 The Food and Drug Administration considers the act of preparing a radiopharmaceutical kit to be:
a   compounding
b   manufacturing.
c   neither, it has its own separate exempt category.

---

10 Regulatory oversight of the compounding actions carried out in a nuclear pharmacy fall under the primary jurisdiction of the:

a   Food and Drug Administration

b   State Board of Medical Examiners

c   State Board of Pharmacy

d   State Division of Nuclear Safety.

References

Abood R. (2005). *Pharmacy Practice and the Law*. Sudbury, MA: Jones and Bartlett.

CardioGen-82 package insert (2000). *Elution of Rubidium-82 Chloride Injection*. Princeton NJ: Bracco Diagnostics; http://www.nuclearonline.org/PI/Cardiogen.pdf.

Kowalsky R, Falen S (2004). *Radiopharmaceuticals in Nuclear Pharmacy and Nuclear Medicine*, 2nd edn. Washington, DC: American Pharmacists Association, pp. 216–217.

Thompson *et al. v.* Western States Medical Center *et al.* (2002) US Supreme Court Case No. 01-344, decided April 29, 2002; http://www.fda.gov/cder/pharmcomp/supremeCourt.pdf (accessed February 26, 2009).

US Food and Drug Administration (1992). *Compliance Policy Guide 7132.16*. [Later renumbered as 460.200] Washington, DC: US Food and Drug Administration; http://www.fda.gov/ora/compliance_ref/cpg/cpgdrg/cpg460-200.html (accessed February 26, 2009).

US Food and Drug Administration (1997). *Modernization Act*. Washington, DC: US Food and Drug Administration; http://www.fda.gov/cder/fdama/default.htm (accessed February 26, 2009).

US Food and Drug Administration (2002). *Compliance Policy Guide*, Ch. 4, Subch. 460.200: *Pharmacy Compounding*. Washington, DC: US Food and Drug Administration; http://www.fda.gov/ora/compliance_ref/cpg/cpgdrg/cpg460-200.html (accessed February 26, 2009).

World Nuclear Association (2009). *Electricity Generation: Nuclear Power Reactors*. London: World Nuclear Association; http://www.world-nuclear.org/how/npreactors.html (accessed February 12, 2009).

Further reading and web sources

International Atomic Energy Association http://www.iaea.org (accessed February 19, 2009).

Radiochemistry Society http://www.Radiochemistry.org; also see *Medical Isotopes: General Concepts* http://www.radiochemistry.org/nuclearmedicine/radioisotopes/01_isotopes.shtml (accessed February 12, 2009).

US Energy Information Administration http://www.eia.doe.gov; see also *World Nuclear Reactors* http://www.eia.doe.gov/cnear/nuclear/page/nuc_reactors/reactsum2.html (accessed February 12, 2009).

6

Radiopharmaceuticals in nuclear medicine

Wendy Galbraith

Learning objectives

- Describe the indication(s) for the different radiopharmaceuticals used in nuclear medicine
- Explain the normal biodistribution of radiopharmaceuticals
- Apply the radiopharmaceutical information to a patient case.

Introduction

The understanding of radiopharmaceutical use, dosage, normal biodistribution, elimination, contraindications, adverse effects, and preparation is essential to providing quality patient care in nuclear medicine. This chapter describes these basics for the commercially available radiopharmaceuticals used in nuclear medicine. It combines information from primary, secondary, and tertiary sources into one resource that can be used to build upon for any nuclear pharmacy practice setting. The chapter is not all inclusive; rather it covers areas about which the pharmacist is frequently called upon to act as a source of information. The preparation sections in the chapter describe radiochemical purity limits where they apply. One term used is relative front (R_f). For paper and thin-layer chromatography, the R_f is the distance the component travels from the origin of the strip relative to the solvent front (mobile phase) of the system. The reader is encouraged to follow up on terms used in the chapter that he or she is unfamiliar with and to seek resources for indications and dosages of radiopharmaceuticals not mentioned in the chapter. This chapter does not address compounding sterile procedures or radiation safety procedures that must be practiced when handling all radiopharmaceuticals.

Radiopharmaceuticals are grouped by the element providing the radioactive component and each is discussed in terms of indications, dosage, pharmacokinetics (uptake, distribution, and elimination), contraindications and adverse effects, and preparation. The manufacturers' published materials are referred to by the brand named package insert for clarity.

Technetium

Technetium-99m bicisate

Figure 6.1 shows ^{99m}Tc-bicisate (^{99m}Tc-N,N'-1,2-ethylenebis-L-cysteine diethyl ester dihydrochloride; ECD; Neurolite).

Indications and dosage

Technetium-99m bicisate (US Pharmacopeia 2008) is indicated as an adjunct to magnetic resonance imaging (MRI) and computer tomography (CT) in the evaluation and localization of stroke and cerebral functional impairment including dementia, head trauma, and epilepsy.

The dosage for cerebral perfusion is 25 mCi, with a range of 15–30 mCi (Neurolite package insert 2003).

Pharmacokinetics

Technetium-99m bicisate is injected intravenously. It has rapid blood clearance because of its lipophilic structure and high first-pass extraction

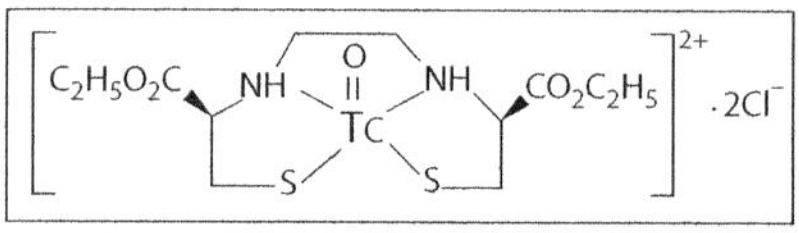

Figure 6.1 Technetium-99m bicisate hydrochloride (Kowalsky & Falen 2004, p. 269).

(60–70%). At five minutes, approximately 5–7% of the administered activity localizes in the brain by passive diffusion (Ziessman *et al.* 2006, p. 425). Brain retention of ^{99m}Tc-bicisate is a result of ester hydrolysis of the complex within the brain and the inability of the charged acid metabolite to exit the brain. Brain washout is 12–14% one hour after injection, then 6% per hour thereafter. This metabolism also occurs outside the brain and is responsible for the rapid urinary excretion of activity. At one hour, normal biodistribution can be seen in the facial muscles, salivary glands, and blood pool (not protein bound). Technetium-99m bicisate is eliminated primarily through the kidneys, with 50% eliminated in the first two hours. Some bowel elimination occurs, with approximately 12% excreted in 48 hours (Kowalsky & Falen 2004, p. 469).

Contraindications and adverse effects

The only contraindication to a ^{99m}Tc-bicisate injection is hypersensitivity to any agent in the kit, and no major precautions exist. No major drug interactions have been reported. The adverse effects occur in less than 1% of patients but include angina, cardiac failure, apnea, headache, nausea, syncope, and rash. The product kit contains the chelate ethylenediaminetetraacetic acid (EDTA) and inconsistent changes in serum calcium and phosphate levels have been observed in less than 2% of patients. Technetium, as free pertechnetate, crosses the placenta and is distributed into breast milk (Neurolite package insert 2003).

Preparation

The ingredients for the Lantheus manufactured product Neurolite can be found in table 6.1. After reduction by stannous chloride, ^{99m}Tc first binds to EDTA as a transchelate molecule. The preparation must stand at room temperature for 30 minutes to allow the formation of ^{99m}Tc-bicisate. The number of technetium atoms, volume of preparation, and conditions of storage must be considered when verifying stability and beyond-use dating if not compounded within the manufacturer's labeling information. Activities from 100–300 mCi have been used in the preparation of the kit with beyond-use dating of up to 24 hours. Package insert preparation specifies 100 mCi of ^{99m}Tc in 2 mL be added to vial B. The second part of kit formulation must be completed in 30 seconds. Vial A is reconstituted (pH 2.7) with 3 mL normal saline and 1 mL is added to vial B (pH 7.6) within 30 seconds. Once the contents of vial A are reconstituted, they immediately begin to undergo hydrolysis into a polar compound and need to be stabilized by buffering. Prior to reconstitution, vial A and vial B are stored at controlled room temperature. The contents of vial A are light sensitive. Radiochemical purity above 90% must be confirmed before administration (Neurolite package insert 2003). Different methods exist for determination of radiochemical

Table 6.1 The components of Neurolite (bicisate) manufactured by Lantheus

Ingredients	Amount	Purpose
Vial A		
Bicisate dihydrochloride	0.9 mg	Ligand
Diethylenediaminetetraacetic acid dihydrate (edetate disodium dihydrate, EDTA)	0.36 mg	Transchelate
Mannitol	24 mg	Solubilizer
Stannous chloride dihydrate	12–72 µg	Reducing agent
Vial B		
Sodium phosphate dibasic heptahydrate	4.1 mg	Buffer
Sodium phosphate monobasic monohydrate	0.46 mg	Buffer
Water for injection	qs 1 mL	Diluent

Source: Neurolite package insert (2003).

purity and include Whatman 3 medium with ethyl acetate as the solvent, with ^{99m}Tc-bicisate having an R_f value of 0.6–1.0 and free pertechnetate having an R_f value of 0–0.19 (Amin 1997; Kowalsky & Falen 2004, pp. 418–419). Older elutions (greater than two hours) of ^{99m}Tc have been used for kit preparation, but elutions older than four hours have resulted in radiochemical purity below 95% and further decreasing over time (Neurolite package insert 2003).

Technetium-99m exametazime

Figure 6.2 shows ^{99m}Tc-exametazime (2-butanone, 3,3′-[(2,2-dimethyl-1,3-dimethylpropyl)amino]bis-dioxime-^{99m}Tc; D,L-hexamethylpropylene amine oxime-^{99m}Tc; Ceretec).

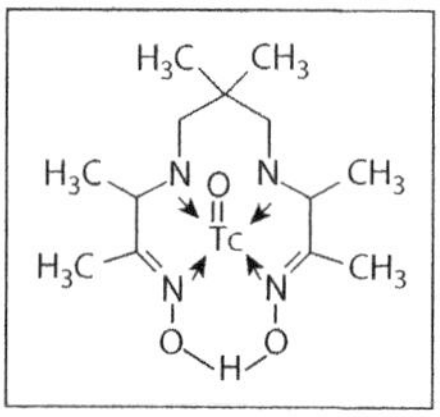

Figure 6.2   Technetium-99m exametazime (Basmadjian 2009).

Indications and dosage

Technetium-99m exametazime (US Pharmacopeia 2008), is indicated as an adjunct to MRI and CT in evaluation and localization of stroke and cerebral functional impairment, including dementia, head trauma, and epilepsy. Unstabilized ^{99m}Tc-exametazime is indicated for the labeling of white blood cells for localization of inflammation.

The dosage for cerebral perfusion is 20–30 mCi stabilized ^{99m}Tc-exametazime administered through a 0.45 μm filter. The dosage of ^{99m}Tc-exametazime-labeled white blood cells is 15–25 mCi unstablized ^{99m}Tc-exametazime (Ceretec package insert 2006).

Pharmacokinetics

Technetium-99m exametazime is injected intravenously and has rapid blood clearance, with approximately 3.5–7% of the activity localizing in the brain by passive diffusion in five minutes because of its lipophilic structure and high first-pass extraction (~80%) (Ziessman 2006, p. 435). Retention in the brain tissue of ^{99m}Tc-exametazime occurs through its intracellular conversion by glutathione oxidation to a hydrophilic compound that diffuses poorly across cell membranes. Brain washout is 12–15% at 15 minutes after injection, but then little more is lost over the next 24 hours. This metabolism also occurs outside the brain and is responsible for the rapid urinary excretion of activity. Normal biodistribution can be seen in the facial muscles, salivary glands, blood pool, gastrointestinal tract, and soft tissue, predominantly in skeletal muscle. Technetium-99m exametazime is eliminated approximately half through the kidneys and half through the bowel at 48 hours (Kowalsky & Falen 2004, p. 467). The lipophilic ^{99m}Tc-exametazime (which is not stabilized by methylene blue) is taken up by leukocytes and selectively retained in neutrophils. The ^{99m}Tc-exametazime-labeled white blood cell elution rate is up to 10% in the first hour. During the first hour following injection of ^{99m}Tc-exametazime-labeled white blood cells, activity is seen in the lungs, liver, spleen, blood pool, bone marrow, and bladder (Ceretec package insert 2006). Bowel activity is routinely visualized after three to four hours and increases with time (Zeissman 2006, p. 396).

Contraindications and adverse effects

The only contraindication to a ^{99m}Tc-exametazime injection is hypersensitivity to any agent in the kit and no major precautions exist. No major drug interactions have been reported with ^{99m}Tc-exametazime. The adverse effects reported are a transient increase in blood pressure in 8% of patients and rash, facial edema, and fever in less than 1%. Technetium, as free pertechnetate, crosses the placenta and is distributed into breast milk (Ceretec package insert 2006).

Preparation

The ingredients for the manufactured product Ceretec can be found in table 6.2 and ^{99m}Tc-exametazime can be prepared as a stabilized or a non-stabilized formulation. The non-stabilized formulation is prepared by adding 54 mCi of ^{99m}Tc in 5 mL and must be used within 30 minutes of preparation. The pH of the non-stabilized ^{99m}Tc-exametazime is 9.0–9.8. The use of 'fresh' pertechnetate is needed. Fresh pertechnetate can be obtained from a generator that has been eluted within two hours from a generator that has been previously eluted within 24 hours. The number of technetium atoms and volume of preparation must be considered when verifying stability and beyond-use dating if not compounded within the manufacturer's labeling information. Activities from 30 mCi to 80 mCi have been used in preparation of the kit for use in labeling white blood cells. When preparing stabilized ^{99m}Tc-exametazime, the stabilizer is prepared first by adding 0.5 mL of 1%

Table 6.2 The components of Ceretec (exametazime) manufactured by GE Healthcare

Ingredients	Amount	Purpose
Reagent vial		
Exametazime	0.5 mg	Ligand
Stannous chloride dihydrate	7.6 µg	Reducing agent
Sodium chloride	4.5 mg	Isotonicity
Methylene blue vial		
Phenothiazin-5-ium,3,7-bis (dimethylamino)-chloride trihydrate	10 mg	Free radical scavenger
Water for injection	1 mL	Diluent
Sodium hydroxide and/or hydrochloric acid	As needed	pH adjustment
Buffer vial		
Monobasic sodium phosphate monohydrate	1.242 mg	Stabilizer
Dibasic sodium phosphate anhydrous	0.639 mg	Stabilizer
Sodium chloride	40.5 mg	Isotonicity
Water for injection	qs 4.5 mL	Diluent

Source: Ceretec package insert (2006).

methylene blue to 4.5 mL phosphate buffer. The kit is reconstituted with 10–54 mCi 'fresh' ^{99m}Tc and after two minutes 2 mL of the stabilizer is added. The pH of stabilized ^{99m}Tc-exametazime is 6.5–7.5 and it has an expiration of four hours. The kit can be stored at controlled room temperature both pre- and postpreparation. Radiochemical purity above 80% must be confirmed before administration. Different methods exist for determination of radiochemical purity and include Whatman 17 medium with ethyl acetate as the solvent, with ^{99m}Tc-exametazime having an R_f value of 0.8–1.0 and free pertechnetate having an R_f value of 0–0.1 (Webber *et al*. 1992; Pandos *et al*. 1999). The methylene blue plus phosphate buffer solution must be used within 30 minutes of mixing. Expiration is influenced by the pH of final preparation, the formation of radiolytic intermediates, and excess stannous ions. The rate of decomposition increases when the pH is greater than 9. When the pH falls into the 4 to 8 range, exametazine is more stable. The new formulation, with methylene blue, was approved in 1995 and provided a method to extend the 30 minute expiration up to four hours. Researchers have been using exametazine for up to six hours. The methylene blue binds free radicals and oxidizes excessive stannous ions (Kowalsky & Falen 2004). The phosphate buffer lowers the pH just below neutral, significantly reducing decomposition. The stabilized ^{99m}Tc-exametazime form is blue and opaque to visualization and must be passed through a filter to remove any particulate matter that may be present in the solution (Kowalsky & Falen 2004).

Technetium-99m disofenin

Figure 6.3 shows ^{99m}Tc-disofenin (*N*-[[(2,6-diisopropylphenyl)carbamoyl]-methyl]iminodiacetic acid; ^{99m}Tc-DISIDA; Hepatolite).

Indications and dosage

^{99m}Tc-Disofenin (US Pharmacopeia 2008) is used in the evaluation of hepatobiliary tract patency, including bile leaks.

Dosage is 5 mCi in patients with normal serum biliruben levels and 5–8 mCi in patients with serum biliruben levels above 5 mg/dL (Hepatolite package insert 2008).

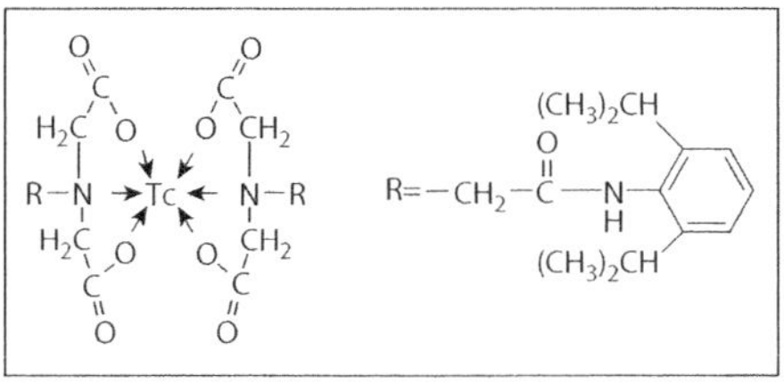

Figure 6.3   Technetium-99m disofenin (Basmadjian 2009).

Pharmacokinetics

Ten minutes after intravenous injection of ^{99m}Tc-disofenin, 80% of the injected dose is taken up in the liver, with approximately 8% remaining in circulation at 30 minutes (US Pharmacopeia 1999, p. 2706). Uptake of this iminodiacetic acid derivative is facilitated by a carrier-mediated, non-sodium-dependent organic anionic pathway and is competitively inhibited by bilirubin. Normal biodistribution is seen in blood, kidneys, and the hepatobiliary system. Elimination is predominantly by the bowel, with approximately 9% elimination via the kidneys by two hours after the injection. With increasing serum bilirubin levels, the renal excretion increases (Hepatolite package insert 2008).

Contraindications and adverse effects

The only contraindication to a ^{99m}Tc-disofenin injection is hypersensitivity to any agent in the kit, and no major precautions exist. Drug interactions have been reported with ^{99m}Tc-disofenin. Merperidine or morphine derivatives will delay intestinal transit of the imaging agent and may result in non-visualization of the bowel (US Pharmacopeia 1999, p. 2707). Hepatic artery infusion of chemotherapeutic agents and total parenteral nutrition result in absent or delayed visualization of the gallbladder in patients with no gall-bladder disease. The adverse effects are rare but include chills, nausea and vomiting, erythema multiforme, and pain at the injection site. Technetium, as free pertechnetate, crosses the placenta and is distributed into breast milk (Hepatolite package insert 2008).

Preparation

The ingredients for the manufactured product Hepatolite can be found in table 6.3. The manufacturer's labeling describes adding 100 mCi ^{99m}Tc in 4 mL of normal saline to the kit. After this, the kit must stand for four minutes at room temperature. The expiration is six hours postlabeling and the kit can be stored at controlled room temperature pre- and postpreparation.

Table 6.3 The components of Hepatolite (disofenin) manufactured by Pharmalucence

Ingredient	Amount	Purpose
Disofenin	20 mg	Ligand
Stannous chloride dihydrate	0.24–0.6 mg	Reducing agent
Sodium hydroxide and/or hydrochloric acid	As needed	pH adjustment

Source: Hepatolite package insert (2008).

The number of technetium atoms and volume of preparation must be considered when verifying stability and beyond-use dating if not compounded within the manufacturer's labeling information. The contents of the vial are light sensitive. Radiochemical purity above 90% must be confirmed before administration. Different methods exist for determination of radiochemical purity and include the two-strip method for determining radiochemical impurities (subtracting from 100% to calculate the percentage purity). The free pertechnetate impurity has an R_f value of 1.0 in a system of silicic acid medium in saturated saline (20% saline) solvent. Hydrolyzed-reduced (HR) pertechnetate radiochemical impurity has an R_f value of 0 in a system of silica gel medium in water solvent (Lecklitner *et al.* 1985).

Technetium-99m macroaggregated albumin

Technetium-99m macroaggregated albumin (^{99m}Tc-MAA) particles are available as MAA-Draximage and as Pumolite.

Indications and dosage

^{99m}Tc-MAA is used in lung perfusion imaging, LeVeen shunt (peritoneal) assessment, venogram scintigraphy, and assessment of right-to-left cardiac shunt.

Dosage is dependent on activity and number of particles. In the adult with non-pulmonary hypertension, the dose is 3–6 mCi with a particle count of 200,000–750,000. The number of particles must be decreased to 100,000 in patients with right-to-left shunt. In children, the particle count and dosage must be decreased, for example 50,000–100,000 particles in patients aged one to five years (Pulmolite package insert 2008).

Pharmacokinetics

The aggregated particles are formed by denaturation of human albumin in a heating and aggregation process (US Pharmacopeia 1999, p. 2697). By light microscopy, more than 90% of the particles are between 10 and 90 μm, while the typical average size is 15–40 μm; none is greater than 150 μm. Immediately after injection, 80% of the administered activity is seen in the pulmonary aveolar capillary bed by physical blockade. The particles undergo erosion and fragmentation to the reticuloendothelial system in 30 minutes, with effective half-life of three hours. More than 75% of the ^{99m}Tc portion is eliminated via the kidneys in the first 24 hours (Pulmolite package insert 2008).

Contraindications and adverse effects

Technetium-99m MAA is contraindicated in patients with hypersensitivity to human serum albumin and severe pulmonary hypertension. A drug interaction with heparin results in the appearance of a perfusion image that is typically observed with pulmonary emboli. A precaution is noted for its use in right-to-left heart shunts as rare instances of hemodynamic and idiosyncratic reactions to ^{99m}Tc-MAA have occurred. Technetium, as free pertechnetate, crosses the placenta and is distributed into breast milk (Pulmolite package insert 2008).

Preparation

The ingredients for the two currently manufactured products can be found in tables 6.4 and 6.5. Manufacturer's labeling specifies different maximum activity of pertechnetate for each kit (50 mCi in 2 mL for Pulmolite [Pulmolite package insert 2008], 100 mCi in 2 mL for MAA Draximage [MAA Draximage package insert 2006]). The labeled product should stand for at least five minutes at room temperature to complete labeling. Product information expiration is six hours. Storage pre- and postpreparation is

Table 6.4 The components of MAA (macroaggregated albumin) manufactured by Draximage

Ingredient	Amount	Purpose
Albumin aggregated	2.5 mg (4×10^6 to 8×10^6 particles)	Ligand
Albumin human	5 mg	Stabilizer
Stannous chloride dihydrate	0.06–0.11 mg	Reducing agent
Sodium chloride	1.2 mg	Isotonicity
Sodium hydroxide and/or hydrochloric acid	As needed	pH adjustment

Source: MAA Draximage package insert (2006).

Table 6.5 The components of MAA (macroaggregated albumin) manufactured by Pharmalucence

Ingredient	Amount	Purpose
Albumin aggregated	1 mg (3.6×10^6 to 6.5×10^6 particles)	Ligand
Albumin human	10 mg	Stabilizer
Stannous chloride dihydrate	2.4–7 µg	Reducing agent
Sodium chloride	10 mg	Isotonicity
Sodium hydroxide and/or hydrochloric acid	As needed	pH adjustment

Source: Pulmolite package insert (2008).

refrigeration at 2–8°C. Activities have been prepared of up to 250 mCi, with radiochemical purity above 90%, at 18 hours when stored at controlled room temperature. The number of technetium atoms and volume of preparation and conditions of storage must be considered when verifying stability and beyond-use dating if not compounded within the manufacturer's labeling information. Radiochemical purity above 90% must be confirmed before administration. Different methods exist for determination of radiochemical purity, and include silica gel medium with normal saline as the solvent, with ^{99m}Tc-MAA having an R_f value of 0 and free pertechnetate having an R_f value of 1.0 (Mallol & Bonino 1997). The USP has specified that 90% of the particles range from 10 to 90 µm, with none greater than 150 µm. Particle sizing is usually performed by microscopic analysis with a sample of labeled preparation on a hemocytometer (Gansbeke *et al.* 1985). Manufactured vials contain 4 to 12 million particles. Particle number must be calculated based on pertechnetate activity added to the kit and time of kit preparation. A pediatric particle table should be consulted when determining pediatric dosages (Pulmolite package insert 2008).

Technetium-99m mebrofenin

Figure 6.4 shows ^{99m}Tc-mebrofenin (^{99m}Tc-(2,2'-[[2-[(3-bromo-2,4,6-trimethylphenyl)-amino]-2-oxoethyl]imino] bisacetic acid); Choletec; Mebrofenin).

Indications and dosage

Technetium-99m mebrofenin (US Pharmacopeia 2008) is an iminodiacetic acid derivative used in the evaluation of hepatobiliary tract patency, including bile leaks.

Dosage is 5 mCi in patients with normal serum biliruben levels and 5–10 mCi in patients with serum biliruben levels greater than 15 mg/L (Choletec package insert 2007).

Pharmacokinetics

After intravenous injection, 80% of the dose will be seen in the hepatobiliary system via liver accumulation in 10 minutes; 17% remains in circulation. This

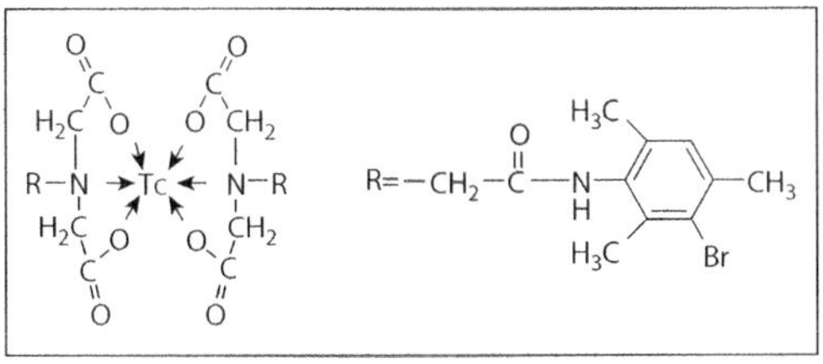

Figure 6.4 Technetium-99m mebrofenin (Basmadjian 2009).

tracer has less competitive binding for bilirubin then the other hepatobiliary tracer disofenin. Uptake of iminodiacetic acids is facilitated by the carrier-mediated, non-sodium-dependent organic anionic pathway and is competitively inhibited by bilirubin. With increasing bilirubin levels, the tracer will increasingly be excreted via the kidneys. Normal biodistribution is seen in blood, kidneys, and the hepatobiliary system. Elimination is predominantly via the bowel, with approximately 1% elimination via the kidneys in the three hours after injection (Choletec package insert 2007).

The only contraindication to a ^{99m}Tc-mebrofenin injection is hypersensitivity to any agent in the kit, and no major precautions exist. Drug interactions have been reported with ^{99m}Tc-mebrofenin. Hepatic artery infusion of chemotherapeutic drugs and total parenteral nutrition result in absent or delayed visualization of the gallbladder in patients with no gallbladder disease. Less then 1% of patients experience chills, nausea, urticaria, and rash at the injection site. Patients who have not eaten for 24 hours or have been on parental feeding will have delayed or non-visualization of the gallbladder and should be pretreated with sincalide to empty the gallbladder. Merperidine or morphine derivatives will delay intestinal transit of the imaging agent and may result in non-visualization of the bowel. Technetium, as free pertechnetate, crosses the placenta and is distributed into breast milk (Choletec package insert 2007).

Preparation

The ingredients for the manufactured product can be found in table 6.6. The manufacturer's labeling states that the maximum activity is 100 mCi, and the minimum volume of reconstitution of the lyophilized powder is 1 mL, with a shelf-life of 18 hours for the Bracco brand (Choletec package insert 2007) and six hours for the Pharmalucence brand (Mebrofenin package insert 2008) at room temperature. In practice, activity can be increased to 200 mCi with a

Table 6.6 The components of Choletec (mebrofenin) manufactured by Bracco Diagnostics and Mebrofenin manufactured by Pharmalucence

Ingredient	Amount	Purpose
Mebrofenin	45 mg	Ligand
Stannous fluoride	0.54–1.03 mg	Reducing agent
Methylparaben	5.2 mg	Preservative
Propylparaben	0.58 mg	Preservative
Sodium hydroxide and/or hydrochloric acid	As needed	pH adjustment

Source: Choletec package insert (2007); Mebrofenin package insert (2008).

shelf-life of 12 hours at room temperature with kit stabilization still well above 90%. Unique properties of this kit are that it contains the preservatives methylparaben and propylparaben. The kit can be stored at controlled room temperature pre- and postpreparation. The number of technetium atoms and volume of preparation must be considered when verifying stability and beyond-use dating if not compounded within the manufacturer's labeling information. Radiochemical purity above 90% must be confirmed before administration. Different methods exist for determination of radiochemical purity and include the two-strip method for determining radiochemical impurities (subtracting from 100% to calculate percent purity). The free pertechnetate impurity has an R_f value of 1.0 in a system of silicic acid medium in saturated saline (20% saline) solvent. The HR-pertechnetate radiochemical impurity has an R_f value of 0 in a system of silica gel medium in water solvent (Kowalsky & Falen 2004, pp. 418–419).

Technetium-99m medronate

Figure 6.5 shows ^{99m}Tc-medronate (^{99m}Tc-methylene diphosphonate; ^{99m}Tc-MDP).

Indications and dosage

Technetium-99m MDP (US Pharmacopeia 2008) is used in skeletal imaging and in assessment of osteomyelitis.

The adult dosage for skeletal imaging is 20–35 mCi (MDP-Bracco package insert 2006).

Pharmacokinetics

Technetium-99m MDP is administered intravenously and skeletal uptake occurs as a function of blood flow to bone and then ion exchange during osteoblastic activity. The diphosphonate compound is exchanged for calcium in formation of the hydroxyapatite crystals (US Pharmacopeia 1997, p. 2718). Three hours after administration, approximately 50% of the activity is excreted via the kidneys and approximately 50% is seen in the skeleton. Soft tissue uptake can increase with decreased renal function or dehydration (MDP-Bracco package insert 2006).

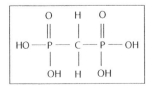

Figure 6.5   Methylene diphosphonate (Basmadjian 2009).

Contraindications, adverse effects, and drug interactions

The only contraindication to a ^{99m}Tc-MDP injection is hypersensitivity to any agent in the kit. Caution should be used in patients with possible or diagnosed hypocalcemia. Drug interactions include iron-containing compounds, amphotericin B, gentamicin, cyclophosphamide, vincristine, and doxorubicin; these can increase renal retention of the radiopharmaceutical. Aluminum-containing antacids will increase liver accumulation.

Adverse effects are rare but include hypotension, dizziness, urticaria, chills, nausea and vomiting, and asthenia. Technetium, as free pertechnetate, crosses the placenta and is distributed into breast milk (MDP Bracco package insert 2006).

Preparation

The ingredients for the four manufactured products can be found in tables 6.7 to 6.10. Manufacturer's labeling indicates different maximum amounts of activity of pertechnetate for each kit: 500 mCi in 0.5 mL for Bracco and Pharmalucence (MDP Bracco package insert 2006; MDP Pharmalucence

Table 6.7 The components of MDP (medronate) manufactured by Bracco and Pharmalucence

MDP

Ingredient	Amount	Purpose
Medronic acid	20 mg	Ligand
Stannous fluoride	0.13–0.38 mg	Reducing agent
Ascorbic acid	1 mg	Stabilizer
Sodium hydroxide and/or hydrochloric acid	As needed	pH adjustment

Source: MDP Bracco package insert (1999); MDP Pharmalucence package insert (2008).

Table 6.8 The components of MDP (medronate) manufactured by Draximage

Ingredient	Amount	Purpose
Medronic acid	10 mg	Ligand
Stannous chloride dihydrate	0.8–1.2 mg	Reducing agent
p-Aminobenzoic acid	2 mg	Stabilizer
Sodium hydroxide and/or hydrochloric acid	As needed	pH adjustment

Source: MDP Draximage package insert (2006).

Table 6.9 The components of MDP (medronate) Multidose manufactured by GE Healthcare		
Ingredient	Amount	Purpose
Medronic acid	10 mg	Ligand
Stannous fluoride	0.17–0.29 mg	Reducing agent
Ascorbic acid	2 mg	Stabilizer
Sodium hydroxide and/or hydrochloric acid	As needed	pH adjustment

Source: MDP Multidose package insert (2006).

Table 6.10 The components of MDP (medronate) Multidose Utilipak manufactured by GE Healthcare		
Ingredient	Amount	Purpose
Medronic acid	30 mg	Ligand
Stannous fluoride	0.51–0.87 mg	Reducing agent
Ascorbic acid	6 mg	Stabilizer
Sodium hydroxide and/or hydrochloric acid	As needed	pH adjustment

Source: MDP Multidose Utilipak package insert (2006).

package insert 2008), 500 mCi in 2 mL for Draximage (MDP Draximage package insert 2006), and no activity specified for the GE Healthcare Medi-Physics brands (Multidose package insert 2006; Multidose Utilipac package insert 2006). The prepared product should stand for at least two minutes at room temperature to complete labeling. Expiration time from all manufactured products is six hours. Storage pre- and postpreparation is at controlled room temperature. In practice, activities up to 800 mCi in kits with 20 mg MDP have been prepared with radiochemical purity above 90% at 12 hours when stored at controlled room temperature. The number of technetium atoms and volume of preparation and conditions of storage must be considered when verifying stability and beyond-use dating if not compounded within the manufacturer's labeling information. Radiochemical purity above 90% must be confirmed before administration. Different methods exist for determination of radiochemical purity and include the two-strip method for determining radiochemical impurities (subtracting from 100% to calculate percent purity). The free pertechnetate impurity has an R_f value of 1.0 in a

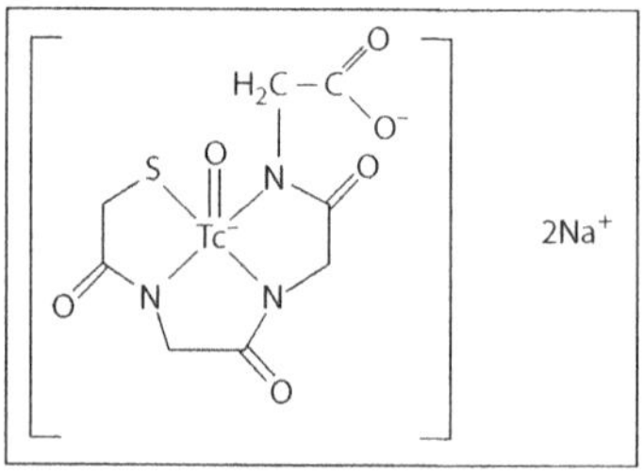

Figure 6.6 Technetium-99m mertiatide (Basmadjian 2009).

system of silica gel medium and acetone solvent. The HR-pertechnetate radio-chemical impurity has an R_f value of 0 in a system of silica gel medium in normal saline (Frier & Hesslewood 1980).

Technetium-99m mertiatide

Figure 6.6 shows ^{99m}Tc-mertiatide ([N-[N-[N-(mercaptoacetyl)-glycyl]-glycyl]glycinato(5-)-N,N',N',S]-oxotechnetate (disodium salt); ^{99m}Tc-mercaptylacetyltriglycine; Mag-3) (Basmadjian 2009).

Indications and dosage

Technetium-99m mertiatide (US Pharmacopeia 2008) is used to evaluate renal function; this includes assessment of effective renal plasma flow, urinary-tract obstruction, split kidney function, and renogram curves.

The adult dosage is 5–10 mCi and the pediatric dosage is 0.1 mCi/kg body weight, with a minimum dosage of 1 mCi (Mag-3 package insert 2005).

Pharmacokinetics

Technetium-99m mertiatide is highly protein bound, which is reversible. Most of the injected activity (90%) is excreted in three hours; 98% undergoes tubular secretion with no reabsorbtion, while 2% is excreted through glomerular filtration. As ^{99m}Tc-mertiatide has a high extraction fraction and is cleared from circulation within a short period, imaging can begin immediately after administration. With decreasing renal function, hepatobiliary excretion will increase (Mag-3 package insert 2005).

Contraindications and adverse effects

The only contraindication to a ^{99m}Tc-mertiatide injection is hypersensitivity to any agent in the kit, and no major precautions exist. No major drug interactions have been reported. The adverse effects are rare but include nausea, vomiting, wheezing, dyspnea, itching, rash, tachycardia, hypertension, shaking, chills, fever, and seizure. Technetium, as free pertechnetate, crosses the placenta and is distributed into breast milk (Mag-3 package insert 2005).

Table 6.11 The components of Mag-3 (mertiatide) manufactured by GE Healthcare

Ingredient	Amount	Purpose
Betiatide	1 mg	Ligand
Sodium tartrate dihydrate	40 mg	Transchelate ligand
Lactose monohydrate	20 mg	Solubilizing agent
Stannous chloride dihydrate	0.05–0.2 mg	Reducing agent
Sodium hydroxide and/or hydrochloric acid	As needed	pH adjustment

Source: Mag-3 package insert (2005).

Preparation

The ingredients for the manufactured product can be found in table 6.11. The preparation of ^{99m}Tc-mertiatide is a transchelation process. A maximum of 100 mCi ^{99m}Tc in 4 to 5 mL is added to the reaction vial with a venting needle placed in the septum. Before removal of the syringe, the plunger must be pulled back 2 mL or more to introduce air into the reaction vial. The air oxidizes excess stannous ion and prevents progressive formation of ^{99m}Tc-labeled impurities Tc(V) to Tc(IV). This venting process is extremely important. The vial must be incubated at 100°C within five minutes of adding the pertechnetate. During heating, the betiatide benzoyl-protecting group is hydrolyzed to mertiatide and the ^{99m}Tc is transferred to the mertiatide ligand from the tartrate transchelate ligand. The product is stored at controlled room temperature both pre- and postpreparation. Betiatide is light sensitive and must be protected from light. Manufacturer's expiration is six hours, but in practice labeling efficiencies have been greater than 90% at 12 hours (Mag-3 package insert 2005). Radiochemical purity above 90% must be confirmed before administration. Different methods exist for determination of radiochemical purity and include the two-strip method for determining radiochemical impurities (subtracting from 100% to calculate percent purity). The free pertechnetate impurity has an R_f value of 1.0 in a system of Whatman 3 medium and acetone solvent. The HR-pertechnetate radiochemical impurity has an R_f value of 0 in a system of silica gel medium in water (Chen *et al.* 1993; Bozkurt *et al.* 2009).

Technetium-99m oxidronate

Figure 6.7 shows sodium oxidronate (sodium hydroxymethylenediphosphonate [HMDP]; TechneScan).

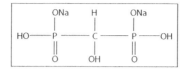

Figure 6.7 Sodium hydroxymethylenediphosphonate (HMDP) (Basmadjian 2009).

Indications and dosage

Technetium-99m oxidronate (US Pharmacopeia 2008), otherwise known as ^{99m}Tc-HMDP, is used in skeletal imaging and in determination of osteomyelitis.

The adult dosage for skeletal imaging is 20–35 mCi (TechneScan package insert 2005).

Pharmacokinetics

Technetium-99m HMDP is administered intravenously and skeletal system uptake occurs as a function of blood flow to bone and ion exchange during osteoblastic activity. The diphosphonate compound is exchanged for calcium in formation of the hydroxyapatite crystals. Two hours after administration, approximately 50% of the activity is excreted via the kidneys and approximately 50% is seen in the skeleton. Soft tissue uptake can increase with decreased renal function or dehydration (TechneScan package insert 2005).

Contraindications, precautions and drug interactions

The only contraindication to a ^{99m}Tc-HMDP injection is hypersensitivity to any agent in the kit. Caution should be used in patients with possible or diagnosed hypocalcemia. Drug interactions include iron-containing compounds, amphotericin B, gentamicin, cyclophosphamide, vincristine, and doxorubicin; these can increase renal retention of the radiopharmaceutical. Aluminum-containing antacids will increase liver accumulation. Adverse effects are rare but include hypotension, dizziness, urticaria, chills, nausea and vomiting, and asthenia. Technetium, as free pertechnetate, crosses the placenta and is distributed into breast milk (TechneScan package insert 2005).

Preparation

The ingredients for the manufactured product can be found in table 6.12. Manufacturer's labeling specifies 300 mCi in 3 mL with an expiration of eight hours after preparation. Storage pre- and postpreparation is at controlled room temperature. In practice, activities up to 500 mCi have been shown to have greater than 90% radiochemical purity for over 12 hours when stabilized with 0.5–2 mg ascorbic acid. The ascorbic acid should be added no more than three minutes after completion of the ^{99m}Tc-HMDP preparation. The number of technetium atoms and volume of preparation and conditions of

Table 6.12 The components of TechneScan (sodium oxidronate) manufactured by Covidien		
Ingredient	**Amount**	**Purpose**
Oxidronate sodium	3.15 mg	Ligand
Stannous chloride dihydrate	0.258–0.343 mg	Reducing agent
Gentisic acid	0.84 mg	Stabilizer
Sodium chloride	30 mg	Isotonicity
Sodium hydroxide and/or hydrochloric acid	As needed	pH adjustment

Source: HMDP package insert (2005).

storage must be considered when verifying stability and beyond-use dating if not compounded within the manufacturer's labeling information. The maximum amount of oxidronate should not exceed 2 mg/dose. Radiochemical purity above 90% must be confirmed before administration. Different methods exist for determination of radiochemical purity and include the two-strip method for determining radiochemical impurities (subtracting from 100% to calculate percent purity). The free pertechnetate impurity has an R_f value of 1.0 in a system of silica gel medium and acetone solvent. The HR-pertechnetate radiochemical impurity has an R_f value of 0 in a system of silica gel medium in normal saline (Frier & Hesslewood 1980).

Technetium-99m pentetate

Figure 6.8 shows ^{99m}Tc-pentetate (^{99m}Tc-[N,N-bis[2-[bis(carboxymethyl) amino]ethyl]-glycinato(5-)] sodium; ^{99m}Tc-diethylenetriaminepentaacetic acid [^{99m}Tc-DTPA]).

Indications and dosage

Technetium-99m DTPA (US Pharmacopeia 2008) is used to evaluate renal function, including glomerular filtration rate, urinary-tract obstruction, split kidney function, and renogram curves. It is also used for lung ventilation studies when aerosolized, cardiac first-pass studies for right and left

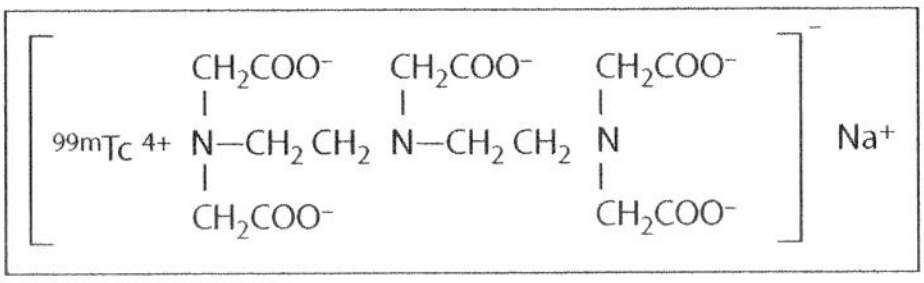

Figure 6.8 Technetium-99m pentetate (Basmadjian 2009).

ventricular ejection fraction determination, and as a conventional brain imaging agent.

The adult dosage is 3–5 mCi for estimation of glomerular filtration rate, 10–15 mCi for renogram, 30 mCi for cardiac first-pass studies, and 35–75 mCi for ventilation studies. Calcium DTPA, 1 mg with 1–2 mCi, is used for CSF studies (see Contraindications and precautions) (Ponto 2008). The pediatric dosage for renal imaging is 0.1 mCi/kg body weight with a minimum dose of 1 mCi.

Pharmacokinetics

Technetium-99m DTPA is rapidly cleared from circulation within the first five minutes and undergoes 100% glomerular filtration; 90% of the injected activity is excreted in four hours, with a biological half-life of 2.5 hours (DTPA Pharmalucence package insert 2008). When administered intrathecally, the activity remains compartmentalized (see Contraindications and precautions).

Contraindications and precautions

The only contraindication to a ^{99m}Tc-DTPA injection is hypersensitivity to any agent in the kit. No major drug interactions have been reported. The adverse effects are rare but include chills, nausea, and uticaria at the injection site (DTPA Pharmalucence package insert 2008). Caution should be used when the calcium DTPA kit preparation is administered intrathecally for evaluation of CSF leaks and ventriculoperitoneal shunt patency. H_2Na_3DTPA was found to cause irreversible blockade of nerve conduction in isolated ischiatic rat nerves, whereas $CaNa_3DTPA$, even in much higher concentrations caused no effect. $CaNa_3DTPA$ prepared for intrathecal administrations requires adherence to all USP standards including no more than 14 endotoxin units per administration (Ponto 2008). Technetium, as free pertechnetate, crosses the placenta and is distributed into breast milk.

Preparation

The ingredients for the two manufactured products can be found in tables 6.13 and 6.14. The preparations of ^{99m}Tc-DTPA from various manufacturers differ in the maximum amount of ^{99m}Tc that can be added to their kits along with the storage conditions and expiration times associated with preparation use (DTPA Draximage package insert 2006; DTPA Pharmalucence package insert 2008) (table 6.15). In practice, the ^{99m}Tc-DTPA expiration can be extended for ventilation studies to 18 hours. In kits that do not have a stabilizer, free pertechnetate has been between 2 and 10% and this shortens the expiration time when used for glomerular filtration rate determination as the free pertechnetate will undergo protein binding and cause underestimation of the filtration rate (Russell *et al.* 1986). Radiochemical purity above

Table 6.13 The components of DTPA (diethylenetriaminepentaacetic acid; pentetate) manufactured by Draximage

Ingredient	Amount	Purpose
Pentetic acid	20 mg	Ligand
p-Aminobenzoic acid	5 mg	Stabilizer
Calcium chloride dihydrate	3.73 mg	Stabilizer
Stannous chloride dihydrate	0.25–0.385 mg	Reducing agent
Sodium hydroxide and/or hydrochloric acid	As needed	pH adjustment

Source: DTPA Draximage package insert (2006).

Table 6.14 The components of DTPA (diethylenetriaminepentaacetic acid; pentetate) manufactured by Pharmalucence

Ingredient	Amount	Purpose
Pentetate calcium trisodium	20.6 mg	Ligand
Stannous chloride dihydrate	0.15–0.3 mg	Reducing agent
Sodium hydroxide and/or hydrochloric acid	As needed	pH adjustment

Source: DTPA Pharmalucence package insert (2008).

Table 6.15 Comparison of two DTPA (diethylenetriaminepentaacetic acid; pentetate) kits showing differences in activity, storage conditions, and expiration time

	Draximage	Pharmalucence
Maximum activity	500 mCi	160 mCi
Volume	2–10 mL	1–8 mL
Incubation time	15 min	1 min
Storage conditions before/after labeling	2–25°C	15–30°C
Expiration time	12 h	6 h (1 h for GFR)

GFR, glomerular filtration rate.

90% must be confirmed before administration. Different methods exist for determination of radiochemical purity and include the two-strip method for determining radiochemical impurities (subtracting from 100% to calculate percent purity). The free pertechnetate impurity has an R_f value of 1.0 in a system of silica gel medium and acetone solvent. The HR-pertechnetate radiochemical impurity has an R_f value of 0 in a system of silica gel medium in normal saline; (Billinghurst 1973; Gansbeke *et al.* 1985).

Sodium pertechnetate

Indication and dosage

Sodium pertechnetate ($Na^{99m}TcO_4$) is used for studies of the brain (20–30 mCi), thyroid (5–10 mCi), salivary system (1 mCi), blood pool (10–30 mCi), direct cystography (1 mCi), and nasolacrimal system (100 µCi) (Technelite package insert 2005; Ultra Technekow package insert 2006).

Pharmacokinetics

When injected intravenously or taken orally, $Na^{99m}TcO_4$ accumulates in thyroid (trapped and released unchanged), salivary glands, choroid plexus, gastric mucosa, intracranial lesions, and blood pool and is excreted via kidneys. Sodium pertechnetate is instilled into the bladder by catheter for cystography studies. When imaging the nasolacrimal system the dose is instilled as an eye drop (Technelite package insert 2005).

Contraindications and precautions

The only contraindication to sodium pertechnetate injection is hypersensitivity to a previous sodium pertechnetate injection. Allergic reactions, including anaphylaxis have occurred. Technetium, as free pertechnetate, crosses the placenta and is distributed into breast milk. Drug interactions have been reported with aluminum-containing antacids, sulfonamides, stannous ion-containing drugs, and other radiopharmaceuticals and result in failure of radiopharmaceutical to leave vascular space and an increased blood pool activity (Technelite package insert 2005).

Preparation and quality control

Sodium pertechnetate is eluted with normal saline from a $^{99}Mo/^{99m}Tc$ generator as a sterile, pyrogen-free solution ready for administration. The radionuclide purity must be less than 0.15 µCi ^{99}Mo per 1 mCi ^{99m}Tc at the time of injection. The radiochemical purity must be greater than 95% sodium pertechnetate and the chemical impurity of alumina must be less than 10 µg/mL. Radiochemical purity above 95% may be determined with silica gel medium and acetone solvent, with sodium pertechnetate having an R_f value of 1.0 and technetium dioxide ($^{99m}TcO_2$) having an R_f of 0.

Technetium-99m pyrophosphate

Indications and dosage

In the past, ^{99m}Tc-labeled pyrophosphate (^{99m}Tc-PYP) was used to evaluate infarcted myocardial tissue and skeletal imaging but it is no longer used for these indications. The kit is utilized mostly for its stannous ion content for labeling red blood cells (RBC) for blood pool imaging, including resting nuclear ventriculography, and to a lesser extent to assess gastrointestinal bleeding and hemangiomas.

The dosage for ^{99m}Tc-labeled RBC is 20–30 mCi administered intravenously.

Pharmacokinetics

When the kit is used to label RBC, typically an *in vivo* method is used. For gastrointestinal bleeds, the *in vivo* method cannot be used because of interference with imaging by the variable amounts of technetium localizing in the gastric mucosa as well as elimination of radioactivity via the urinary tract. With *in vivo* RBC labeling, ^{99m}Tc diffuses across the RBC membrane and is reduced by the previously injected stannous ion, whereupon it binds to hemoglobin and this prevents it from diffusing back out of the cell. Approximately 78% of the injected activity remains in the blood pool. The biological half-life of ^{99m}Tc-labeled RBC is approximately 80 days for the *in vivo* method (PYP package insert 2008).

Contraindications, precautions, and interactions

The only contraindication to a PYP injection is hypersensitivity to any agent in the kit. *In vivo* labeling of RBC can be affected by many drugs and processes, including dipyridamole, recent iodinated contrast agent administration, or dialysis. Therapies directed against the white blood cell (WBC) membrane in patients with chronic lymphocytic leukemia or non-Hodgkin's lymphoma may result in a poor label. Extreme deviations in amounts of stannous ion or sodium pertechnetate can result in a poor label. Technetium, as free pertechnetate, crosses the placenta and is distributed into breast milk (PYP package insert 2008).

Preparation

The ingredients for the manufactured products can be found in tables 6.16 and 6.17 (TechneScan PYP 2005; PYP package insert 2008). Preparation of

Table 6.16 The components of PYP (pyrophosphate) manufactured by Pharmalucence

Ingredient	Amount	Purpose
Sodium pyrophosphate	12 mg	Ligand
Stannous chloride dihydrate	2.8–4.9 mg	Reducing agent
Sodium hydroxide and/or hydrochloric acid	As needed	pH adjustment

Source: PYP package insert (2008).

Table 6.17 The components of Technescan PYP (pyrophosphate) manufactured by Covidien

Ingredient	Amount	Purpose
Sodium pyrophosphate	11.9 mg	Ligand
Stannous chloride dihydrate	3.2–4.4 mg	Reducing agent
Sodium hydroxide and/or hydrochloric acid	As needed	pH adjustment

Source: TechneScan PYP package insert (2005).

^{99m}Tc-labeled RBC utilizing stannous ion from the PYP manufactured kits can be performed two ways. The *in vivo* method is used more often and involves first administering 10–20 µg Sn^{2+}/kg body weight intravenously and then 20–30 mCi sodium pertechnetate 20–30 minutes later. The modified *in vivo* method uses the same first step, but in the second step 2 mL of the patient's blood is drawn into the sodium pertechnetate syringe where the labeling takes place *in vitro*. The ^{99m}Tc-labeled RBC are then reinjected into the patient.

Technetium-99m red blood cells

Indications and dosage

The principal application of *in vitro* labeled blood pool agents is assessment of gastrointestinal bleeding. Blood pool agents are also used in myocardial ventriculography for assessment of wall motion abnormalities and for measurement of ventricular ejection fraction and volume.

The adult dosage of labeled RBC is 20–40 mCi administered intravenously.

Pharmacokinetics

Following intravenous injection, the ^{99m}Tc-labeled RBC distribute in the blood pool with an estimated biological half-life of 29 hours; 95% of ^{99m}Tc remains bound to RBC 24 hours after injection (UltraTag package insert 2005).

Contraindications and precautions

The only contraindication to a ^{99m}Tc-labeled RBC injection is hypersensitivity to any agent in the kit, and no major precautions exist. No major drug interactions have been reported. Technetium, as free pertechnetate, crosses the placenta and is distributed into breast milk (UltraTag package insert 2005).

Preparation

The ingredients for the manufactured product can be found in table 6.18. Anticoagulated blood (2 mL) is added to the reaction vial and allowed to react for five minutes. Syringe I contents are added and the vial is gently inverted four to five times. The contents of syringe II are added and again the vial is gently inverted four or five times. Sodium pertechnetate 10–100 mCi is added and allowed to react for 20 minutes. The labeled RBC should be administered within 30 minutes of labeling. Storage of the kit is at controlled room temperature. Since sodium hypochlorite is light sensitive, it should be protected from light if taken out of the manufacturer's packaging. Radiochemical purity can be determined by centrifuging the labeled product and removing the plasma from the labeled RBC. The percentage tagging efficiency can be calculated by dividing the RBC activity by the RBC activity plus the plasma activity. Usual labeling efficiencies are greater than 95% (UltraTag package insert 2005).

Table 6.18 The components of UltraTag (red blood cell labeling) manufactured by Covidien

Ingredient	Amount	Purpose
Stannous chloride dihydrate	50–105 µg	Reducing agent
Sodium citrate dihydrate	3.67 mg	Stabilizer
Dextrose anhydrous	5.5 mg	Stabilizer
Sodium hydroxide	As needed	pH adjustment
Syringe I		
Sodium hypochlorite	0.6 mg	Oxidant
Sterile water for injection	qs 0.6 mL	Diluent
Sodium hydroxide	As needed	pH adjustment
Syringe II		
Citric acid monohydrate	8.7 mg	Cell sequestration, pH adjustment
Sodium citrate dihydrate	32.5 mg	Cell sequestration, pH adjustment
Dextrose anhydrous	12 mg	Cell sequestration, stabilizer
Sterile water for injection	qs 1 mL	Diluent
Sodium hydroxide	As needed	pH adjustment

Source: UltraTag package insert (2005).

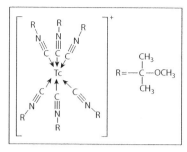

Figure 6.9   Technetium-99m sestamibi (Basmadjian 2009).

Technetium-99m sestamibi

Figure 6.9 shows ^{99m}Tc-sestamibi (^{99m}Tc-methoxyisobutylisonitrile; ^{99m}Tc-MIBI; technetium (1+)-^{99m}Tc-hexakis(1-isocyano-2-methoxy-2-methylpropane; hexakis(2-methoxy-2methylpropyl isocyanide) ^{99m}Tc-technetium (1+); Cardiolite; Miraluma; Sestamibi).

Indications and dosage

Technetium-99m sestamibi (US Pharmacopeia 2008), is used in myocardial perfusion imaging to assess the severity and localization of myocardial infarction and myocardial ischemia, to determine left ventricular ejection fraction, to assess ventricular wall motion, and to assess coronary artery disease. ^{99m}Tc-Sestamibi is also used to assess hyperparathyroidism and in detection and localization of breast carcinoma after a mammogram (Cardiolite package insert 2003).

Dosages are 8–15 mCi for myocardial perfusion at rest and 24–45 mCi under stress (3× rest), 25 mCi for breast imaging, and 20 mCi for parathyroid imaging.

Pharmacokinetics

Technetium-99m sestamibi is injected intravenously and has a high volume of distribution. It has low protein binding and is rapidly cleared from the blood. It accumulates in myocytes in relation to blood flow, with a first-pass extraction efficiency of approximately 65% as a result of lipophilicity through passive diffusion and approximately 1.2% of the injected activity accumulates in the myocyte mitochondria owing to the overall cationic 1+ structure. Normal distribution is hepatobiliary, cardiac, salivary glands, and thyroid. It is eliminated through the biliary system into the intestines. At 48 hours, 27% of the injected activity is eliminated via the kidneys and 33% via the bowels. The effective half-life is three hours in the myocardium and 28 minutes in the liver. A certain amount of liver and bowel clearance must have occurred before cardiac imaging may proceed (Cardiolite package insert 2003).

Contraindications and adverse effects

The only contraindication to a ^{99m}Tc-sestamibi injection is hypersensitivity to any agents in the kit, and no major precautions exist. No major drug interactions have been reported with sestamibi. The most frequent adverse effect is a metallic or bitter taste after injection. Adverse effects less frequently reported are flushing, headache, nausea, skin rash, angina, and ST segment changes. Technetium, as free pertechnetate, crosses the placenta and is distributed into breast milk (Cardiolite package insert 2003).

Preparation

The ingredients for the manufactured product can be found in table 6.19 (Cardiolite package insert 2003; Sestamibi package insert 2008). After reduction by stannous chloride, ^{99m}Tc first binds to citrate as a transchelate molecule. The solution must be heated at $100°C$ for 10 minutes to accelerate the formation of ^{99m}Tc-sestamibi. The number of technetium atoms, volume of preparation and length of heating must be considered when verifying stability and beyond-use dating if not compounded within the manufacturer's labeling information. Activities from 150 mCi to 600 mCi have been used in preparation of the kit. Package insert preparation specifies 150 mCi of ^{99m}Tc in 3 mL, shake vigorously, and then boil for 10 minutes; this has a shelf-life of six hours. Pre- and postpreparation storage is at room temperature, $15–25°C$, protected from light. Radiochemical purity above 90% must be confirmed before administration. Different methods exist for determination of radiochemical purity and include Whatman 17 medium with ethyl acetate as the solvent, with ^{99m}Tc-sestamibi having an R_f value of 0.2–1.0 and free pertechnetate having an R_f value of 0–0.1 (Patel *et al.* 1995).

Table 6.19 The components of Cardiolite (sestamibi; 5 mL vial) manufactured by Lantheus and Sestamibi (10 mL vial) manufactured by Covidien

Ingredient	Amount	Purpose
Tetrakis (2-methoxy isobutyl isonitrile) copper (I) tetrafluoroborate	1 mg	Chelate
Sodium citrate dihydrate	2.6 mg	Transchelate
Mannitol	20 mg	Solubilizing agent
L-Cysteine hydrochloride monohydrate	1 mg	Accelerator
Stannous chloride dihydrate	25–75 µg	Technetium reducing agent

Source: Cardiolite package insert (2003); Sestamibi package insert (2008).

Figure 6.10 *meso*-2,3-Dimercaptosuccinic acid (DMSA) (Basmadjian 2009).

Technetium-99m succimer

Figure 6.10 shows succimer (*meso*-2,3-dimercaptosuccinic acid [DMSA]).

Indications and dosage

Technetium-99m succimer [99mTc-DMSA] (US Pharmacopeia 2008), is used in the evaluation of parenchymal disorders including renal cortex scarring.

The adult dosage is 3–5 mCi; the pediatric dosage is 0.05 mg/kg body weight, with a minimum of 0.3 mCi.

Pharmacokinetics

Technetium-99m DMSA activity is cleared from the plasma with a half-life of approximately 60 minutes, and 50% of the injected activity concentrates in the renal cortex. Approximately 16% of the activity is excreted in the urine within two hours. At six hours, approximately 20% of the dose is concentrated in each kidney (DMSA package insert 2004).

Contraindications, adverse effects, and drug interactions

The only contraindication to a 99mTc-DMSA injection is hypersensitivity to any agent in the kit, and no major precautions exist. Drug interactions with 99mTc-DMSA include aluminum chloride, which causes a decrease in renal distribution and an increased hepatic distribution. Captopril has caused decreased renal uptake. The adverse effects are rare and include instances of syncope, fever, nausea, and maculopapular skin rash. Technetium, as free pertechnetate, crosses the placenta and is distributed into breast milk (DMSA package insert 2004).

Preparation

The ingredients for the manufactured product can be found in table 6.20. Sodium pertechnetate, 40 mCi in 2 mL, is added to the DMSA vial, and the preparation must stand at room temperature for 10 minutes prior to use. The kit must be stored under refrigeration before preparation; after reconstitution, it has an expiration time of four hours at controlled room temperature. The contents of the vial are light sensitive (DMSA package insert 2004). Technetium-99m DMSA has been shown to adsorb to plastic syringes to varying degrees and this can be decreased with dilution. Radiochemical purity

Table 6.20 The components of DMSA (succimer; dimercaptosuccinic acid) manufactured by GE Healthcare

Ingredient	Amount	Purpose
Dimercaptosuccinic acid	1 mg	Ligand
Ascorbic acid	0.7 mg	Trans-chelate
Inositol	50 mg	Solubilizing agent
Stannous chloride dihydrate	0.38–0.46 mg	Reducing agent
Sodium hydroxide and/or hydrochloric acid	As needed	pH adjustment

Source: DMSA package insert (2004).

above 90% must be confirmed before administration. Different methods exist for determination of radiochemical purity and include the two-strip method for determining radiochemical impurities (subtracting from 100% to calculate percent purity). The free pertechnetate impurity has an R_f value of 1.0 in a system of silica gel medium and acetone solvent. The HR-pertechnetate radiochemical impurity has an R_f value of 0 in a system of silica gel medium in normal saline (Mallol & Bonino 1997).

Technetium-99m sulfur colloid

Indication and dosage

Technetium-99m sulfur colloid (^{99m}Tc-SC) (US Pharmacopeia 2008) is used in the evaluation of liver and spleen (1–8 mCi), bone marrow (3–12 mCi), gastroesophageal motility (150–300 µCi orally), pulmonary aspiration (300–500 µCi orally), LeVeen shunts (1–3 mCi intraperitoneal), lymphoscintigraphy (0.4–1.0 mCi), and profuse gastrointestinal bleeding (10 mCi).

Pharmacokinetics

Intravenously injected ^{99m}Tc-SC is selectively concentrated in the reticuloendothelial system by phagocytic cells of the liver (80–90% of injected dose), spleen (5–10%), and bone marrow (1–10%) within 15 minutes (Sulfur Colloid package insert 2008).

Contraindications, adverse effects, and drug interactions

The only contraindication to a ^{99m}Tc-SC injection is hypersensitivity to any agent in the kit, and no major precautions exist. Drug interactions include antacids, resulting in diffuse pulmonary accumulation, and chemotherapy (carmustine, lomustine), resulting in an irregular distribution of activity in liver and a shift of activity from liver to spleen and/or to bone marrow. Adverse effects include cardiopulmonary arrest, seizures, anaphylaxis, hypotension, dyspnea, abdominal pain, fever, chills, bronchospasm, nausea, vomiting, perspiration, redness, urticaria, numbness, dizziness, and burning at the injection site. Technetium, as free pertechnetate, crosses the placenta and is distributed into breast milk (Sulfur Colloid package insert 2008).

Preparation

The ingredients for the manufactured product can be found in table 6.21. As much as 500 mCi in 3 mL can be used in preparation of the kit. The pertechnetate is added to the reaction vial followed by 1.5 mL of syringe A. The preparation is heated at 100°C for five minutes and then cooled for a minimum of three minutes before 1.5 mL of syringe B is added. Particle size formation is affected by the length of heating. Storage pre- and postpreparation is at controlled room temperature. The manufacturer's expiration is six hours. Particle size of prepared kit is 0.1–1.0 μm For lymphoscintigraphy, the preparation must be filtered with a 0.1 μm filter for a particle range of 30–100 nm. Technetium-99m SC is the only technetium kit in which pertechnetate is not reduced. Radiochemical purity above 92% must be confirmed before administration. Different methods exist for determination of radiochemical purity and include silica gel medium with normal saline as the solvent, with ^{99m}Tc-SC having an R_f value of 0 and free pertechnetate having an R_f value of 1.0 (Pauwels & Jeitsma 1977; Zimmer & Patel 1977).

Table 6.21 The components of Sulfur Colloid manufactured by Pharmalucence

Ingredient	Amount	Purpose
Sodium thiosulfate anhydrous	2 mg	Ligand
Edetate disodium	2.3 mg	Stabilizer
Gelatin	18.1 mg	Colloid formation
Vial A		
0.148 M Hydrochloric acid	1.8 mL	pH adjustment
Vial B		
Sodium biphosphate anhydrous	44.28 mg	pH adjustment
Sodium hydroxide	14.22 mg	pH adjustment

Source: Sulfur Colloid package insert (2008).

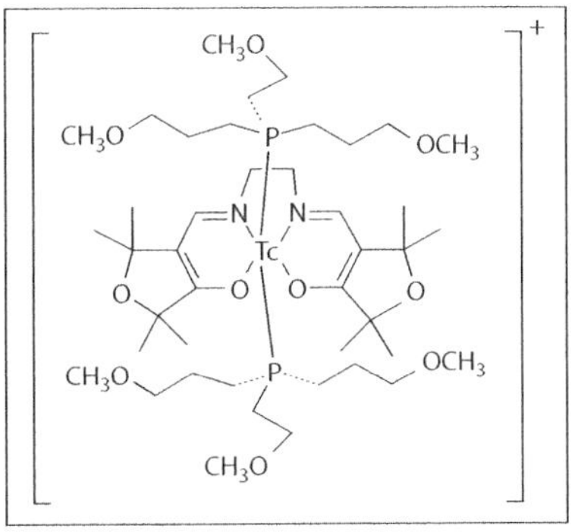

Figure 6.11 Technetium-99m tetrofosmin (Basmadjian 2009).

Technetium-99m tetrofosmin

Figure 6.11 shows ^{99m}Tc (^{99m}Tc-6,9-bis(2-ethoxyethyl)-3,12-dioxa-6,9-diphosphatetradecane; Myoview).

Indications and dosage

Technetium-99m tetrofosmin (US Pharmacopeia 2008) is used in myocardial perfusion imaging to assess the severity and localization of myocardial infarction and myocardial ischemia, to determine left ventricular ejection fraction, to assess ventricular wall motion, and to assess coronary artery disease.

Dosage is 8–15 mCi for myocardial perfusion at rest and 24–45 mCi under stress (3× rest).

Pharmacokinetics

Technetium-99m tetrofosmin is injected intravenously and has a high volume of distribution. It has low protein binding and is rapidly cleared from the blood. It accumulates in myocytes in relation to blood flow with a first-pass extraction efficiency of approximately 60% owing to lipophilicity through passive diffusion. Approximately 1.2% of the injected activity accumulates in the myocyte cytoplasm as a result of the overall cationic 1+ structure. Normal biodistribution is hepatobiliary, cardiac, salivary glands, and thyroid. It is eliminated through the biliary system into the intestines, and through the renal system. At 48 hours, 40% of the injected activity is eliminated via the kidneys and 26% via the bowels. A certain amount of liver and bowel clearance must have occurred before cardiac imaging may proceed (Myoview package insert 2006).

Contraindications and adverse effects

The only contraindication to a ^{99m}Tc-tetrofosmin injection is hypersensitivity to any agents in the kit, and no major precautions exist. No major drug interactions have been reported with tetrofosmin. Adverse effects are rare and include angina, flushing, dyspnea, headache, vomiting, abdominal discomfort, and hypotension. Technetium, as free pertechnetate, crosses the placenta and is distributed into breast milk (Myoview package insert 2006).

Preparation

The ingredients for the manufactured product can be found in table 6.22. When preparing the kit, special attention must be given to removal of nitrogen gas from the vial with a vented needle and to avoid the addition of technetium at a concentration greater than 30 mCi/mL. After reduction by stannous chloride, ^{99m}Tc first binds to gluconate as a transchelate molecule. The solution must stand at room temperature for 15 minutes to allow the formation of ^{99m}Tc-tetrofosmin. The number of technetium atoms, volume of preparation, storage conditions, and concentration must be considered when verifying stability and beyond-use dating if not compounded within the manufacturer's labeling information. Activities from 240 mCi to 600 mCi have been used in preparation of the kit, with greater than 90% radiochemical purity at 12 hours after preparation. The package insert preparation specifies 240 mCi of ^{99m}Tc in 8 mL with an expiration of 12 hours at controlled room temperature. The kit must be stored refrigerated before preparation and the contents should be protected from light. Radiochemical purity above 90% must be confirmed before administration. Different methods exist for determination of radiochemical purity and include Whatman 17 medium with ethyl acetate as the solvent, with ^{99m}Tc-tetrofosmin having an R_f value of 0.2–1.0 and free pertechnetate having an R_f value of 0–0.1 (Patel et al. 1998). A new radiochemical quality control method using a silica cartridge for the stationary phase and 70:30 methanol:water as the mobile phase has identified an unknown complex formed in compounding if the proper venting does not take place when adding the technetium to the kit (Hammes et al. 2004). The unknown complex has been shown to have the same biodistribution and elimination as ^{99m}Tc-tetrofosmin but has no retention in cardiac tissues.

Table 6.22 The components of Myoview (tetrofosmin) manufactured by GE Healthcare

Ingredient	Amount	Purpose
Tetrofosmin	0.23 mg	Ligand
Stannous chloride dihydrate	5–15.8 µg	Reducing agent
Disodium sulphosalicylate	0.32 mg	Stabilizer
D-Gluconate	1 mg	Transchelate
Sodium hydrogen carbonate	1.8 mg	Stabilizer

Source: Myoview package insert (2006).

Technetium-99m tetrofosmin has been shown to adsorb to plastic syringes to varying degrees and has been shown to have slight myocardial redistribution six hours after administration.

Carbon

Carbon-14 urea

Indications and dosage

Carbon-14 urea (US Pharmacopeia 2008) is used as an *in vitro* test in the detection of gastric urease for the diagnosis of *Helicobacter pylori* in the human stomach. The test is not used frequently, but has been recommended to document *H. pylori* eradication following specific antibiotic therapy. A capsule form contains 1 mg urea labeled with 37 kBq (1 μCi) ^{14}C (PYtest package insert 1997).

Pharmacokinetics

Following ingestion of the capsule by the patient, respiratory excretion of ^{14}C peaks between 10 and 15 minutes and declines thereafter, with a biological half-life of approximately 15 minutes. The ^{14}C-urea that comes into contact with *H. pylori* in the stomach is hydrolyzed into ^{14}C-carbon dioxide ($^{14}CO_2$) and ammonia. The $^{14}CO_2$ enters the bloodstream and is exhaled by the patient. The ^{14}C-urea that is not hydrolyzed by *H. pylori* is excreted in the urine, with a half-life of approximately 12 hours. Approximately 10% of the ^{14}C remains in the body at 72 hours and is gradually excreted, with a biological half-life of 40 days. The patient takes the ^{14}C-urea capsule with 20 mL of warm water and then drinks 20 mL more warm water. A breath sample is collected at 10 minutes (PYtest package insert 1997).

Contraindications and drug interactions

While there are no contraindications or known adverse effects, there are drug interactions that decrease the sensitivity of the test. Antibiotics, proton pump inhibitors, sucralfate, and bismuth preparations are known to suppress *H. pylori*. Ingestion of antibiotics or bismuth within four weeks and proton pump inhibitors or sucralfate within two weeks prior to performing the test may give false-negative results. If the test is used to determine eradication, it should be performed no sooner than one month after completion of therapy (Balon *et al.* 2002).

Preparation

Carbon-14 is a pure beta emitter with a physical half-life of 5730 years and maximum beta energy of 160 keV. To measure pure beta emissions, ^{14}C is counted in a liquid scintillation counter (LSC). The patient's $^{14}CO_2$-containing breath sample is most typically collected in a mylar balloon and mailed to the manufacturer for counting. Alternatively, if the location has a liquid scintillation counter for the detection of pure beta emitters, the patient's sample can be collected directly into the breath collection fluid, but a safety trap must be used to prevent patient ingestion of the collection fluid. The breath collection fluid has thymolphthalein as an indicator and is a blue color as long as the pH is greater then 7. The patient's CO_2 is trapped by the collecting fluid, releasing hydrogen ions and reducing the pH to less than 7, which turns the collection fluid mixture colorless (Abrams 2000). The color change of the collection fluid (from blue to colorless) indicates the end-point of transfer, at which point 1 mmol of CO_2 has been trapped in the collection fluid. The liquid scintillation cocktail (10 mL) is then added to the collection fluid and the sample is counted in the LSC (PYtest package insert 1997). The PYtest is exempt from the Clinical Laboratory Improvement Act as the Act does not consider breath to be a specimen. In addition, no radioactive material license is needed to order or handle the 1 µCi of ^{14}C. This was published in the *Federal Register* as exempt from distribution as a radioactive drug and became effective January 1998 (National Archives and Records Administration 1997).

Chromium

Chromium-51 sodium chromate

Indications and dosage

Chromium-51 sodium chromate (US Pharmacopeia 2008) is used to label RBC *in vitro*. The reinjected labeled RBC are used to determine RBC volume or mass and used indirectly to determine plasma volume. In the past, ^{51}Cr-labeled RBC have been used to determine RBC survival rates, RBC sequestration, and in gastrointestinal bleeding to quantify the blood loss (US Pharmacopeia 1999, pp. 2590–2591).

For RBC volume or mass determination, 10–30 µCi of ^{51}Cr as ^{51}Cr-labeled RBC is administered intravenously (Chromatope package insert 2005). Note the activity required to label the RBC is generally greater; for example, for RBC volume or mass determination, 100–150 µCi of ^{51}Cr is added to approximately 40 mL whole blood in approximately 8 mL Anticoagulant Citrate Dextrose solution (A-C-D package insert 1994; Kowalsky & Falen 2004, p. 755).

Pharmacokinetics

In vitro, the hexavalent ^{51}Cr readily penetrates the erythrocyte and binds to hemoglobin. Unbound ^{51}Cr is reduced to the trivalent state by the addition of

100 mg ascorbic acid, so no further binding occurs *in vivo*. When the ^{51}Cr-labeled RBC are administered intravenously, the labeled cells have a biological half-life of 25–35 days. This shortened survival time, compared with the 120 day true lifespan of RBC, reflects the elution of ^{51}Cr from the cells, at a rate of 1% per day, and the cell damage that occurs during the blood withdrawal and labeling procedure. The labeled cells circulate and are taken up in the reticuloendothelial tissues, with the majority in the spleen. Cells sequestered by the spleen will release ^{51}Cr back into the plasma (US Pharmacopeia 1999, p. 2591).

Contraindications and precautions

There are no known contraindications for ^{51}Cr, but caution should be exercised when it is administered to a nursing woman since ^{51}Cr is excreted in human milk. No adverse reactions have been reported with use of ^{51}Cr (Chromatope package insert 2005).

Preparation

Chromium-51 decays by electron capture with a primary gamma emission of 320 keV and a physical half-life of 27.7 days. It is essential that the user adheres to strict aseptic procedures during the preparation, withdrawal, and administration of the labeled RBC. Most hospital nuclear medicine departments will perform the labeling procedure and analysis in their own facility. The manufacturer's package insert or other appropriate literature must be consulted for specific methods of labeling RBC. Other drugs needed for the procedure include ACD and ascorbic acid. A plasma volume study using ^{125}I-labeled human serum albumin (HSA) will usually be performed at the same time as estimation of RBC volume or mass. The analysis is very dependent on accurate measurement techniques and should be completely mapped out before beginning the procedure. Certification under the Clinical Laboratory Improvement Act is required by most facilities to perform the procedure. The ^{51}Cr is supplied as a single-dose vial in a concentration of 100 μCi/mL (Chromate 2005) and a multiple dose vial containing 6 mg/mL benzyl alcohol as the preservative in a concentration of 200 μCi/mL (Chromatope package insert 2005). Both products should be stored at controlled room temperature.

Fluorine

Fluorine-18 fludeoxyglucose

Figure 6.12 shows the structure of ^{18}F-2-fluoro-2-deoxy-D-glucose (fludeoxy-glucose FDG); ^{18}F-FDG; Metatrace FDG).

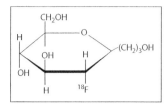

Figure 6.12   2-Fluoro-2-deoxy-D-glucose (Basmadjian 2009).

Indications and dosage

Fluorine-18 FDG is an intravenous, diagnostic radiopharmaceutical used for PET imaging. It is indicated for assessment of abnormal glucose metabolism, diagnoses of cancer or to assist in the evaluation of malignancy in patients with known cancer. It is also indicated for the identification of viable left ventricular myocardium and for the identification of regions of abnormal glucose metabolism in the brain, commonly those associated with epileptic seizure foci.

The dosage for adults is 5–10 mCi, which is administered intravenously over 30 seconds for malignancy, cardiology, and brain imaging. In pediatrics, the recommended dose is 2.6 mCi, but the optimal dosage should be a fraction of the adult dosage based on the child's body size or weight (Metatrace FDG package insert 2002).

Pharmacokinetics

Fluorine-18 FDG is a glucose analog that concentrates in cells that rely upon glucose as an energy source, or in cells whose dependence on glucose increases under pathophysiological conditions. Fluorine-18 FDG is transported through the cell membrane by facilitative glucose transporter proteins and is phosphorylated within the cell to ^{18}F-FDG 6-phosphate by the enzyme hexokinase. Once phosphorylated, it cannot exit until it is dephosphorylated by glucose-6-phosphatase. Therefore, the retention and clearance of ^{18}F-FDG reflect a balance involving glucose transporter, hexokinase, and glucose-6-phosphatase activities. Regions of 'increased ^{18}F-FDG uptake' correlate with increased glucose metabolism. Regions of decreased/absent uptake reflect the absence of glucose metabolism. Background activity reflects normal glucose uptake by cells. When administered intravenously, ^{18}F-FDG readily distributes to all tissues. Within 33 minutes, a mean of 3.9% of the injected dose can be measured in the urine. Bladder activity two hours after injection indicates that a mean of 20.6% of the injected activity is present. After background clearance, peak imaging is at 30–40 minutes after injection (Metatrace FDG package insert 2002). For cardiac viability imaging, the uptake of ^{18}F-FDG must be enhanced by administering 50 g of glucose one hour prior to the cardiac scan. The heart primarily uses fatty acids for its metabolism needs. After a glucose load, insulin is released and the result is an increase in glucose metabolism in preference to fatty acids in the myocardium. In the ischemic heart, areas of ischemic muscle switch to anaerobic glycolysis, with glucose as the principal substrate. The increase in ^{18}F-FDG uptake in myocardial ischemic areas after a glucose load is 2.5 times higher than if the patient is fasting (Kowalsky & Falen 2004).

Contraindications and drug interactions

There are no known contraindications or adverse effects for ^{18}F-FDG. Drug interactions are those that may compete with glucose metabolism and include insulin or glucose. In all cases except myocardial viability, ^{18}F-FDG imaging is performed in the fasting state to minimize competitive inhibition of ^{18}F-FDG uptake by glucose. A minimum fast of four hours is recommended prior to initiation of the study (Metatrace FDG package insert 2002). Though sources differ on the exact level, most agree that a plasma glucose concentration above 200 mg/dL warrants a delay of the study until this falls below 200 mg/dL. Diabetic patients should be counseled to take their diabetic control medication and have a morning meal no fewer than four hours prior to their appointment time (Bogsrud & Lowe 2006). Insulin will facilitate the entry of glucose into muscle, adipose tissue, and the liver. Administering insulin at the same time as ^{18}F-FDG should be avoided because it tends to increase glucose accumulation in skeletal muscle and less is available for accumulation in tumors (Coleman 1999). Diabetic patients are best imaged early in the morning before the first meal, and insulin or oral hypoglycemic medication should be titrated appropriately the night before the study. The type of insulin and duration should be considered when scheduling a diabetic patient. Blood sugar can be controlled with oral hypoglycemic drugs four hours before the study or a patient can be rescheduled to a suitable time before the next injection if using a long-acting insulin (Gorospe *et al.* 2005).

Preparation

Fluorine-18 decays by positron (β^+) emission with a mean energy of 250 keV and has a half-life of 109.8 minutes. The photons useful for diagnostic imaging are the 511 keV gamma photons, resulting from the annihilation interaction of the emitted positron with an electron. The ^{18}F-FDG is produced in an automated radiochemical synthesis unit from ^{18}F produced in a cyclotron by proton bombardment of enriched $H_2{}^{18}O$. The half-life of ^{18}F requires that the isotope is produced and synthesized into ^{18}F-FDG within hours of administration to the patient. The operation of a cyclotron and the synthesis of ^{18}F-FDG are closely regulated by standards described in the USP with proposed new good manufacturing procedures by the FDA.

Gallium

Gallium-67 citrate

Indications and dosage

Gallium-67 citrate (US Pharmacopeia 2008) has been used in a variety of tumor and inflammatory studies. It is indicated for the diagnostic imaging of Hodgkin's disease, lymphomas, bronchogenic carcinoma, and for chronic inflammatory abcesses. Imaging with ^{67}Ga is ordered most frequently for suspected recurrence of lymphoma and for monitoring the effects of therapeutic regimens (Kowalsky & Falen 2004, pp. 316, 704).

The adult dosage for ^{67}Ga-citrate is 5–10 mCi administered intravenously. The pediatric dosage should be a fraction of the adult dose based on the child's body size or weight.

Pharmacokinetics

After intravenous injection, the citrate complex dissociates in the blood and ^{67}Ga becomes bound to plasma transferrin. Elimination from the body is slow, with 25% via the kidneys in the first 24 hours and rising to 35% of the injected dose via the kidneys and bowel at seven days (Kowalsky & Falen 2004, p. 696); 85% of the ^{67}Ga activity has a biological half-life of 25 days. Normal localization is in the liver, spleen, gastrointestinal tract, kidneys (renal cortex), skeleton, and bone marrow. Localization in these organs is non-specific and the exact mechanism of ^{67}Ga localization in infection and tumors is not clear. The theory is that ^{67}Ga bound to transferrin passes into the leukocyte or tumor, where it binds to lactoferrin. Because of the slow excretion of ^{67}Ga, imaging is typically performed 48–72 hours after injection. Imaging up to 96 hours has been performed to distinguish tumor from the normal bowel accumulation, which will clear over time (Kowalsky & Falen 2004, p. 705). Daily laxatives and/or enemas are recommended during the first week after injection until the final images are obtained, in order to cleanse the bowel of radioactive material and minimize the possibility of false-positive studies (Gallium 67-BMS package insert 2005).

Contraindications, precautions, adverse effects, and drug interactions

There are no known contraindications for ^{67}Ga. However, as ^{67}Ga contains 9 mg/mL (0.9%) benzyl alcohol as a preservative, it should be used with caution in newborns, particularly infants born prematurely, and individuals with impaired liver function (Gallium 67-BMS package insert 2005). Hiller (1986) showed that gasping syndrome significantly decreased when benzyl alcohol use was discontinued in newborns of very low birth weight (less than 1 kg; less than 1 month old), and those less than 27 weeks of gestational age. A dosage of 0.5 mCi 14 days after ^{67}Ga calibration would contain approximately 44 mg benzyl alcohol. It would be prudent to avoid use in this patient group, but the risks and benefits should be discussed on a case-by-case basis. Gallium is excreted in breast milk. It has been recommended that nursing be resumed when the infant's ingested effective dose equivalent is below 100 mrem, which would be approximately three weeks after administration of ^{67}Ga. Because of the difficulty of maintaining the maternal milk over such an extended period of time, complete cessation of nursing is usually recommended (US Pharmacopeia 1999, p. 1539). Adverse effects are rare, but occurrences of hypersensitivity reactions or allergic reactions, skin rash, and nausea have been reported in association with ^{67}Ga use (Gallium 67-BMS package insert 2005). Many drugs and conditions alter the distribution of ^{67}Ga and are taken into consideration when interpreting the results of a study. These include antineoplastic agents, iron, intravenous calcium gluconate, corticosteroids, glucocorticoids, doxorubicin, phenytoin, antibiotics, drugs that may induce nephritis (e.g. allopurinol and non-steroidal anti-inflammatory drugs), and amiodarone (US Pharmacopeia 1999, p. 1540). Therapy with radiation can also alter distribution and should not have contrast (radiography, CT, or gadolinium imaging) during the time needed for the ^{67}Ga scan (Shackett 2009, p. 105).

Preparation

Gallium-67 is produced in a cyclotron by the proton irradiation of enriched zinc oxide and has a physical half-life of 78.3 hours. The principal mode of decay is by electron capture, with three primary photon emissions of 93, 184 and 300 keV. The ^{67}Ga is supplied as a ready to use, multiple dose vial, with a calibration concentration of 2 mCi/mL and expiration 14 days after calibration. Storage is at controlled room temperature (Gallium 67-BMS package insert 2005).

Indium

Indium-111 chloride

Indium-111 chloride is not indicated for direct administration. It is used to radiolabel proteins and antibodies that are then used for imaging: capromab pendetide (ProstaScint), ibritumomab tiuxetan (Zevalin), and penetreotide (OctreoScan). It is produced in a cyclotron by the proton irradiation of cadmium-112 (^{112}Cd). At the time of calibration, it contains not more than 0.075% ^{114m}In and ^{65}Zn combined. At the time of expiration, it contains not more than 0.15% ^{114m}In and ^{65}Zn combined (Indium-111 package insert 2007). The impurity ^{114m}In has a physical half-life of 49.5 days and a small abundance of gamma and beta emissions in the ranges 190–725 keV gamma and 358 keV beta. The ^{65}Zn has a physical half-life of 244 days, with primary gamma energy of 1.15 MeV and a primary beta maximum emission energy of

1.3 MeV (Firestone & Shirley 1996). The ^{111}In is supplied in hydrochloric acid with a low pH (1.0–1.4) and any necessary dilution should be with the same concentration of acid. If it is diluted with sterile water for injection or normal saline, the ^{111}In comes out of solution and sticks firmly to the wall of the vial or syringe (Welch & Welch 1975). Caution should be used when increasing the pH of commercially available ^{111}In, as in rinsing the manufacturer's vials with normal saline, which has resulted in colloidal formation and loss of activity. The ^{111}In will remain in solution above pH 3.4 if it is complexed with a weak chelating agent such as sodium acetate, tartrate, or citrate (Kowalsky & Falen 2004, p. 315). Since most radiopharmaceuticals require a pH above 3, the labeling procedure with ^{111}In includes buffering the solution with a weak chelating agent. The ^{111}In is supplied as single-dose vials and should be stored at controlled room temperature (Indiclor package insert 2005; Indium-111 package insert 2006).

Indium-111 pentetate

Figure 6.13 shows ^{111}In-pentetate (disodium[N,N-bis[2-(carboxymethyl) amino]glycinato(5-)]-indate (2-)-^{111}In; ^{111}In-DTPA; Indium DTPA).

Indications and dosage
Indium-111-pentetate (^{111}In-DTPA) is used in radionuclide cisternography to study the flow of CSF in the brain, particularly to diagnose normal pressure hydrocephalus. It is also used to localize CSF leaks, to test the patency of CFS shunts, and to detect and quantify CSF rhinorrhea. In infants, ^{111}In-DTPA has been used to evaluate CSF dynamics and patency of the cerebral ventricular system (US Pharmacopeia 1999, p. 1698). It has also been used for liquid gastric emptying studies when dual isotope is preferred.

The adult dosage for CSF evaluation is 500 μCi slowly administered intrathecally into the subarachnoid space of the lumbar spine, usually administered by an interventional radiologist. In dual-isotope liquid gastric emptying studies, 100 μCi is administered orally with 4 fluid ounces (114 mL) water.

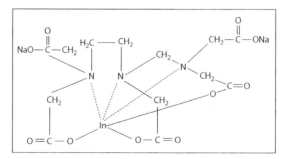

Figure 6.13 Indium-111 pentetate (Indium DTPA package insert 2006).

The activity when measured in a dose calibrator is subject to geometry differences. The plastic syringe reading must be multiplied by a correction factor to lower the reading given from the dose calibrator's manufacturer's ^{111}In setting for an accurate assay.

Pharmacokinetics

After intrathecal administration, ^{111}In-DTPA diffuses to the basal cisterns within two to four hours and subsequently will be apparent in the sylvian and cerebral cisterns (US Pharmacopeia 1999, p. 1699). In normal individuals, the radiopharmaceutical will ascend to the parasagittal region within 24 hours, with simultaneous partial or complete clearance of activity from the basal cisterns and sylvian regions. The radiopharmaceutical does not normally enter the cerebral ventricles. Approximately 65% of the administered dose is excreted by the kidneys within 24 hours; this increases to 85% in 72 hours. Images are obtained 4 and 24 hours after administration. Patients with CSF leaks may have imaging at one to two hours; nasal packs (pledgets) are usually used to confirm the presence of CSF rhinorrhea (Indium DTPA package insert 2006).

Contraindications and precautions

There are no known contraindications to the use of ^{111}In-DTPA. Adverse effects have been seen in less than 0.4% of patients and are aseptic meningitis and pyrogenic reactions. Extreme care must be exercised to assure aseptic conditions for intrathecal injections (Indium DTPA package insert 2006).

Preparation

Indium-111 is produced in a cyclotron by the proton irradiation of [112]Cd. It has a half-life of 67.9 hours, with electron capture as the primary mode of decay. The principal photon emissions are at 171 and 245 keV. At calibration time, the impurity of [114m]In, with a half-life of 49.5 days, and [65]Zn, with a half-life of 244 days, must be less than 0.06% each. The concentration of each radionuclide contaminant changes with time (Indium DTPA package insert 2006). ^{111}In-DTPA is ^{111}In complexed to disodium pentetate (ratio 1:1), with a pH of 7. The rate of formation of ^{111}In-DTPA is slow and requires heating to complete the complexation. Once the ^{111}In-DTPA complex is formed, it is very stable and will not allow *in vivo* ligand exchange with transferrin (Welch & Welch 1975). It is supplied as a ready-to-use single-dose vial with a concentration of 1 mCi/mL and a total activity of 1.5 mCi on the day of calibration (Indium DTPA package insert 2006). Currently, GE Healthcare is only manufacturer of ^{111}In-DTPA in the USA.

Indium-111 oxyquinoline

Figure 6.14 shows ^{111}In-oxyquinoline (Indium oxine).

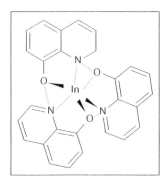

Figure 6.14   Indium-111 oxyquinoline (Basmadjian 2009).

Indications and dosage

Indium-111 oxyquinoline (US Pharmacopeia 2008) is indicated for labeling of leukocytes for infection imaging.

The adult dosage of ^{111}In-oxyquinoline-labeled leukocytes is 500–800 µCi. It should only be used in children after considering the use of ^{99m}Tc-labeled leukocytes. The activity when measured in a dose calibrator is subject to geometry differences. The plastic syringe reading must be multiplied by a correction factor to lower the reading given from the dose calibrator's manufacturers ^{111}In setting for an accurate assay.

Pharmacokinetics

Indium-111 oxyquinoline is ^{111}In complexed relatively weakly with 8-hydroxyquinoline (ratio 1:3). When it is incubated with leukocytes *in vitro* (free of plasma, which contains transferrin), the lipophilic ^{111}In-oxyquinoline passively diffuses into the leukocyte cell membrane. Intracellularly, the ^{111}In will bind to cytoplasmic proteins, trapping the ^{111}In inside the cell and releasing the oxyquinoline to diffuse back out of the cell. The labeled leukocytes are then reinjected to permit the imaging of inflammatory sites based on normal physiological properties of leukocytes (US Pharmacopeia 1999, p. 1696). After intravenous administration of the labeled leukocytes, approximately 60% of the activity will distribute equally to the spleen and liver, with some activity in the bone marrow. Part of normal biodistribution is lung accumulation immediately after injection, with a biological half-life of 15 minutes and almost no activity left in the lungs at four hours. The clearance of ^{111}In-oxyquinoline-labeled leukocytes from the blood is slow. Imaging is usually performed 18 to 24 hours after administration. The renal and bowel elimination of the labeled leukocytes is 1% of the injected activity in the first 24 hours. Clearance from whole blood and biological distribution can be affected by the condition of the injected cells and the labeling techniques used (Indium Oxine package insert 2006).

Contraindications, adverse effects, and drug interactions

As ^{111}In is excreted in breast milk, temporary discontinuation of nursing for 24 hours is recommended. Altered biodistribution of ^{111}In-oxyquinoline-labeled leukocytes can occur when the patient has had long-term antibiotic or corticosteroid treatment, or is currently on hyperalimentation (US Pharmacopeia 1999, p. 1697).

Preparation

Indium-111 is produced in a cyclotron by the proton irradiation of ^{112}Cd. It has a physical half-life of 67.9 hours, with electron capture as the primary mode of decay. The principal photon emissions are at 171 and 245 keV. The impurity of ^{114m}In, with a half-life of 49.5 days, should not be more than 1 μCi/mCi ^{111}In at time of calibration (Indium oxine package insert 2006) ^{111}In-oxyquinoline is supplied in a single-dose vial at a concentration of 1 mCi/mL, with a total activity of 1 mCi at the time of calibration and can be stored at controlled room temperature. After leukocyte labeling, the cells should be reinjected as quickly as possible, preferably within one hour. After three hours, the labeled leukocyte cells begin to lose their chemotaxis and this can lead to false-negative results (US Pharmacopeia 1999, p. 1698). Currently, ^{111}In-oxyquinoline is only manufactured by one company and is produced once a week with a Wednesday calibration. Leukocyte labeling efficiency can decrease with increasing plasma concentration because ^{111}In preferentially complexes with transferrin in plasma and will disassociate from the oxyquinoline. Leukocyte-labeling efficiency will decrease with a decreased patient leukocyte blood count. The recommended amount of leukocytes for an average labeling efficiency of 77% with ^{111}In-oxyquinoline is 3×10^8 to 4×10^8 cells (Indium Oxine package insert 2006). The ^{111}In-oxyquinoline should not be administered directly. It is only to be used for the *in vitro* radiolabeling of leukocytes. The manufacturer's package insert or other appropriate literature should be consulted for the specific method of separating and labeling leukocytes (US Pharmacopeia 1999, p. 1698).

Indium-111 capromab pendetide

Indications and dosage

Indium-111 capromab pendetide (^{111}In-ProstaScint) is indicated for use in patients with biopsy-proven and clinically localized prostate cancer who are at high risk for metastasis. It is also indicated for use in patients after prostatectomy who have a high clinical suspicion of occult recurrent or residual prostate cancer.

Dosage is 0.5 mg capromab pendetide labeled with 5–6 mCi ^{111}In administered intravenously over 5 to 20 minutes with vital signs monitored. The activity when measured in a dose calibrator is subject to geometry differences. The plastic syringe reading must be multiplied by a correction factor to lower the reading given from the dose calibrator's manufacturer's ^{111}In setting for an accurate assay.

Pharmacokinetics

Capromab pendetide is an intact IgG murine monoclonal antibody that reacts with prostate-specific antigen, a glycoprotein expressed by the prostate epithelium. Capromab is conjugated by the manufacturer to a bifunctional chelating compound, GYK-DTPA (capromab pendetide) and the resulting ^{111}In-capromab pendetide formed during labeling with ^{111}In by the end user is very stable *in vivo*. After intravenous administration, ^{111}In-capromab pendetide has a very slow clearance from the vasculature and a very small volume of distribution. The biological half-life is 67 (±11) hours and approximately 10% of the administered activity is excreted renally within 72 hours. Normal activity is seen in the liver, spleen, and bone marrow. Normal activity has also been seen in the bowel, blood pool, kidneys, bladder, and genitalia. Imaging has been performed immediately after administration and at 30 minutes for blood pool imaging. Localization imaging is performed at 72 hours. Some patients may require imaging 120 hours after administration. The patient must complete a bowel-cleansing preparation prior to the three-day imaging procedure. Blood pool imaging using ^{99m}Tc-labeled RBC is performed to help identify vasculature during imaging (ProstaScint package insert 1997).

Contraindications, precautions, and adverse effects

Indium-111 capromab pendetide is contraindicated in patients who are hypersensitive to the product or any other murine product. It can only be used by physicians who have completed specific training from the manufacturer in image interpretation. This program is called Partners in Excellence or PIE. Adverse effects include anaphylaxis, increases in bilirubin, and hypotension. The administration of a murine antibody may induce human anti-mouse antibodies (ProstaScint package insert 1997) and this may interfere with diagnostic tests that employ murine-based immunoassay techniques, such as for the tumor marker prostate-specific antigen. Formation of human anti-mouse antibodies also may alter the biodistribution of murine-based diagnostic imaging agents or therapeutic agents.

Preparation

The kit is ordered from the manufacturer and is composed of (a) the antibody in 1 mL of phosphate-buffered saline, which must be refrigerated,

Table 6.23 The components of ProstaScint (capromab pendetide) manufactured by EUSA Pharma

Ingredient	Amount	Purpose
Reaction vial (10 mL)		
Capromab pendetide	0.5 mg	Ligand
Sodium phosphate	As needed	pH adjustment
Buffer vial		
Sodium acetate	82 mg	Chelating agent
Glacial acetic acid	As needed	pH adjustment (5–7)

Source: ProstaScint package insert (1997).

(b) a vial of acetate buffer, and (c) a 0.22 μm Millex GV low protein binding sterile filter (Millipore filter) (table 6.23). The 5 mCi/0.5mL (at time of calibration) ^{111}In chloride (pH approximately 1 to 1.4) must be purchased separately and can be stored at controlled room temperature, 20–25°C. The ^{111}In is produced in a cyclotron by the proton irradiation of ^{112}Cd and has a half-life of 67.9 hours, with electron capture as the primary mode of decay. The principal photon emissions are at 171 and 245 keV. The impurities of ^{114m}In, with a half-life of 49.5 days and primary gamma energies of 192, 558 and 724 keV, and ^{65}Zn, with a half-life of 243.9 days and a primary gamma energy of 1.15 MeV, must be less than 0.06% each (US Pharmacopeia 2008). The following is a brief description of the labeling process from the manufacturer's product information (ProstaScint package insert 1997). First, 0.1 mL of acetate buffer is added to the ^{111}In chloride. This step produces the intermediate species, indium acetate, which keeps the indium soluble at the pH necessary for antibody labeling. The ^{111}In chloride (at least 7 mCi) is added to the antibody. This step takes 30 minutes for the complexation of ^{111}In to the pendetide bifunctional chelate at room temperature. After 30 minutes incubation, 1.9 mL of the acetate buffer is added to the mixture to complete the preparation. The preparation is drawn into a syringe and pushed through the 0.22 μm Millex GV sterile filter into another syringe or sterile vial (to remove any translucent particulates). The quality control is performed by mixing a 1 μL sample with a 1 μL 0.05 mmol/L DTPA solution (letting it stand until dry) and placing a small sample on silica gel paper and developing in normal saline. The ^{111}In-ProstaScint reference value is 0 and the impurity of ^{111}In complex with DTPA has a reference value of 1.0. Radiochemical purity must be greater than 90%. The manufacturer's end-use dating is eight hours.

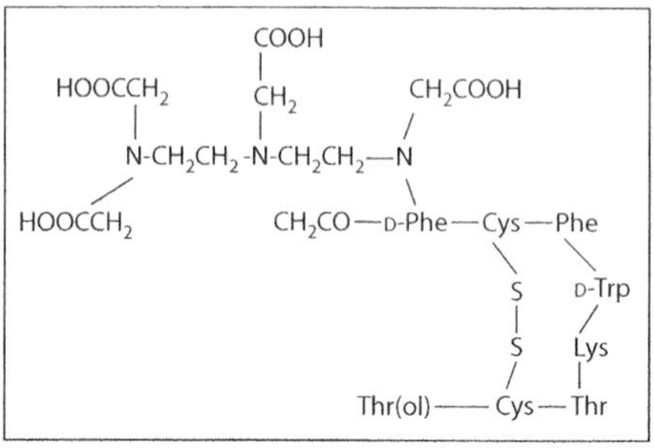

Figure 6.15 Indium-111 -pentetreotide (Basmadjian 2009).

Indium-111 pentetreotide

Figure 6.15 shows ^{111}In-pentetreotide (N-(diethylenetriamine-N,N,N', N'-tetraacetic acid-N'-acetyl)-D-phenylalanyl-L-hemicystyl-L-phenylalanyl-D-tryptophyl-L-lysyl-L-threonyl-L-hemicystyl-L-threoninol cyclic(2,7)disulfide; Octreoscan).

Indications and dosage

Indium-111 pentetreotide (US Pharmacopeia 2008) is an agent for the scintigraphic localization of primary and metastatic neuroendocrine tumors bearing somatostatin receptors (Octreoscan package insert 2006).

The adult dosage is 10 µg pentetreotide labeled with 6 mCi ^{111}In and administered intravenously. The pediatric dosage is 10 µg pentetreotide labeled with 0.14 mCi/kg body weight ^{111}In or a minimum of 1 mCi (Balon *et al.* 2001). The activity when measured in a dose calibrator is subject to geometry differences. The plastic syringe reading must be multiplied by a correction factor to lower the reading given from the dose calibrator's manufacturer's ^{111}In setting for an accurate assay.

Pharmacokinetics

Indium-111 pentetreotide is a conjugate of the bifunctional chelate DTPA, and octreotide, a long-acting analog of the human hormone somatostatin. When labeled with ^{111}In, the product ^{111}In-pentetreotide binds to somatostatin receptors throughout the body (Octreoscan package insert 2006; Intenzo *et al.* 2007). After intravenous administration, ^{111}In-pentetreotide is cleared rapidly from the blood, with 30% of the administered activity remaining in the blood pool at 10 minutes. Normal biodistribution occurs in the pituitary gland, thyroid gland, spleen, liver, and urinary bladder. Elimination is almost entirely via the kidneys, with 50% of the administered activity recovered in the urine by six hours and 85% within 24 hours. Bowel excretion is only about 2% of the administered dose. The biological half-life of ^{111}In-pentetreotide is six hours. Imaging is performed at 24 hours. Some patients may require imaging 48 hours after administration (Octreoscan package insert 2006).

Contraindications, adverse effects, and drug interactions

Indium-111 pentetreotide is contraindicated in patients who have a hypersensitivity to ^{111}In-pentetreotide or octreotide (Sandostatin). Many precautions should be considered before ^{111}In-pentetreotide administration. In patients suspected of having insulinoma, an intravenous infusion of glucose should be available because of the potential for inducing severe hypoglycemia. Indium-111 pentetreotide should not be administered together with solutions for total parenteral nutrition. Patients receiving octreotide (Sandostatin) therapy should suspend medication 48 hours before administration of the radiopharmaceutical. Patients taking Sandostatin Depot should have the ^{111}In-pentetreotide administration three days before their monthly injection (Balon *et al.* 2001). Delayed imaging may be necessary for patients with decreased renal function. Adverse effects were reported in less than 1% of patients and include dizziness, headache, hypotension, changes in liver enzymes, joint pain, and nausea (Octreoscan package insert 2006).

Preparation

Indium-111 is produced in a cyclotron by the proton irradiation of ^{112}Cd; it has a physical half-life of 67.9 hours, with electron capture as the primary mode of decay. The principal photon emissions are 171 and 245 keV. Pentetreotide is labeled by adding at least 7 mCi of ^{111}In-chloride to the lyophilized mixture and incubating at room temperature for 30 minutes. The activity of the ^{111}In-chloride supplied with the kit depends on the day received. Currently, the activity received on Monday and Tuesday product is precalibrated for 3.3 mCi on Friday. Activities received on Wednesday, Thursday, and Friday are precalibrated for 3.3 mCi on Sunday. The activity on Friday is 5.38 mCi, which is not enough for an adult dosage, and imaging would have to be on Saturday, an inconvenient day for most clinics. The lowest acceptable activity days are Tuesday and Thursday at 6.87 mCi. In order to present a consistent product in terms of specific activity of the pentetriotide injected, all the available ^{111}In is added on Tuesday and Thursday, and on Monday and Wednesday a portion is added that is sufficient to ensure that the patient receives at least 6 mCi of activity while still receiving all or nearly all of the 10 μg pentetreotide for binding. The ^{111}In-chloride should not be diluted before the labeling process is complete and the final preparation should not be diluted to more than 3 mL (Octreoscan package insert 2006). Radiochemical purity above 90% must be confirmed before administration. In a chromatography system of instant

Table 6.24 The components of Octreoscan (pentetreotide) manufactured by Covidien

Ingredient	Amount	Purpose
Reaction vial (10 mL)		
Pentetreotide	10 µg	Ligand
Gentisic acid	2 mg	Stabilizer
Ascorbic acid	0.37 mg	Stabilizer
Trisodium citrate buffer	4.9 mg	Buffer
Inositol	10 mg	Stabilizer
Indium vial (10 mL)		
^{111}In-chloride sterile solution in 0.02 M HCl	3.3 mCi/3.3 mL (Friday & Sunday)	Tracer
Ferric chloride	3.85 µg	Weak chelating agent

Source: Octreoscan package insert (2006).

thin-layer chromatography with silica gel medium and normal saline solvent, ^{111}In-pentetreotide has an R_f value of 0 and ^{111}In has an R_f value of 1.0 (Zimmer 1994). The OctreoScan kit should be stored refrigerated at 2–8°C (36–46°F). After reconstitution, the preparation should be stored at or below 25°C (77°F). Expiration is six hours after preparation with storage at room temperature (Octreoscan package insert 2006) (table 6.24).

Iodine

Iodine-123 sodium iodide

Indications and dosage

Iodine-123 sodium iodide (^{123}I-radioiodide; Sodium Iodide I-123) (US Pharmacopeia 2008) is indicated for diagnostic studies of the thyroid.

The adult dosage for a thyroid function test is 100–400 µCi administered orally. The lower portion of the range (100 µCi) is recommended for uptake studies alone, and the higher portion (400 µCi) for thyroid imaging (Sodium Iodide I-123 package insert 2005). The pediatric minimum dosage is 10 µCi for uptake studies and 50 µCi for thyroid imaging (US Pharmacopeia 1999, p. 2600).

Pharmacokinetics

The action of radioiodide is based on the accumulation and retention of iodine as required for the synthesis of thyroid hormones. Thyroid retention of any radioactive iodide permits quantification of organ uptake and imaging of the anatomical distribution in thyroid tissue. Radioiodide is also concentrated in functioning papillary/follicular thyroid cancer and metastases. Radioiodide is readily absorbed from the gastrointestinal tract. Normal distribution is in the choroid plexus, gastric mucosa, salivary glands, nasal mucosa and lactating breast tissue. In the thyroid, radioiodide is removed from the blood by thyroid epithelial cells via active transport. In the follicular colloid tissue, the iodide is oxidized to iodine and bound to tyrosyl residues of thyroglobulin. Thyroid uptake is usually increased in hyperthyroidism and in goiters with impaired hormone synthesis. Uptake is usually decreased in hypothyroidism. In the euthyroid patient, 5–30% of the administered activity is concentrated in the thyroid gland at 24 hours and it has an effective half-life of eight hours. The biological half-life in the thyroid compartment for euthyroid patients is 80 days and for hyperthyroid patients is 5 to 40 days. The normal range of urinary excretion in 24 hours is reported to be 37–75% of the administered dose, varying with thyroid and renal function. Less than 2% of the administered activity is excreted via the bowel and salivary glands at 48 hours. Imaging is usually performed at four hours after administration and then again 18 to 24 hours after administration (US Pharmacopeia 1999, p. 2599; Sodium Iodide I-123 package insert 2005).

Contraindications and drug interactions

Patients with a hypersensitivity to iodide should not receive the product. Drugs that could decrease the radioiodide uptake include the recent intake of stable iodine in any form, or the use of thyroid or antithyroid drugs and amiodarone. The patient should have not had a diagnostic study with radiographic contrast medium within four weeks of ^{123}I-radioiodide administration. Lithium increases radioiodide uptake (US Pharmacopeia 1999, p. 2600).

Preparation

Iodine-123 is a cyclotron-produced radionuclide that decays to [123]Te by electron capture and has a physical half-life of 13.2 hours, with a primary photon energy of 159 keV. The capsule preparations of ^{123}I-radioiodide may contain small amounts of radionuclide contaminants with longer physical half-lives (e.g. [125]I, [121]Te). The ratio of these isotopes at expiration is large enough to increase the radiation dose to the patient. Capsules expire 24 hours after calibration. The ^{123}I isotope is preferable to ^{131}I for diagnostic studies because of its lower radiation dose and better imaging properties. Iodine-123 is supplied as 100 μCi and 200 μCi capsules for use Tuesday through Thursday. The capsules are easily dissolvable in 5 mL purified water USP for patients who cannot swallow capsules. In order to assay the patient dose accurately, a National Institute of Standards and Testing calibrated capsule is required for the dose calibrator channel setting for the appropriate capsule geometry. Capsules should be stored at controlled room temperature (Sodium Iodide I-123 package insert 2005).

Iodine-123 iobenguane

Indications and dosage

Iodine-123 iobenguane (^{123}I-*meta*-iodobenzylguanidine sulfate [^{123}I-mIBG]; AdreView) is indicated for use in the detection of primary or metastatic pheochromocytoma or neuroblastoma as an adjunct to other diagnostic tests.

For adults and children weighing over 70 kg, the recommended dosage is 10 mCi administered intravenously over one to two minutes. For smaller children, the dosage is weight based and a chart is supplied in the manufacturer's product information. The typical pediatric dosage is 5 mCi with a minimum dosage of 1 mCi (AdreView package insert 2008).

Pharmacokinetics

Iodine-123 iobenguane is a physiological analog of the guanidines. In adrenergic nerves, guanidines are believed to share the same transport pathway as norepinephrine and to accumulate in, and displace norepinephrine from, intraneuronal storage granules. Similarly, ^{123}I-mIBG is concentrated in chromaffin granules in adrenergic neurons (US Pharmacopeia 1999, p. 1749).

After intravenous administration ^{123}I-mIBG is rapidly cleared from the blood and accumulates mainly in the liver, and to a lesser degree in the lungs, heart, spleen, and salivary glands. The majority of the ^{123}I-mIBG activity is excreted unaltered by the kidneys via glomerular filtration. In patients with normal renal function, 40–50% of the administered activity is eliminated within 24 hours (US Pharmacopeia 1999, p. 1748) and 70–90% of the administered dose is recovered unaltered in urine within four days. Only a small amount ($< 1\%$) of the administered activity is eliminated via the bowel. Imaging is carried out 18 to 24 hours after administration (AdreView package insert 2008).

Contraindications, precautions, adverse effects, and drug interactions

Iodine-123 iobenguane is contraindicated in patients with a known hypersensitivity to iobenguane or iobenguane sulfate. Radioiodide is excreted into human breast milk. The AdreView product information suggests that nursing women should consider interrupting nursing for 10 half-lives or six days. Adverse reactions have been mostly isolated occurrences but included dizziness, rash, pruritus, flushing, or injection site hemorrhage. Drugs that block norepinephrine uptake or deplete norepinephrine stores may decrease ^{123}I-mIBG uptake in neuroendocrine tumors. When possible, these drugs should be discontinued for at least five biological half-lives before ^{123}I-mIBG administration. Examples include antihypertensives that deplete norepinephrine stores or inhibit reuptake (e.g. reserpine, labetalol: discontinue 72 hours before); antidepressants that inhibit norepinephrine transporter function (e.g. amitriptyline and derivatives, imipramine and derivatives, selective serotonin reuptake inhibitors: discontinue 48 hours before), and sympathomimetic amines (e.g. phenylephrine, phenylpropanolamine, pseudoephedrine, ephedrine: discontinue 24 hours before) (US Pharmacopeia 1999, p. 1748; AdreView package insert 2008). The package insert also states that 'AdreView contains benzyl alcohol which may cause serious reactions in premature or low birth-weight infants,' and that 'safety and effectiveness have not been established in pediatric patients < 1 month of age.' AdreView contains 10.3 mg/mL benzyl alcohol. Hiller (1986) showed that gasping syndrome significantly decreased when benzyl alcohol use was discontinued in newborns of very low birth weight (< 1 kg; less than one month old), and those less than 27 weeks of gestational age. It would be prudent to avoid use in this patient group, but the risks versus benefits should be discussed on a case-by-case basis. Thyroid protection with potassium iodide or potassium perchlorate should be administered orally at least one hour before ^{123}I-mIBG administration and should continue six days after administration (US Pharmacopeia 1999, p. 1748; AdreView package insert 2008).

Preparation

The ingredients for the manufactured product can be found in table 6.25. Iodine-123 is a cyclotron-produced radionuclide that decays to ^{123}Te by electron capture and has a physical half-life of 13.2 hours, with a primary photon energy of 159 keV. AdreView (iobenguane I-123 injection) is supplied as a single-dose, ready-to-use radiopharmaceutical for intravenous administration. AdreView can be stored at controlled room temperature. As per the manufacturer's product information, 'This product does not contain a

Table 6.25 The components of AdreView (iobenguane; mIBG) manufactured by GE Healthcare

Ingredient	Amount	Purpose
Iobenguane sulfate	0.4 mg	Ligand
Iodine-123	10 mCi	Tracer
Sodium dihydrogen phosphate dihydrate	92 mg	Stabilizer
Disodium hydrogen phosphate dihydrate	14 mg	Stabilizer
Benzyl alcohol (1%)	51.5 mg	Stabilizer

Source: AdreView package insert (2008).

preservative.' It is currently only available Tuesday through Thursday and expires 24 hours after calibration (AdreView package insert 2008). In order to assay the patient dosage accurately, a National Institute of Standards and Testing calibrated vial provides the appropriate vial geometry for the dose calibrator channel setting. The dose is typically measured using the vial subtraction method.

Iodine-125 iodohydroxybenzenesulfonate

Indications and dosage

Iodine-125 iodohydroxybenzensulfonate (^{125}I-HBS; Iotrex) is for use in the GliaSite Radiation Therapy System (RTS, Proxima) for intracavitary brachytherapy of malignant gliomas in the brain. The total amount of Iotrex required depends upon the GliaSite balloon volume and the patient's previous radiation history of the resected tumor margins (Iotrex package insert 2001).

Mechanism of action

Iotrex is the radiation source, a component of the RTS, which is intended to deliver intracavitary radiation therapy (brachytherapy) in patients with malignant brain tumors following tumor resection surgery. The RTS is an inflatable balloon catheter that is placed into a resected cavity in the brain after surgical removal of a brain tumor (Kowalsky & Falen 2004, p. 784). The Iotrex solution is instilled in the GliaSite inflatable balloon and remains for a fixed period of time (usually three to six days) to deliver a radiation dose of 40–60 Gy (Kowalsky & Falen 2004, p. 784). Studies have indicated that less than 0.8% of the ^{125}I radioactivity may diffuse out of the GliaSite balloon over a seven day period. Iodine-125 is rapidly cleared via the kidneys and 93% of systemic ^{125}I is found in the urine in the first two hours.

Contraindications and precautions

Iotrex is contraindicated for use in any device other than the GliaSite RTS device. Iotrex is not to be administered to patients who are pregnant or lactating and should not be administered to patients with other serious concurrent infections or medical illnesses that would jeopardize its safe administration. It is only to be used by physicians who are licensed for liquid brachytherapy sources and devices (Nuclear Regulatory Commission 2006) and have received training by the manufacturer in the use of the GliaSite RTS. In order to assay the patient dosage accurately, a National Institute of Standards and Testing calibrated 5 mL Becton Dickinson syringe is available for the dose calibrator channel setting for the appropriate syringe geometry. Alternatively, the manufacturer's product information specifies channel settings that are only for use on two models of Capintec dose calibrators (CRC-12 and CRC-35R) (Iotrex package insert 2001).

Preparation

Iodine-125 is produced in a reactor by neutron activation of ^{124}Xe. It has a half-life of 59.4 days and decays by electron capture, with the primary photon emissions of 27 and 31 keV X-rays and 35.5 keV gamma radiation. Iotrex is supplied as single-dose vials containing 195 mCi in 1 mL at time of calibration or as prefilled syringes with volume and activity based on patient prescription (Iotrex package insert 2001).

Iodine-125 iothalamate

Indications and dosage

Iodine-125 iothalamate (Glofil) is indicated for non-imaging evaluation of glomerular filtration in the diagnosis or monitoring of patients with renal disease.

Iodine-125 iothalamate has been administered using two types of protocol. The Sigman protocol uses a continuous intravenous infusion of 20–100 µCi. The Cohen protocol (Cohen *et al.* 1969) uses a single intravenous injection of 10–30 µCi (Glofil package insert 1969).

Mechanism of action and pharmacokinetics

The renal clearance of ^{125}I-iothalamate closely approximates that of inulin. Inulin clearance is regarded as the standard for measuring glomerular filtration rate (Kowalsky & Falen 2004, p. 640). After intravenous administration, ^{125}I-iothalamate is cleared by glomerular filtration without tubular secretion or reabsorption. Following infusion administration of ^{125}I-iothalamate, the effective half-life is approximately 1.6 hours. Iodine-125 iothalamate is not used as an imaging agent because the photon emissions of ^{125}I are not strong enough to penetrate the body. After ^{125}I-iothalamate administration, blood samples are collected at approximately 60, 120, and 180 minutes. Urine samples are collected at 120 and 180 minutes. The samples are counted *in vitro* in a well gamma detector. The glomerular filtration rate is calculated from the total counts in the urine divided by the mean counts in the plasma, taking into account the patient's body surface area (Glofil package insert 1969).

Contraindications and precautions

Iodine-125 iothalamate is contraindicated in patients hypersensitive to the product. The Glofil product contains benzyl alcohol as a preservative. Hiller (1986) showed that gasping syndrome significantly decreased when benzyl alcohol use was discontinued in newborns of very low birth weight (< 1 kg; less than one month old), and those less than 27 weeks of gestational age. It would be prudent to avoid use in this patient group, but the risks versus benefits should be discussed on a case-by-case basis. Thyroid protection with potassium iodide or postassium perchlorate should be administered orally at least 24 hours before ^{125}I-iothalamate administration. The procedure using ^{125}I-iothalamate for estimating glomerular filtration rate is challenging and the technique is rarely used in nuclear medicine.

Preparation

Iodine-125 is produced in a reactor through neutron activation of [124]Xe. It has a half-life of 59.4 days and decays by electron capture, with the primary photon emissions of 27 and 31 keV X-rays and 35.5 keV gamma radiation. Glofil is supplied as a ready-to-use, sterile multidose vial containing approximately 1 mg/mL sodium iothalamate and with 0.9% benzyl alcohol as a preservative. The radioactive concentration of the material is 250–300 µCi/mL as of the calibration date. The manufacturer's product information states that the dosage can be calculated by the manufacturer's calibration concentration and be based on volume without assay in a dose calibrator. The product should be refrigerated upon receipt at 2–8°C (Glofil package insert 1969).

Iodine-125 human serum albumin

Indications and dosage

Iodine-125 human serum albumin (^{125}I-HSA; Jeanatope I-125; Iotrex [Iotrex package insert 2001]; RISA) is indicated for the non-imaging evaluation of total blood and plasma volume (Jeanatope I-125 package insert 2009).

For plasma volume determination, the dosage is 5–10 µCi. In order to assay the patient dosage accurately, a National Institute of Standards and Testing calibrated vial provides the appropriate vial geometry for the dose calibrator channel setting. The activity is typically measured using the vial subtraction method.

Mechanism of uptake, biodistribution, elimination

Following intravenous injection, ^{125}I-HSA is uniformly distributed throughout the intravascular pool similarly to the patient's serum albumin within 10 minutes; extravascular distribution takes place more slowly. Labeled albumin also can be detected in the lymphatic system and in certain body tissues within 10 minutes of injection, but maximum distribution of radioactivity throughout the extravascular space does not occur until two to four days after administration. The administered radioactivity is excreted almost entirely in the urine, only around 2% of the total dose ultimately appearing in the feces. The biological half-life of labeled albumin is dependent upon a number of factors, and published studies have varied considerably in their reporting of this figure from below 10 days to 20 days. One important factor affecting the biological half-life is the initial rate of excretion, and this depends in part on the quality of the labeled albumin. With Jeanatope I-125, the biological half-life in normal individuals has been reported to be approximately 14 days (Jeanatope I-125 package insert).

Contraindications and precautions

Cross-sensitivity may occur in patients sensitive to HSA-containing products, and allergic reactions are possible. Radioiodide crosses the placenta and is distributed in breast milk. Thyroid protection with potassium iodide or potassium perchlorate should be administered orally at least 24 hours before ^{125}I-HSA administration (US Pharmacopeia 1999, p. 2454). The procedure using ^{125}I-HSA for *in vitro* plasma volume determination is challenging. Most hospital nuclear medicine departments will perform the plasma determination procedure and analysis in their own facility. The manufacturer's package insert or other appropriate literature must be consulted for specific methods for the procedure. A RBC volume or mass study using ^{51}Cr-labeled RBC will usually be performed at same time as the plasma volume determination. The analysis is very dependent on accurate measurement techniques and should be completely mapped out before beginning the procedure. Clinical Laboratory Improvement Act certification is required by most facilities to perform the procedure.

Preparation

Iodine-125 is produced in a reactor by neutron activation of ^{124}Xe. It has a physical half-life of 59.4 days and decays by electron capture, with the primary photon emissions of 27 and 31 keV X-rays and 35.5 keV gamma radiation. Iodine-125 HSA is supplied as a sterile multidose vial for intravenous use. Each milliliter provides approximately 10 mg protein (normal HSA), 16 mg guanidine hydrochloride for isotonicity, and 9 mg benzyl alcohol as a preservative. The stabilizers acetyl tryptophanate and sodium caprylate have a concentration of less than 0.0089 mol/L. The pH has been adjusted to 7.2–7.8 with sodium hydroxide or hydrochloric acid. Jeanatope I-125 is prepared from blood that was non-reactive when tested for hepatitis B surface antigen and human immunodeficiency virus antibody. The concentration of Jenatope I-125 is 1 mCi/mL and the product should be stored refrigerated (Jeanatope I-125 package insert).

Iodine-131 iobenguane

Indications and dosage

Iodine-131 iobenguane (^{131}I-*meta*-iodobenzlyguanidine sulfate [^{131}I-mIBG]) is indicated for use in the detection of primary or metastatic pheochromocytoma or neuroblastoma as an adjunct to other diagnostic tests.

The recommended dose in adults is 0.5 mCi. In obese patients with body surface area over $1.7\,m^2$, the dose should be $0.3\,mCi/m^2$ up to a maximum of $1.0\,mCi$ administered by slow intravenous injection over 15 to 30 seconds or longer (I-131 mIBG package insert 2008). Since ^{123}I-mIBG is now commercially available as AdreView, the diagnostic use of ^{131}I-mIBG in children is not recommended.

Pharmacokinetics

The pharmacokinetics of ^{131}I-mIBG is the same as for ^{123}I-mIBG (see ^{123}I-mIBG). The major difference is that the decreased activity administered results in the need for more time for background activity to be excreted renally before imaging can begin. Imaging ^{131}I-mIBG usually is 48 hours after intravenous administration. The use of thyroid protection beginning one day prior to administration and continuing for five days after administration is extremely important because of the beta particle decay profile of [131]I (I-131 mIBG package insert 2008).

Contraindications, adverse effects, and drug interactions

Iodine-131 mIBG is contraindicated in patients with a known hypersensitivity to iobenguane or iobenguane sulfate. It is also contraindicated in patients with renal failure. Adverse effects include hypotension, nausea, and vomiting (I-131 mIBG package insert 2008). The drug interactions that apply for ^{123}I-mIBG also apply for ^{131}I-mIBG (see ^{123}I-mIBG).

Preparation

Iodine-131 is a reactor fission by-product of uranium 235; it decays by beta and gamma emission and has a physical half-life of 8.02 days. The principal beta particle has a mean energy of 192 keV and the primary photon that is useful for detection and imaging is 363 keV. Iodine-131 mIBG is supplied frozen in a single-dose vial, ready for administration after to the three hours of thawing. Each 2 mL glass vial contains 1.15 mCi in 0.5 mL at the time of calibration. The drug should be stored frozen at a temperature of -20 to $-10°C$ and expires six hours after thawing (I-131 mIBG package insert 2008).

Iodine-131 sodium iodide

Indications and dosage

Iodine-131 sodium iodide (^{131}I-radioiodide; Sodium Iodide I 131) is indicated for both diagnostic studies of the thyroid and for therapeutic applications for thyroid disorders.

The adult dosage for a diagnostic thyroid function test is 10–30 µCi orally. The therapeutic dosage of ^{131}I depends on the thyroid disorder and can range from a whole-body scan with 2–5 mCi, to the treatment of thyroid carcinoma with 200 mCi. The dosage is administered orally in capsule or liquid form. There is no sterile pyrogen-free form currently commercially available for intravenous administration.

Pharmacokinetics

The action of radioiodide is based on the accumulation and retention of iodine as required for the synthesis of thyroid hormones. Thyroid retention of any radioactive iodide permits quantification of organ uptake and imaging of anatomical distribution in thyroid tissue. Radioiodide is also concentrated in functioning papillary/follicular thyroid cancer and metastases. Radioiodide is readily absorbed from the gastrointestinal tract. Normal distribution is largely to the thyroid and kidneys, and to a lesser extent the choroid plexus, gastric mucosa, salivary glands, nasal mucosa, and lactating breast tissue. In the thyroid, radioiodide is removed from the blood by thyroid epithelial cells via active transport. In the follicular colloid tissue, the iodide is oxidized to iodine and bound to tyrosyl residues of thyroglobulin. Thyroid uptake is usually increased in hyperthyroidism and in goiters with impaired hormone synthesis. Uptake is usually decreased in hypothyroidism. The biological half-life in the thyroid gland for euthyroid patients is 80 days and for hyperthyroid patients is 5 to 40 days. The normal range of urinary excretion in 24 hours is reported to be 37–75% of the administered dose, varying with thyroid and renal function. Imaging with millicurie amounts of ^{131}I-radioiodide is usually performed 18 to 24 hours after administration (US Pharmacopeia 1999, p. 2603; Sodium Iodide I 131 package insert 2005).

Contraindications, adverse effects, and drug interactions

Iodine-131 is contraindicated in pregnant women. Iodine-131 crosses the placenta and may cause severe and irreversible hypothyroidism in the neonate. The fetal thyroid begins to concentrate iodine during the twelfth week of gestation. Since the dose is administered orally, patients with vomiting and diarrhea should not receive ^{131}I.

Adverse events associated with sodium iodide include hypersensitivity reactions, radiation toxicities, and metabolic events. Immediate adverse reactions typically are related to hypersensitivity, such as anaphylaxis, rash, hives, and bronchospasm. Radiation adverse events related to the dose include bone marrow depression, leukopenia, thrombocytopenia, acute leukemia, anemia, blood dyscrasia, chromosomal abnormalities, radiation sickness, and death. Delayed radiation toxicity includes radiation thyroiditis, gastritis, and sialadenitis. Metabolic adverse events include hypothyroidism and exaggerated hyperthyroidism caused by radiation thyroiditis. Tenderness and swelling of the neck, pain on swallowing, sore throat, and cough may occur about the third day after treatment. Drugs that could decrease the ^{131}I uptake include the recent intake of stable iodine in any form, or the use of thyroid or antithyroid drugs and amiodarone. The patient should have not had a diagnostic study with radiographic contrast medium within four weeks of ^{131}I administration. Lithium increases ^{131}I uptake (Sodium Iodide I 131 package insert 2005).

Preparation

Iodine-131 is a reactor fission by-product of uranium 235. Iodine-131 decays by beta and gamma emission and has a physical half-life of 8.02 days. The principal beta particle has a mean energy of 192 keV and the primary photon that is useful for detection and imaging is at 363 keV. Iodine-131 is available in hard gelatin capsule and liquid form and is for oral administration only. Iodide oxidizes at room temperature to iodine. The commercial preparations contain stabilizers (e.g. EDTA) and a reducing agent (i.e. sodium thiosulfate) to increase the stability (Sodium Iodide I 131 package insert 2005). For diluting oral preparations, a solution of purified water USP containing 0.2% sodium thiosulfate should be used. The use of acidic solutions below pH 7.5 will stimulate the volatilization of iodine. High concentration iodine solutions are used to compound capsules on-site in the nuclear pharmacy. Iodine should always be handled in a negative-pressure charcoal-filtered glove box to protect the worker. Air monitoring and bioassay programs should be in place before any type of iodine compounding procedure is started.

Iodine-131 tositumomab

Indications and dosage

Iodine-131 tositumomab (Bexxar) is indicated as a single-course treatment in patients with relapsed non-Hodgkin's lymphoma who are refractory to rituximab. This regimen should not be used as initial therapy (Bexxar package insert 2005).

Treatment with ^{131}I-tositumomab is a two-step regimen consisting of an initial step to determine the patient dosage (dosimetric step) and the therapy step 7 to 14 days later (therapeutic step) (Bexxar therapeutic regimen). Both steps require a 450 mg predose of tositumomab in 50 mL normal saline administered intravenously over one hour. In the dosimetric step, 5 mCi of ^{131}I-tositumomab in 30 mL normal saline is administered intravenously over 20 minutes. The patient's therapeutic dosage is then based on the patient's elimination rate of the dosimetric step: a high dose for a patient with fast elimination and a low dose for one with slow elimination. The treatment goal is to expose the lymphoma to 75 cGy (65 cGy if platelet count is below 100,000 cells/μL [100×10^9 cells/L]) of radiation. The dosage for the therapeutic step will vary for each patient depending on the information obtained from the dosimetric step (Bexxar package insert 2005).

Pharmacokinetics

Tositumomab is a murine monoclonal antibody directed against the CD20 antigen, which is found in high density on normal mature B lymphocytes and on greater than 90% of B cell non-Hodgkin's lymphomas. Tositumomab possesses all the cytotoxic properties of antibodies for cell death, namely induction of apoptosis, complement-dependent cytotoxicity, and antibody-dependent cellular cytotoxicity. Iodine-131 tositumomab is a radioiodinated derivative of tositumomab with a covalent linkage to ^{131}I. Iodide-131 has beta particle decay properties that result in localized therapeutic radiation and destruction of cells. The beta particle effective path length in tissue is approximately 1 mm and so it can have cytotoxic effects on cells not reached by the antibody. This effect is called 'crossfire' (Kowalsky & Falen 2004, p. 768; Bexxar package insert 2005). The tositumomab administered as a predose before each step is given to decrease the spleen uptake and increase the terminal half-life of ^{131}I-tositumomab, thus increasing the amount available for uptake by the tumor cells. The median total body effective half-life of ^{131}I-tositumomab, as measured by total body gamma camera counts, in 980 patients with non-Hodgkin's lymphoma was 67 hours (range 28–115 hours). Elimination of ^{131}I-tositumomab occurs by decay and excretion in the urine, with 67% of the administered activity excreted after five days; 98% of the clearance was accounted for in the urine (Bexxar package insert 2005).

Contraindications, precautions, adverse effects, and drug interactions

The Bexxar therapeutic regimen is contraindicated in patients with known hypersensitivity to murine proteins or any other component of the Bexxar therapeutic regimen. Serious hypersensitivity reactions, including some with fatal outcome, were reported during and following administration of the Bexxar therapeutic regimen. The therapeutic regimen is contraindicated in patients with more than 25% lymphoma marrow involvement, platelet count less than 100,000 cells/µL, or neutrophil count less than 1500 cells/µL. The most common adverse reactions associated with the Bexxar therapeutic regimen are severe or life-threatening cytopenias. The time to nadir is four to seven weeks and the duration of cytopenia is approximately 30 days. Because of the variable nature in the onset of cytopenia, complete blood counts should be obtained weekly for 10–12 weeks. Patients who have received murine proteins should be screened for human anti-mouse antibodies. No formal drug interaction studies have been performed. Because of the frequent occurrence of severe and prolonged thrombocytopenia, the potential benefits of medications that interfere with platelet function and/or anticoagulation should be weighed against the potential increased risk of bleeding and hemorrhage. During administration, the same 0.22 µm low protein-binding in-line filter must be used for both the predose of tositumomab and the ^{131}I-tositumomab dose (Bexxar package insert 2005). Vials of ^{131}I-tositumomab may contain free iodine in the head space after thawing. A charcoal venting system is recommended to avoid airborne ^{131}I.

Preparation

The components of the Bexxar therapy will only be shipped to individuals who are participating in the manufacturer's certification program or have been certified by the manufacturer in the preparation and administration of the Bexxar therapeutic regimen. The training and product information has detailed directions for the preparation, administration, imaging, and dosage calculations, and these should be read completely before dispensing. Iodide-131 is a reactor fission by-product of ^{235}U. Iodide-131 decays by beta and gamma emission and has a physical half-life of 8.02 days. The principal beta particle has a mean energy of 192 keV and the primary photon that is useful for imaging during the dosimetric step is at 363 keV. Iodine-131 tositumomab is supplied as a single-dose, preservative-free liquid for intravenous administration. Both the dosimetric and the therapeutic doses must contain 35 mg tositumomab. The dosimetric dosage form is supplied at nominal protein and activity concentrations of 0.1 mg/mL tositumomab and 0.61 mCi/mL ^{131}I at calibration. The therapeutic dosage form is supplied at nominal protein and activity concentrations of 1.1 mg/mL tositumomab and 5.6 mCi/mL ^{131}I at calibration. Both the dosimetric regimen and the therapeutic regimen are shipped with a vial of cold tositumomab, 14 mg/mL, which should be used to bring the total amount of tositumomab to 35 mg. The ^{131}I-tositumomab must be in a final volume of 20 mL to reduce radiolysis, and the dispensed activity must be within 5% of the written directive. For the predose, 450 mg tositumomab is diluted to a total volume of 50 mL using normal saline. The diluted tositumomab may be used for up to 24 hours when stored refrigerated at 2–8°C (36–46°F) and for up to eight hours at room temperature. The ^{131}I-tositumomab must be stored in a freezer at a temperature of −20°C or below until it is removed for thawing prior to administration to the patient. Thawed dosimetric and therapeutic doses of ^{131}I-tositumomab are stable for up to eight hours at 2–8°C (36–46°F) or at room temperature (Bexxar package insert 2005).

Phosphorus

Phosphorus-32 chromic phosphate

Indications and dosage

Phosphorus-32 (^{32}P) chromic phosphate (Phosphocol) has been used in the past for intracavitary instillation for the treatment of peritoneal or pleural effusions caused by metastatic disease, and may be injected interstitially for the treatment of cancer (Phosphocol package insert 2008). More recently

^{32}P-chromic phosphate has been used for radiation synovectomy with intra-articular injections into the synovial space in joints for diseases such as rheumatoid arthritis and hemophiliac arthropathy (Siegel *et al.* 1994). It is not intended for intravascular use.

The dosage range for intraperitoneal or intrapleural instillation is 6–20 mCi (Phosphocol package insert 2008). The dosage for radiation synovectomy is usually less than 1 mCi (Kowalsky & Falen 2004, p. 784).

Pharmacokinetics

Phosphorus-32 is a pure beta emitter. The beta emissions have a maximum range of 8 mm, but an average range of 2 mm, and result in localized therapeutic radiation and destruction of cells. The local irradiation causes mesothelial fibrosis and fibrosis of small blood vessels (Baker *et al.* 1987, p. 86). Phosphorus-32 chromic phosphate is an insoluble suspension and when instilled in a cavity causes local scarring, which is effective in the palliative treatment of painful symptoms resulting from accumulation of fluid in these cavities (Kowalsky & Falen 2004, p. 783).

Contraindications, precautions, and adverse effects

Phosphorus-32 chromic phosphate is not for intravascular use and it should not be used in the presence of ulcerative tumors or where there are exposed cavities or evidence of loculation. It may increase the risk for leukemia in certain situations. There have been two reports of children who developed acute lymphocytic leukemia 10 months after intra-articular injections. Careful administration of ^{32}P-chromic phosphate is required to avoid placing the dose into loculations, bowel lumen, or the body wall. Intestinal fibrosis or necrosis and chronic fibrosis of the body wall have been reported as consequences of unrecognized misplacement of the therapeutic agent. Adverse effects include transitory radiation sickness, bone marrow depression, pleuritis, peritonitis, nausea, and abdominal cramping (Phosphocol package insert 2008). Visual inspection of the injection is recommended to avoid any accidental intravenous administration of ^{32}P-chromic phosphate. Phosphorus-32 sodium phosphate (see ^{32}P-sodium phosphate discussion) is clear and colorless, whereas ^{32}P-chromic phosphate is a green cloudy suspension intended for intracavitary therapy only (US Pharmacopeia 1999, p. 2617).

Preparation

Phosphorus-32 is produced in a reactor by neutron activation of ^{35}S. It has a half-life of 14.3 days and decays to ^{32}S by beta particle emission, with an average energy of 695 keV. Phosphorus-32 chromic phosphate suspension is commercially available as Phosphocol and is supplied as a multidose vial with 2% benzyl alcohol added as preservative. The insoluble suspension has an average particle size of 1–2 μm, a concentration of 5 mCi/mL at calibration and a total activity of 15 mCi (Kowalsky & Falen 2004, p. 783; Phosphocol package insert 2008). Phosphocol should be stored at controlled room temperature. In order to assay the patient dose accurately, a National Institute of Standards and Testing calibrated vial provides the appropriate vial geometry for the dose calibrator channel setting. The dosage is typically measured using the vial subtraction method with attention to volume correction.

Phosphorus-32 sodium phosphate

Indications and dosage

Phosphorus-32 sodium phosphate (Sodium P-32) is used primarily in the therapy of polycythemia vera (Sodium P-32 package insert 2000). It has been used in the past for palliative treatment of bone pain in patients with metastases from carcinomas of the prostate, lung, and breast (Baker *et al.* 1987, p. 85).

The adult dose for polycythemia vera is 2.3 mCi/m^2 body surface, not to exceed 5 mCi. Subsequent doses are based on the patient's initial response (US Pharmacopeia 1999, p. 2617).

Pharmacokinetics

Phosphorus-32 is a pure beta emitter. The beta emissions result in localized therapeutic radiation and destruction of cells. Phosphorus-32 sodium phosphate localizes in rapidly proliferating hematopoietic cells in the bone and bone marrow, where the ^{32}P radiation has a maximum range of 8 mm, but an average range of 2 mm. Subsequent radiation damage to these cells halts their reproduction (Baker *et al.* 1987, p. 84; US Pharmacopeia 1999, p. 2616). Upon intravenous administration, ^{32}P-sodium phosphate diffuses rapidly from the circulation to the extra- and intracellular fluids, and normal distribution is in the bone marrow, liver, and spleen; 10% of the administered activity is eliminated in the urine within 24 hours after administration with a very small percentage eliminated via the bowel. The biological half-life for the whole body is 39 days (US Pharmacopeia 1999, p. 2616).

Contraindications, precautions, and adverse effects

For polycythemia vera, ^{32}P-sodium phosphate should not be administered when the leukocyte count is below 5000 cells/μL or the platelet count is below 150,000 cells/μL. Adverse effects include leukopenia, thrombocytopenia, and anemia (US Pharmacopeia 1999, p. 2617). Phosphorus-32 sodium phosphate should not be administered for intracavitary use. Visual inspection of the injection is recommended to avoid the accidental intravenous administration of ^{32}P-chromic phosphate, which is a green cloudy suspension rather than clear and colorless as is ^{32}P-sodium phosphate (US Pharmacopeia 1999, p. 2617).

Preparation

Phosphorus-32 is produced in a reactor by neutron activation of ^{35}S. It has a half-life of 14.3 days and decays to ^{32}S by beta particle emission, with a maximum energy of 1.7 MeV and an average energy of 695 keV. Sodium P-32 is supplied as a single-dose vial with a concentration of 0.67 mCi/mL at calibration and a total activity of 5 mCi per vial. It should be stored at controlled room temperature (Sodium P-32 package insert 2000). In some instances, autoradiolysis may cause the normally colorless solution to turn a pale yellow, but this has no effect on its therapeutic application (Baker *et al.* 1997, p. 84). In order to assay the patient dose accurately, a National Institute of Standards and Testing calibrated vial provides the appropriate vial geometry for the dose calibrator channel setting. The activity is typically measured using the vial subtraction method with attention to volume correction.

Rubidium

Rubidium-82 chloride

Indications and dosage

Rubidium-82 chloride (Cardiogen) is used in PET imaging to assess myocardial perfusion, ischemia, and heart function.

The usual adult dosage for a single intravenous administration of ^{82}Rb is 40 mCi, with a range of 30–60 mCi. The dosage is administered at a rate of 50 mL/min, not to exceed a cumulative volume of 200 mL. The maximum activity is 60 mCi per administration and no more than 120 mCi in the two administration protocols. Rubidium-82 from the Cardiogen-82 generator system (Rubidium Rb 82 Generator) should only be administered with the automated infusion system that is labeled for use with the generator (Cardiogen package insert 2000).

Pharmacokinetics

Following intravenous administration, ^{82}Rb rapidly clears the blood and is extracted by myocardial tissue in a manner analogous to potassium. Areas of myocardial infarction can be detected with ^{82}Rb chloride injection within two to seven minutes after injection as photon-deficient or 'cold areas' on the myocardial scan. Uptake is also observed in kidney, liver, spleen, and lung. Rubidium-82 has a physical half-life of 75 seconds and decays to stable ^{82}Kr, which is readily eliminated (US Pharmacopeia 1999, p. 2536; Cardiogen package insert 2000; Kowalsky & Falen 2004, p. 28).

Contraindications, precautions, and adverse effects

There are no known contraindications to ^{82}Rb chloride. Caution should be used when given to patients with congestive heart failure because of the transitory increase in circulatory volume load. Before using the ^{82}Rb from the generator system, the full preparation instructions for the ^{82}Rb generator and the ^{82}Rb automatic infusion system should be consulted.

Preparation

Rubidium-82 is the decay product of ^{82}Sr and decays by positron emission. The two imaging photons at 511 keV (traveling in directly opposite directions) are a result of the annihilation phenomena that occurs when an emitted positron collides with an orbiting electron. Strontium-82 has a physical half-life of 25 days, which enables a single generator to be used for one month at a given site. Strontium-82 is produced in an accelerator by high-energy proton irradiation of ^{85}Rb. The ^{82}Sr is adsorbed on a hydrous stannic oxide column; when the column is rinsed with normal saline for infusion, the ^{82}Rb that has been produced is eluted. Rubidium-82 has a very short half-life of 75 seconds. The automated infusion system is calibrated to deliver a measured activity to the patient based on the decayed ^{82}Sr without requiring physical measurment in a dose calibrator. Quality assurance must be performed on the infusion system once a day to ensure that the radionuclide contaminants ^{82}Sr and ^{85}Sr are within acceptable limits. The ^{82}Rb generator should be stored at controlled room temperature (Cardiogen package insert 2000).

Samarium

Samarium-153 lexidronam

Indications and dosage

Samarium-153 lexidronam (Quadramet) is a therapeutic agent consisting of radioactive ^{153}Sm and a tetraphosphonate chelate, ethylenediaminetetra-methylenephosphonic acid (EDTMP). It is used for the palliative treatment of bone pain of skeletal metastases. It is indicated for relief of pain in patients with confirmed osteoblastic metastatic bone lesions that enhance on nuclear medicine bone scan.

The adult dosage is 1 mCi/kg body weight, administered intravenously over a period of one minute (Quadramet package insert 2003).

Pharmacokinetics

Samarium-153 decays by beta and gamma emission. The beta emissions result in localized therapeutic radiation and destruction of cells. The exact mechanism of bone pain palliation is not known but ^{153}Sm-EDTMP has an affinity for bone and concentrates in bone metastases similar to the ^{99m}Tc-diphosphonate bone imaging agents and their association with hydroxyapatite cells (Kowalsky & Falen 2004, p. 781) Samarium-153 EDTMP clears rapidly from the blood, with 15% of the administered activity remaining

30 minutes and 1% remaining five hours after administration. Distribution is primarily to the sites of bone metastatic lesions, where approximately 65% of the administered activity is found. Elimination is renally, with approximately 35% of the administered activity in the urine by six hours (Quadramet package insert 2003).

Contraindications, precautions, and adverse effects

Samarium-153 EDTMP is contraindicated in patients who have known hypersensitivity to EDTMP or similar phosphonate compounds. Because of the potential for bone marrow suppression, blood counts should be monitored weekly beginning two weeks after [153]Sm-EDTMP administration and continuing for at least eight weeks or until recovery of adequate bone marrow function. Some patients have reported a transient increase in bone pain shortly after injection (flare reaction). This is usually mild and self-limiting and occurs within 72 hours of administration (Quadramet package insert 2003).

Preparation

Samarium-153 is a product of neutron irradiation of samarium-152 and decays by beta and gamma emissions, with a physical half-life of 46.7 hours. The primary beta emission energies are at 810, 710, and 640 keV, with an average beta energy of 233 keV; the primary gamma photon is at 103 keV (Kowalsky & Falen 2004, p. 329). The average particle range of [153]Sm is approximately 3 mm in tissue and 1.7 mm in bone. Samarium-153 EDTMP is supplied as a ready-to-use, single-dose vial with a calibration of 50 mCi/mL in 100 and 150 mCi vials. The commercial product Quadramet should be stored frozen until use and has an expiration of 56 hours postcalibration (Friday 8 pm EST) or eight hours after thawing (Quadramet package insert 2003). In order to assay the patient dosage accurately, a National Institute of Standards and Testing calibrated vial provides the appropriate vial geometry for the dose calibrator channel setting. The dose is typically measured using the vial subtraction method with attention to volume correction. Although [152]Sm decays to stable europium-153, the product contains a radionuclide impurity of europium-154, which has a half-life of 8.5 years and a primary gamma energy of 123 keV. A waste disposal program specific for this radionuclide of long half-life must be in place before [153]Sm is ordered.

Strontium

Strontium-89 chloride

Indications and dosage

Strontium-89 chloride (Metastron) is used for the palliative treatment of bone pain of skeletal metastases.

The adult dosage of ^{89}Sr-chloride is 40–60 µCi/kg, with a maximum of 4 mCi administered intravenously over one to two minutes (Metastron package insert 2006).

Pharmacokinetics

Strontium-89 is a pure beta emitter. The beta emissions result in localized therapeutic radiation and destruction of cells. The exact mechanism of bone pain palliation is not known. Following intravenous administration, ^{89}Sr distributes similarly to calcium, clearing rapidly from the blood and selectively localizing in bone mineral. Uptake of strontium by bone occurs preferentially in sites of active osteogenesis in hydroxyapatite cells, not in bone marrow cells. The retained ^{89}Sr delivers a radiation dose sufficiently large to produce a palliative effect; 12–90% of the administered activity is distributed to metastatic bone lesions depending on the extent of disease (US Pharmacopeia 1999, p. 2633). The remaining activity is eliminated: 66% renal and 33% bowel. Urinary excretion is highest in the first 48 hours after administration (Metastron package insert 2006).

Contraindications, precautions, adverse effects, and drug interactions

Strontium-89 chloride should not be used in patients with platelet counts below 60,000 cells/µL and white cell counts below 2400 cells/µL. It is recommended that the patient's peripheral blood cell counts be monitored at least once every other week for three to four months after ^{89}Sr administration. The nadir of platelet depression in most patients is found between 12 and 16 weeks following administration, returning to preadministration levels six months after treatment. Repeated administrations of ^{89}Sr-chloride should be based on an individual patient's response to therapy, current symptoms, and hematological status, but intervals less than 90 days are generally not recommended (Metastron package insert 2006). A calcium-like flushing sensation has been observed in patients following rapid (less than 30 second injection) administration. A small number of patients have reported a transient increase in bone pain at 36 to 72 hours after injection. Saturation of bone-binding sites by calcium medications may cause decreased uptake of ^{89}Sr. Calcium-containing products should be discontinued two weeks prior to and two weeks after administration of ^{89}Sr-chloride (US Pharmacopeia 1999, p. 2633).

Preparation

Strontium-89 is a product of neutron activation of enriched ^{88}Sr and decays by beta emission, with a physical half-life of 50.5 days, to stable yttrium-89. The maximum beta energy is 1.463 MeV with an average energy of 583 keV (Kowalsky & Falen 2004, p. 327). The maximum particle range of ^{89}Sr in tissue is approximately 8 mm. Metastron is supplied as a ready-to-use, single-dose vial with a calibration of 1 mCi/mL. The expiration is 28 days postcalibration and the product should be stored at controlled room temperature. In order to assay the patient dose accurately, a National Institute of Standards and Testing calibrated vial provides the appropriate vial geometry for the dose calibrator channel setting. The activity is typically measured using the vial subtraction method with attention to volume correction.

Thallium

Thallous-201 chloride

Indications and dosage

Thallous-201 chloride (Thallium Covidien; Thallium GE; Thalium Lantheus) is used most frequently in myocardial perfusion imaging to assess coronary artery disease. It is also used to assess myocardium survival or viability in patients who are stable following an acute myocardial infarction and are being considered for possible reperfusion procedures. Thallium-201 is used infrequently in parathyroid disorders and tumor imaging.

The adult dosage is 2–4 mCi. The pediatric dosage for tumor imaging is 30 μCi/kg body weight, with a maximum of 3 mCi (US Pharmacopeia 1999, p. 2783).

Pharmacokinetics

Thallium accumulates in the cells of the myocardium and other tissues in a manner analogous to that of potassium. The initial biodistribution is primarily related to regional blood flow. Ischemic myocytes take up less thallium than non-ischemic myocytes in proportion to the relative change in blood flow. When administered intravenously, thallium rapidly clears from the blood, with normal distribution in the heart, liver, and, to a lesser extent, the renal and testicular systems. At 10 minutes after administration, 4% of the administered activity is in the heart. Imaging should begin within 10 minutes of ^{201}Tl administration because thallium is not fixed in the myocardium but redistributes, and imaging should be completed by 30 minutes after administration (Kowalsky & Falen 2004, p. 527). Elimination is slow, with only 4–8% of the administered activity eliminated in the urine within 24 hours (US Pharmacopeia 1999, p. 2782). The biological half-life is approximately 10 days (Kowalsky & Falen 2004, p. 528).

Contraindications, precautions, adverse effects, and drug interactions

Thallium is distributed into breast milk. Adverse effects are rare but include allergic reactions, blurred vision, hypotension, nausea, and sweating. Drug interactions that have been reported to decrease ^{201}Tl accumulation in the heart include digitalis glycosides and intravenous propranolol. Food increases thallium distribution to the abdomen, including stomach, liver, spleen, and intestines, which may interfere with cardiac imaging (US Pharmacopeia 1999, p. 2782; Thallium Covidien package insert 2006).

Preparation

Thallium-201 is produced in a cyclotron by proton irradiation of ^{203}Tl. It has a physical half-life of 73.1 hours and decays by electron capture to mercury-201. The primary photons used for imaging are the X-rays from mercury-201 of 68–80 keV. Thallium-201 also has characteristic primary gamma photons of 135 and 167 keV. Thallium-201 chloride is supplied in a multiple-dose, ready-to-use vial with a concentration of 1 or 2 mCi/mL at calibration. Commercially supplied ^{201}Tl contains 0.9% benzyl alcohol as a preservative (Thallium Lantheus package insert 2004; Thallium Covidien package insert 2006; Thallium GE package insert 2006). It is recommended that ^{201}Tl be administered close to calibration time to minimize the effect of higher levels of radionuclide contaminants ^{200}Tl (physical half-life 26 hours, primary gamma energy of 367 keV) and ^{202}Tl. Thallium-201 chloride has an expiration five days postcalibration (Thallium Covidien package insert 2006).

Xenon-133

Indications and dosage

Xenon-133 gas (Xenon 133) is used for the evaluation of pulmonary function and for imaging the lungs. It has been used in the past for assessment of cerebral blood flow.

The adult dosage of ^{133}Xe is 10–20 mCi administered by inhalation from a closed respirator system or spirometer that traps the exhaled ^{133}Xe. The minimum pediatric dosage is 2 mCi (US Pharmacopeia 1999, p. 2985; Xenon 133 package insert (Lantheus) 2003; Xenon 133 package insert (Covidien) 2006).

Pharmacokinetics

When administered by inhalation, ^{133}Xe gas is distributed in the lungs in a manner similar to that of air and can identify the regions of the lung that are aerated. Ventilation imaging is performed as the patient inhales the ^{133}Xe. Successive images are obtained while the patient holds their breath (15 to 35 second single-breath-hold image) and during phases of breathing (four to five minutes rebreathing and washout from lungs) (US Pharmacopeia 1999, p. 2984). Xenon passes through the airways into the alveoli. It diffuses easily, passing through cell membranes and exchanging freely between blood and tissue. It passes into the pulmonary venous circulation via capillaries. Most of the xenon that passes through the peripheral circulation returns to the lungs and is exhaled (Xenon 133 package insert (Covidien) 2006). Clearance from the lungs is rapid and lung outlines are not seen in normal patients three to five minutes after initiation of washout phase (Saha 1987, p. 16). Because xenon is lipid soluble, radioactivity has been noted in the liver during the washout phase of a ventilation study, especially in patients with fatty liver infiltration (US Pharmacopeia 1999, p. 2985).

Contraindications, precautions, adverse effects, and drug interactions

There are no known contraindications or adverse effects for ^{133}Xe (Xenon 133 package insert (Covidien) 2006). Patients receiving total parenteral nutrition therapy will have the appearance of radioactivity in the liver (Hladik *et al.* 1987, p. 211).

Preparation

Xenon-133 is a by-product of the fission of ^{235}U. The physical half-life is 5.24 days, with a beta emission of 100 keV and a primary photon emission of 81 keV. At the time of calibration, the radionuclide impurities are ^{133m}Xe, ^{131m}Xe, ^{85}Kr, and ^{131}I. Xenon-133m is responsible for the expiration date of 14 days after calibration. The ^{133}Xe gas is supplied in single-dose 10 and 20 mCi calibrated glass vials and stored at controlled room temperature. Storage in a vented negative pressure exhaust hood with regulatory considerations for leaks should be considered. The patient administration system includes a CO_2 absorber (Soda Sorb), moisture absorber (Drierite), charcoal trap or exhaust system, expansion device (breathing bag), bacterial filter, face mask and tubing, and a source of oxygen (Xenon 133 package insert (Covidien) 2006).

Yttrium-90 and indium-111 ibritumomab tiuxetan

Indications and dosage

Yttrium-90 ibritumomab (^{90}Y-ibritumomab tiuxetan; Zevalin) is indicated as a single-course treatment in patients with relapsed non-Hodgkin's lymphoma who are refractory to rituximab.

Treatment with ^{90}Y-ibritumomab is a two-step regimen consisting of an initial 'imaging' step to determine the localization of ibritumomab and the 'treatment' step seven to nine days later. Both steps require a 250 mg/m^2 predose of rituximab (Rituxan) administered intravenously at a rate of 50 mg/h within four hours of the radiolabeled ibritumomab. In the imaging step, 5 mCi ^{111}In-ibritumomab in 10 mL is administered intravenously over 20 minutes. In the treatment step, 0.4 mCi/kg ^{90}Y-ibritumomab (0.3 mg/kg for platelet counts between 100,000 and 149,000 cells/μL) up to a maximum dose of 32 mCi is administered intravenously over 10 minutes (Zevalin package insert 2005).

Pharmacokinetics

Ibritumomab is a murine monoclonal antibody directed against the CD20 antigen, which is found in high density on normal mature B lymphocytes and on greater than 90% of B cell non-Hodgkin's lymphomas. Ibritumomab possesses all the cytotoxic properties of antibodies for cell death, namely induction of apoptosis, complement-dependent cytotoxicity, and antibody-dependent cellular cytotoxicity. The radiolabeled derivative of ibritumomab has a covalent link to ^{90}Y. Yttrium-90 is a pure beta emitter, which results in localized therapeutic radiation and destruction of cells. The beta particle effective path length in tissue is approximately 5 mm and so it can have cytotoxic effects on cells not reached by the antibody. This effect is called 'crossfire' (Kowalsky & Falen 2004, p. 768; Zevalin package insert 2005). Indium-111 ibritumomab permits gamma camera imaging, performed at 24 and 48 hours, to confirm the normal biodistribution of the antibody prior to the therapy treatment with ^{90}Y-ibritumomab. Abnormal distributions to the lung and kidney will exclude treatment with ^{90}Y-ibritumomab. The mean effective half-life for ^{90}Y-ibritumomab activity in blood is 30 hours. Over seven days, a median of 7.2% of the injected activity is excreted in urine (Zelvalin package insert 2005).

Contraindications, precautions, adverse effects, drug interactions

The Zevalin therapeutic regimen is contraindicated in patients with known type I hypersensitivity or anaphylactic reactions to murine proteins or to any component of the product, including rituximab, yttrium chloride, and indium chloride. The Zevalin therapeutic regimen should not be administered to patients with more than 25% lymphoma marrow involvement, a platelet count less than 100,000 cells/µL, a neutrophil count less than 1500 cells/µL, or to patients with a history of failed stem cell collection. Severe cutaneous and mucocutaneous reactions have occurred (onset three days to four months), including erythrema multiforme and Stevens–Johnson syndrome. Yttrium-90 ibritumomab should not be administered to patients with altered biodistribution of ^{111}In-ibritumomab. The Zevalin therapeutic regimen may cause severe, and potentially fatal, infusion reactions. These severe reactions typically occur during the first rituximab infusion, with time to onset of 30 to 120 minutes. Because the Zevalin therapeutic regimen includes the use of rituximab (Rituxan), the prescribing information contained in the package insert for this product should be followed except for dose. The most common severe adverse events reported with the Zevalin therapeutic regimen were thrombocytopenia (61% of patients with platelet counts less than 50,000 cells/µL) and neutropenia. For all patients, the median time to nadir was seven to nine weeks, and the median duration of cytopenia was 22 to 35 days. Weekly monitoring for cytopenia and its complications (e.g. febrile neutropenia, hemorrhage) for up to three months after administration is necessary. Caution should be exercised in treating patients with drugs that interfere with platelet function or coagulation following the Zevalin therapeutic regimen. Patients who have received murine proteins should be screened for human anti-mouse antibodies as they may alter ibritumomab biodistribution. The most common toxicities reported are neutropenia, thrombocytopenia, anemia, gastrointestinal symptoms (nausea, vomiting, abdominal pain, and diarrhea), increased cough, dyspnea, dizziness, arthralgia, anorexia, anxiety, and ecchymosis. The dose of ^{90}Y-ibritumomab must not exceed 32 mCi regardless of the patient's weight. A 0.22 μm low-protein-binding filter should be in-line between the syringe and the infusion port prior to injection of ^{111}In-ibritumomab and ^{90}Y-ibritumomab (Zevalin package insert 2005).

Preparation

Yttrium-90 is the daughter product of ^{90}Sr, a fission by-product of ^{235}U. It decays by pure beta emission and has a physical half-life of 64.1 hours. The principal beta particle has a maximum energy of 2.27 MeV and a mean energy of 750–935 keV (Kowalsky & Falen 2004, p. 328; Zevalin package insert 2005). The Zevalin therapy regimen is supplied as two separate and distinctly labeled kits that contain all of the non-radioactive ingredients necessary to compound a single dose of ^{111}In-ibritumomab and a single dose of ^{90}Y-ibritumomab. Changing the ratio of any of the reactants in the radiolabeling process may adversely impact the therapeutic results. The product information has detailed directions and worksheets for the preparation that should be read completely before compounding and dispensing ^{111}In-ibritumomab and ^{90}Y-ibritumomab. Ibritumomab tiuxetan, the antibody covalently bound to a tiuxetan-α bifunctional chelate, is supplied as 3.2 mg in 2 mL normal saline and must be stored refrigerated (Zevalin package insert 2005). Both radionuclides (^{111}In and ^{90}Y) must be buffered with sodium acetate prior to the addition of ibritumomab tiuxetan to avoid pH instability and colloidal formation (Kowalsky & Falen 2004, p. 328). For ^{111}In-ibritumomab labeling, at least 6 mCi of ^{111}In-chloride (purchased separately) is added to the reaction vial and must stand at room temperature for exactly 30 minutes. The product is then brought to a final volume of 10 mL with supplied formulation buffer containing 750 mg HSA. Indium-111 ibritumomab should be stored at 2–8°C and expires 12 hours after labeling. For ^{90}Y-ibritumomab labeling, at least 40 mCi of ^{90}Y-chloride (supplied by MDS Nordion when the Zevalin therapy regimen kit is ordered) is added to the reaction vial and this must stand at room temperature for exactly five minutes. The product is then brought to a final volume of 8 to 10 mL (depending on dispensing syringe size and activity measurement protocols) with supplied formulation buffer, containing 750 mg HSA. The ^{90}Y-ibritumomab should be stored at 2–8°C and expires eight hours after labeling. The radiochemical purity of ^{111}In-ibritumomab and

^{90}Y-ibritumomab must be determined prior to administration to be greater than 95% (Zevalin package insert 2005). In order to assay the patient dose accurately, a National Institute of Standards and Testing calibrated vial is required for the dose calibrator channel setting for the appropriate vial and syringe geometry settings. The dose is typically measured in the syringe with specific attention to changes in type of syringe, type of needle, and total volume in syringe (Siegel *et al.* 2004).

Summary

Some of the radiopharmaceuticals discussed in this chapter are used infrequently in the clinical setting (e.g. ^{125}I-iothalamate). Radiopharmaceuticals that are not commercially available but still have a vital place in patient care have not been discussed (e.g. ^{99m}Tc-glucoheptonate for renal flow and scarring). The practice of nuclear pharmacy is a discipline that uses multiple sources of information and processes with one goal, to provide the most appropriate radiopharmaceutical in the highest quality for improving the health of the patient. The student is encouraged to become familiar with current guidelines from the Society of Nuclear Medicine and the American College of Radiology as sources for the radiopharmaceutical evaluation process.

Self-assessment questions

1   An order is received for a blood pool imaging procedure. What radiopharmaceuticals would be appropriate for this indication?
2   Why is ^{99m}Tc-white blood cell imaging of the abdomen performed within one to two hours after administration?
3   A patient has received ^{99m}Tc-tetrofosmin. The images reveal no cardiac uptake but otherwise normal biodistribution. What step in the preparation of the kit would have the potential to change the mechanism of uptake for ^{99m}Tc-tetrofosmin?

References

Abrams DN (2000). Pharmaceutical interference with the [^{14}C]carbon urea breath test for the detection of *Helicobacter pylori* infection. *J Pharm Sci* 3: 228–233.

A-C-D package insert (1994). *A-C-D Solution Modified*. Princeton, NJ: Bracco Diagnostics.

AdreView package insert (2008). *AdreView (Iobenguane I 123 Injection) for Intravenous Use*. Arlington Heights, IL: GE Healthcare, Medi-Physics.

Amin KC *et al.* (1997). A rapid chromatographic method for quality control of technetium-99m-bicisate. *J Nucl Med Technol* 25: 49–51.

Baker WJ *et al.* (1987). Therapeutic applications of radiopharmaceuticals. In: Hladik III WB *et al.* eds. *Essentials of Nuclear Medicine Science*. Baltimore, MD: Williams & Wilkins.

Balon HR *et al.* (2001). Procedure guideline for somatostatin receptor scintigraphy with (111)In-pentetreotide. *J Nucl Med* 42: 1134–1138.

Balon HR *et al.* (2002). *Society of Nuclear Medicine Procedure Guidelines: Nuclear Medicine Procedure Guideline for C-14 Urea Breath Test.* Reston, VA: Society of Nuclear Medicine.

Basmadjian GP (2009). http://medchem.ouhsc.edu/ (accessed May 16, 2009).

Bexxar package insert (2005). *Bexxar (Tositumomab and Iodine I 131 Toditumomab).* Research Triangle Park, NC: GlaxoSmithKline.

Billinghurst MW (1973). Chromatographic quality control of ^{99m}Tc-labeled compounds. *J Nucl Med* 14: 793–797.

Bogsrud TV, Lowe VJ (2006). Normal variants and pitfalls in whole-body PET imaging with ^{18}F FDG. *Appl Radiol June*,16–30.

Bozkurt MF *et al.* (2009). Quality control of instant kit ^{99m}Tc-mercapto acetyl triglycine with inter- and intra-operator measurements. *J Hellen Soc Nucl Med* 12: 59–62.

Cardiogen-82 package insert (2000). *CardioGen Rubidium Rb 82 Generator.* Princeton, NJ: Bracco Diagnostics.

Cardiolite package insert (2003). *Cardiolite and Miraluma Kit for the Preparation of Technetium Tc99m Sestamibi for Injection.* Billerica, MA: Bristol-Myers Squibb Medical Imaging (now Lantheus).

Ceretec package insert (2006). Ceretec Kit for the Preparation of Technetium Tc99m Exametazime Injection. Arlington Heights, IL: GE Healthcare, Medi-Physics.

Chen F *et al.* (1993). A simple two-strip method to determine the radiochemical purity of ^{99m}Tc-mercaptoacetylglycine. *Eur J Nucl Med* 20: 334–338.

Choletec package insert (2007). *Choletec Kit for the Preparation of Tc99m Mebrofenin.* Princeton, NJ: Bracco Diagnostics.

Chromate package insert (2005). *Sodium Chromate Cr 51 Injection.* St. Louis, MO: Mallinckrodt (now Covidien).

Chromatope package insert (2005). *Chromatope Sodium Chromate Cr 51 Injection USP.* Princeton, NJ: Bracco Diagnostics.

Cohen ML *et al.* (1969). A simple reliable method of measuring glomerular filtration rate using single low dose sodium iothalamate ^{131}I. *Pediatrics* 43: 407.

Coleman RE (1999). PET in lung cancer. *J Nucl Med* 40: 814–820.

DMSA package insert (2004). *DMSA Kit for the Preparation of Technetium Tc99m Succimer Injection.* Arlington Heights, IL: GE Healthcare, Medi-Physics.

DTPA Draximage package insert (2006). *DTPA Kit for the Preparation of Technetium Tc99m Pentetate Injection.* Kirkland, Canada: Draximage.

DTPA Pharmalucence package insert (2008). *DTPA Kit for the Preparation of technetium Tc99m Pentetate for Injection.* Bedford, MA: Pharmalucence.

Elhendy A *et al.* (1998). Safety of dobutamine-atropine stress myocardial perfusion scintigraphy. *J Nucl Med* 39: 1662–1666.

Firestone RB, Shirley VS (eds.) (1996). *Table of Isotopes,* 8th edn. New York: John Wiley & Sons for The Ernest O. Lawrence Berkeley National Laboratory; http://ie.lbl.gov/education/isotopes.htm (updated 1998, 1999) (accessed 20 May 2009).

Frier M, Hesslewood SR (1980). *Quality Assurance of Radiopharmaceuticals: A Practical Guide to Hospital Practice. [Special Issue of Nuclear Medicine Communications.]* New York: Chapman & Hall.

Gallium 67-BMS package insert (2005). *Gallium Citrate Ga 67 Injection.* Billerica, MA: Bristol-Myers Squibb Medical Imaging (now Lantheus).

Gansbeke BV *et al.* (1985). Comparative study of quality control procedures for technetium 99m radiopharmaceuticals. *J Radioanal Nucl Chem* 92: 323–332.

Glofil package insert (1969). *Glofil- I-125.* Friendswood, TX: Iso-tex Diagnostics.

Gorospe L *et al.* (2005). Whole-body PET/CT: spectrum of physiological variants, artifacts and interpretive pitfalls in cancer patients. *Nucl Med Commun* 26: 671–687.

Hammes R *et al.* (2004). A better method of quality control for ^{99m}Tc-tetrofosmin. *J Nucl Med Technol* 32: 72–78.

HDP package insert (2005). *TechnScan HDP Kit Preparation of Technetium Tc99m Oxidronate.* St. Louis, MO: Mallinckrodt (now Covidien).

Hepatolite package insert (2008). *Hepatolite Kit for the Preparation of Technetium Tc99m Disofenin for Injection.* Bedford, MA: Pharmalucence.

Hiller JE (1986). Benzyl alcohol toxicity: impact on mortality and intraventricular hemorrhage among very low birth weight infants. *Pediatrics* 77: 500–506.

Hladik III WB *et al.* (1987). Iatrogenic alterations in the biodistribution of radiotracers as a result of drug therapy: reported instances. In: Hladik III WB *et al.* eds. *Essentials of Nuclear Medicine Science.* Baltimore, MD: Williams & Wilkins.

[131I-] mIBG package insert (2008). *I-131 mIBG iobenguane sulfate I-131 Injection Diagnostic.* Bedford, MA: Pharmalucence.

Indiclor package insert (2006). *Indiclor High Purity Indium Chloride In-111 Sterile Solution.* Arlington Heights, IL: GE Healthcare, Medi-Physics.

Indium-111 package insert (2007). *Indium In 111 Chloride Sterile Solution.* St. Louis, MO: Mallinckrodt (now Covidien).

Indium DTPA package insert. (2006). *Indium DTPA In 111 Pentetate Disodium.* Arlington Heights, IL: GE Healthcare, Medi-Physics.

Indium Oxine package insert (2006). *Indium In 111 Oxyquinoline Solution.* Arlington Heights, IL: GE Healthcare, Medi-Physics.

Intenzo CM *et al.* (2007). Scintigraphic imaging of body neuroendocrine tumors. *Radiographics* 27: 1355–1369.

Iotrex package insert (2001). *Iotrex Sodium 3-(^{125}I)-iodo-4-hydroxybenzenesulfonate for GliaSite Radiation Therapy System.* Alpharetta, GA: Proxima Therapeutics.

Jeanatope package insert (2009). *Jeanatope I-125 (Iodinated I-125 Albumin Injection USP).* Friendswood, TX: Iso-tex Diagnostics.

Kowalsky R, Falen S (2004). *Radiopharmaceuticals in Nuclear Pharmacy and Nuclear Medicine,* 2nd edn. Washington, DC: American Pharmacists Association.

Lecklitner ML *et al.* (1985). Failure of quality control to detect errors in the preparation of technetium-99m disofenin (DISIDA). *Clin Nucl Med* 10: 468–474.

MAA Draximage package insert (2006). *MAA Kit for the Preparation of Technetium Tc99m Albumin Aggregated Injection.* Kirkland, Canada: Draximage.

Mag-3 package insert (2005). *TechneScan Mag-3 Kit Preparation of Technetium Tc99m Mertiatide.* St. Louis, MO: Mallinckrodt (now Covidien).

Mallol J, Bonino C (1997). Comparison of radiochemical purity control methods for Tc99m radiopharmaceuticals used in hospital radiopharmacies. *Nucl Med Commun* 18: 419–422.

MDP Draximage package insert (2006). *MDP Kit for the Preparation of Technetium Tc99m Medronate Injection.* Kirkland, Canada: Draximage.

MDP Multidose package insert (2006). *MDP Multidose Kit for the Preparation of Technetium Tc99m Medronate Injection.* Arlington Heights, IL: GE Healthcare, Medi-Physics.

MDP Multidose Utilipak package insert (2006). *MDP Multidose Kit for the Preparation of Technetium Tc99m Medronate Injection.* Arlington Heights, IL: GE Healthcare, Medi-Physics.

MDP Pharmalucence package insert (2008). *MDP Kit for the Preparation of Technetium Tc99m Medronate for Injection.* Bedford, MA: Pharmalucence.

MDP-Bracco package insert (2006). *MDP-Bracco Kit for the Preparation of Technetium Tc99m Medronate.* Princeton, NJ: Bracco Diagnostics.

Mebrofenin package insert (2008). *Mebrofenin Kit for the Preparation of Technetium Tc99m Mebrofenin.* Bedford, MA: Pharmalucence.

Metastron package insert (2006). *Metastron (Strontium-89 Chloride Injection).* Arlington Heights, IL: GE Healthcare, Medi-Physics.

Metatrace FDG package insert (2002). *FDG Fludeoxyglucose F 18 Injection, USP.* Knoxville, TN: Petnet Pharmaceuticals.

Myoview package insert (2006). *Myoview Kit for the Preparation of Technetium Tc99m Tetrofosmin for Injection.* Arlington Heights, IL: GE Healthcare, Medi-Physics.

National Archives and Records Administration (1997). Exempt distribution of a radioactive drug containing one microcurie of carbon-14 urea. *Fed Regist* 62: 63634–63640.

Neurolite package insert (2003). *Neurolite Kit for the Preparation of Technetium Tc99m Bicisate for Injection.* Billerica, MA: Bristol-Myers Squibb Medical Imaging (now Lantheus).

Nuclear Regulatory Commission (2006). *Code of Federal Regulations, Title 10*, Part 35.490. Washington, DC: Nuclear Regulatory Commission; http://www.nrc.gov/reading-rm/doc-collections/cfr/ (accessed September 3, 2009).

Octreoscan package insert (2006). *OctreoScan Kit for the Preparation of Indium In-111 Pentetreotide.* St. Louis, MO: Mallinckrodt (now Covidien).

Pandos G *et al.* (1999). Validation of a column method for technetium-99m exametazime quality control. *J Nuc Med Techol* 27: 3063–3008.

Patel M *et al.* (1995). A miniaturized rapid paper chromatographic procedure for quality control of technetium-99m sestamibi. *Eur J Nucl Med* 22: 14161–14419.

Patel M *et al.* (1998). Modified preparation and rapid quality control test for technetium-99m-tetrofosmin. *J Nuc Med Technol* 26: 2692–2673.

Pauwels EK, Jeitsma RI (1977). Radiochemical quality control of Tc-99m labeled radiopharmaceuticals: some daily practice guidelines. *Eur J Nucl Med* 2: 971–1003.

Phosphocol package insert (2008). *Phosphocol P32 Chromic Phosphate P 32 Suspension.* St. Louis, MO: Mallinckrodt (now Covidien).

Ponto JA (2008). Special safety considerations in preparation of technetium Tc99m DTAP for cerebrospinal fluid-related imaging procedures. *J Am Pharm Assoc* 48: 413–416.

ProstaScint package insert (1997). *ProstaScint kit (Capromab Pendetide) Kit for the Preparation of Indium In 111 Capromab Pendetide.* Princeton, NJ: Cytogen (now EUSA Pharma).

Pulmolite package insert (2008b). *Pulmolite Kit for the Preparation of Technetium Tc99m Albumin Aggregated for Injection.* Bedford, MA: Pharmalucence.

PYP package insert (2008). *PYP Kit for the Preparation of Technetium Tc99m Pyrophosphate Injection.* Bedford, MA: Pharmalucence.

PYtest package insert (1997). *PYtest ^{14}C-urea Capsules.* Draper, UT: Ballard Medical Products.

Quadramet package insert (2003). *Quadramet (Samarium Sm 153 Lexidronam Injection).* Princeton, NJ: Cytogen (now EUSA Pharma).

Russell CD, Rowell K, Scott JW (1986). Quality control of technetium Tc99m DTPA: correlation of analytic tests with *in vivo* protein binding in man. *J Nucl Med* 27: 560–562.

Saha GB (1987). Normal biodistribution of diagnostic radiopharmaceuticals. In: Hladik III WB *et al.* eds. *Essentials of Nuclear Medicine Science.* Baltimore, MD: Williams & Wilkins.

Sestamibi package insert (2008). *Sestamibi Kit for the Preparation of Technetium Tc99m Sestamibi for Injection.* St. Louis, MO: Mallinckrodt (now Covidien).

Shackett P (2009). *Nuclear Medicine Technology: Procedures and Quick Reference*, 2nd edn. Philadelphia, PA: Lippincott, Williams & Wilkins.

Siegel HJ *et al.* (1994). Hemarthrosis and synovitis associated with hemophilia: clinical use of ^{32}P chromic phosphate synoviorthesis for treatment. *Radiology* 190: 257–261.

Siegel JA *et al.* (2004). Accurate dose calibrator activity measurement of ^{90}Y-ibritumomab tiuxetan. *J Nucl Med* 45: 450–454.

Sodium Iodide 131 package insert (2005). *Kit for the Preparation of Sodium Iodide I 131 Capsules and Solution USP Therapeutic–Oral.* Kirkland, Canada: Draximage.

Sodium Iodide I-123 package insert (2005). *Sodium Iodide I-123 Capsules.* Arlington Heights, IL: GE Healthcare, Medi-Physics.

Sodium P-32 package insert (2000). *Sodium Phosphate P 32 Solution.* St. Louis, MO: Mallinckrodt (now Covidien).

Sulfur colloid package insert (2008). *Sulfur Colloid Kit for the Preparation of Technetium Tc99m Sulfur Colloid Injection Diagnostic for Intravenous and Oral Use.* Bedford, MA: Pharmalucence.

Technelite package insert (2005). *TechneLite Technetium Tc99m Generator.* Billerica, MA: Bristol-Myers Squibb Medical Imaging (now Lantheus).

Technescan PYP package insert (2005). *TechnScan PYP Kit for Preparation of Technetium Tc99m Pyrophosphate Injection.* St. Louis, MO: Mallinckrodt (now Covidien).

Thallium Covidien package insert (2006). *Thallous Chloride Tl-201 Injection.* St. Louis, MO: Mallinckrodt (now Covidien).

Thallium GE package insert (2006). *Thallous chloride Tl 201 Injection.* Arlington Heights, IL: GE Healthcare, Medi-Physics.

Thallium Lantheus package insert (2004). *Thallous Chloride Tl 201 Injection.* Billerica, MA: Bristol-Myers Squibb Medical Imaging (now Lantheus).

Ultra TechneKow package insert (2006). *Ultra-TechneKow DTE (Technetium Tc-99m Generator for the Production of Sodium Pertechnetate.* St. Louis, MO: Mallinckrodt (now Covidien).

Ultratag package insert (2005). *UltraTag RBC Kit for Preparation of Technetium Tc99m-Labeled Red Blood Cells.* St. Louis, MO: Mallinckrodt (now Covidien).

US Pharmacopeia (1999). *Drug Information,* Vol I: *Drug Information for the Health Care Professional,* 19th edn. Englewood, CO: Micromedex.

US Pharmacopeia (2008). *US Pharmacopeia 31/National Formulary 26.* Rockville, MD: US Pharmacopeia.

Webber DI *et al.* (1992). Use of a single-strip chromatography system to assess the lipophilic component in technetium-99m exametazime preparations. *J Nucl Med Technol* 20: 29–32.

Welch MJ, Welch TJ (1975). Solution chemistry of carrier free indium. In: Subramanian G *et al.* eds. *Radiopharmaceuticals.* Reston, VA: Society of Nuclear Medicine, pp. 73–79.

Xenon 133 package insert (Covidien) (2006). *Xenon Xe 133 Gas.* St. Louis, MO: Mallinckrodt (now Covidien).

Xenon 133 package insert (Lantheus) (2003). *Xenon Xe 133 Gas.* Billerica, MA: Bristol-Myers Squibb Medical Imaging (now Lantheus).

Zevalin package insert (2005). *Zevalin Ibritumomab Tiuxetan In-111 Zevalin Kit and Y-90 Zevalin Kit.* Waltham, MA: Biogen Idec.

Ziessman HA *et al.* (2006). *Nuclear Medicine: The Requisites in Radiology.* Philadelphia, PA: Elsevier Mosby.

Zimmer AM (1994). An update of miniaturized chromatography procedures for newer radio-pharmaceuticals. In: Hladik WB III, eds. *Correspondence Continuing Education Courses for Nuclear Pharmacists and Nuclear Medicine Professionals,* vol. 3(5). Albuquerque, NM: University of New Mexico, pp. 1–11.

Zimmer AM, Pavel DG (1977). Rapid miniaturized chromatographic quality-control procedures for Tc-99m radiopharmaceuticals. *J Nucl Med* 18: 1230–1233.

7

Positron emission tomography: overview and radiopharmaceuticals

Edward M. Bednarczyk

Learning objectives

- Describe the differences between positron and gamma emitting radioisotopes
- List radiopharmaceuticals widely used in human imaging
- Discuss the use of these radiopharmaceuticals in human imaging
- Describe challenges to synthesis of PET radiopharmaceuticals
- Describe the regulatory process available for new PET radiopharmaceuticals.

Table 7.1 Isotopes used in positron emission tomography

Isotope	Decay half-life (min)	Energy (keV)
^{15}O	2.0	511
^{82}Rb	1.27	511
^{13}N	9.97	511
^{62}Cu	9.74	511
^{11}C	20.4	511
^{18}F	109	511
^{120}I	81	511
^{68}Ge	271 days	(Calibration source)

Introduction

For the uninitiated, PET suggests a technology that images positrons. While this technique does rely on radioisotopes that decay by positron emission (also called β^+ decay), in fact what is imaged are the paired 511 keV photons that result from the annihilation reaction that occurs with the encounter of a positron and an electron (matter and antimatter). The relatively high energy of these photons typically allows for better penetration of tissue than that seen with lower-energy gamma emitters such as ^{99m}Tc used in single photon emission computed tomography (SPECT). This, along with the detection of co-incident photons, routine attenuation correction, correction for scattered photons, and random coincident photons contributes to a higher intrinsic resolution for PET when compared with SPECT imaging. Table 7.1 lists many of the positron-emitting isotopes used in PET, including all of the isotopes commonly used in clinical PET imaging. A review of the table reveals that, in addition to the uniform, high-energy of the emitted photons, the decay half-lives of these isotopes is relatively short, and that many of the isotopes are forms of atoms commonly found in a variety of physiological and therapeutic molecules. Labeling with ^{11}C or ^{18}F can produce a radiopharmaceutical that behaves identically to the unlabeled form. While the advantages of this are immediately obvious, the limitations such as the metabolic fate often are not. Another potential limitation is that all of the emitted photons are at the same energy, making multiple *simultaneous* studies virtually impossible with PET.

Scanners and coincidence imaging

Unlike single-, double-, or triple-headed cameras used in planar or SPECT imaging, current PET cameras utilize a circular array of detector crystals.

Since the photons given off in an annihilation reaction are emitted with equal energy and in opposite directions (180°), these detectors are paired to detect coincident events occurring on opposite sides of the detector array.

Image resolution

Attenuation correction

In addition to detection of coincident photons arriving at opposite sides of the scanner, PET scanners also incorporate an estimate of attenuation of the emitted photons by passing an external 511 keV source around the patient (typically ^{68}Ge). In combined PET/CT units, this correction of photon attenuation (often called a transmission scan) is accomplished using X-rays from the CT source.

Coincidence detection

As noted above, crystal arrays used in PET are essentially paired to detect coincident photons. The image is then tomographically reconstructed to show the distribution of activity within the field of view. Several factors can impact the quality of the data used in reconstruction. These include the distance the emitted positron travels in tissue prior to the annihilation event with an electron, and scattering of the photons as they travel along their line of flight. Scattering of photons occurs through the Compton and photoelectric effects (see Chapter 2). Various software approaches are applied in the reconstruction of the image to minimize these influences.

Ring diameter

The distance that photons travel from their point of origin will magnify all of the previously noted scattering effects. This creates some inherent limitations if a uniform camera is to be used for all imaging studies. One solution that has been applied is the use of cameras of smaller diameters, decreasing the effect of distance on image resolution. This approach is seen in small-bore cameras used in animal imaging and in specialty cameras limited to brain imaging in humans.

Image fusion

Interpretation of the localization of tracer uptake can often be enhanced by combining molecular imaging data with anatomical data. This fusion of imaging types can be accomplished by co-registering images from studies acquired at different times and from multiple platforms using third party software. Currently, most new PET cameras are being sold as devices with anatomical (currently limited to CT) scanners coupled to PET cameras, giving the appearance of a single device. In reality, these new scanners are two separate machines; however, these configurations simplify image co-registration and fusion by limiting temporal changes (both scans are acquired sequentially), eliminating proprietary restrictions of data files, and utilizing fusion software optimized for the hardware.

Image analysis

Clinically, PET scans can be read subjectively as in other nuclear medicine studies, with 'hotter' regions corresponding to areas of increased tracer localization. In many cases, it is helpful to have more objective criteria for assessing an image. The first basic step in this process is to define the region of the image that is of interest: a tumor or region of the brain, for example. This is done by defining a region either manually or by using a predefined algorithm. This process can be greatly facilitated through the use of anatomical images, where available. A simple approach to image assessment would be through measurement of a standardized uptake value. The 'standardization' portion of this approach corrects minimally for injected dose, with better approaches correcting for patient weight or body mass index. This then provides a corrected value for activity within a region that can be compared with activity in reference regions that are assumed to be normal. A variety of more sophisticated models for analyzing uptake has been developed, ranging from multicompartmental analysis to graphical techniques (Logan *et al.* 1996).

Radiopharmaceuticals

Numerous tracers have been developed for imaging with PET. Most of these have had limited use as research tracers, and it is well beyond the scope of this book to give even limited mention of each of these. The purpose of this chapter will be to discuss those that have bridged the gap into at least limited clinical use. In some cases, radiopharmaceuticals that were once very commonly used have fallen out of favor. These will see limited discussion, commensurate with their current clinical application rather than previous experience. For an exhaustive listing of imaging tracers, readers are encouraged to consult the *Molecular Imaging and Contrast Database* (National Institutes of Health 2004–2009).

The radiopharmaceuticals are grouped in the discussion below by their clinical applications.

Glucose metabolism: radiolabeled fluorodeoxyglucose

Fluorine-18 fluorodeoxyglucose (2-deoxy-2-[^{18}F]fluoro-D-glucose [^{18}F-FDG]) is currently the most widely used radiopharmaceutical in PET. The association of this metabolic tracer with PET has become so close that, unfortunately, it has almost become synonymous with PET.

Uptake

Fluorine-18 FDG is a glucose analog that utilizes the same uptake pathway into cells as glucose, via the glucose transporter-1 (GLUT1). Once transported into a cell, ^{18}F-FDG undergoes phosphorylation in identical fashion to glucose. Following phosphorylation, the differences between ^{18}F-FDG and glucose become relevant as the ^{18}F-FDG cannot proceed any further metabolically, effectively becoming 'trapped' within cells and thereby serving as a marker of metabolic activity within tissue.

Normal distribution and elimination

Fluorine-18 FDG is taken up into tissue in proportion to metabolic demand. The brain, as a relatively obligate user of glucose, shows high uptake as does the liver. Fluorine-18 FDG is renally eliminated, with the kidneys and bladder showing substantial activity.

Applications

Heart studies

In the heart, ^{18}F-FDG is used primarily to differentiate living from dead tissue within dysfunctional myocardium, often referred to as 'hibernating' myocardial tissue. Briefly, normal myocardial tissue utilizes free fatty acids as a preferred metabolic substrate. In conditions of severe ischemia, myocardial cells switch to glucose as a preferred substrate, presumably because the glucose pathway requires less oxygen per molecule of ATP produced. Imaging patients with ^{18}F-FDG in conjunction with assessment of myocardial blood flow allows for these regions to be identified. Areas of low flow that show preserved or increased metabolism demonstrate myocytes that have survived sufficiently that they can recover function following procedures to improve perfusion. In order to allow for identification of normal myocardial tissue, patients are typically given a glucose load prior to ^{18}F-FDG. In patients with impaired glucose tolerance, this is generally done in combination with insulin, and where appropriate (i.e. with intravenous administration of glucose and insulin) potassium (often referred to as a GIK regimen).

Neurology

While numerous brain imaging studies have utilized ^{18}F-FDG, clinical application has been limited to three areas: as part of the diagnosis of dementia, in seizure disorders, and in the management of brain tumors.

Dementia

Regional reductions in cerebral glucose have been shown to occur in characteristic patterns for several of the dementias. The most extensively studied of these is Alzheimer's disease, where a characteristic reduction in metabolism is observed in the temporoparietal regions of the brain early in the illness, with later extension to the frontal cortex. The sensory motor cortex is generally spared. While these metabolic changes precede anatomical changes observable with CT or MRI, and become very distinctive as the disease advances, findings prior to the establishment of a clinical diagnosis are less specific. This has limited the general application of ^{18}F-FDG in Alzheimer's disease; however, comparison of individual images with population-derived statistical parameters has been used early in disease to bring both sensitivity and specificity into a clinically useful range.

Seizure disorders

Brain imaging with ^{18}F-FDG shows a seizure focus as a hypometabolic region when imaged interictally, and a hypermetabolic zone when ^{18}F-FDG is administered ictally (Theodore *et al.* 1988). Imaging with ^{18}F-FDG is not used as part of the primary diagnostic workup but rather in patients for whom localization of the seizure focus is desired prior to surgical resection of the focus.

Oncology

Cell proliferation requires energy; therefore, increased uptake of ^{18}F-FDG in neoplastic disorders is not surprising. The use of ^{18}F-FDG in oncology has rapidly emerged as its predominant application in clinical imaging. It can be argued that this use of ^{18}F-FDG has in itself led to the proliferation of PET/CT devices. In essence, ^{18}F-FDG is used to detect increased metabolic activity associated with solid tumors. While increased metabolism is suggestive of malignancy, PET is not used as a primary diagnostic test. It is used in conjunction with anatomical imaging.

Tumor staging, recurrence

An extremely important application of ^{18}F-FDG is to assist in the identification of metastatic lesions in a given patient. This serves both to guide surgical resection, by identifying additional tissue for removal, and also in initial staging of disease to assist in defining a course of therapy.

Response to therapy

While identification of cancer recurrence is important, an emerging application of ^{18}F-FDG is in assessing response to chemotherapy. Typically, anatomical imaging is used to define response and is assessed by reductions in tumor size in comparison with baseline imaging. There is growing evidence that metabolic changes precede anatomical changes, and in fact may be predictive of response to therapy. Currently, it is assumed that reduced or eliminated

^{18}F-FDG uptake in tumors corresponds to or is predictive of cell death. This has important implications for both cancer research and clinical management of patients. Ongoing studies will expand our understanding of this information.

Brain tumors

The brain is an obligate user of glucose, and ^{18}F-FDG use in neuroimaging was among the first and the most widely documented application of this radiopharmaceutical. In spite of this, ^{18}F-FDG has found clinical utility in the evaluation of tumors in brain tissue, particularly after surgical resection or radiation therapy where normal brain anatomy is disrupted and the differentiation of living from necrotic tumor creates some diagnostic challenges. While use after intervention is relatively common, limited uptake of ^{18}F-FDG in low-grade brain tumors, along with advances in anatomical imaging techniques such as MRI, has limited its use.

Limitations of imaging with fluorodeoxyglucose

While ^{18}F-FDG is currently an indispensible tool in the management of many types of cancer, it is by no means without limitations. The first of these is the non-specific nature of the uptake. Numerous conditions can increase metabolism including healing tissue (such as that seen after surgery), inflammation, and movement. Metabolically active tissue such as brown fat can also show increased uptake of glucose, as can benign masses, although typically at a lower rate than malignancies. The normal distribution of ^{18}F-FDG also limits its use in some tumor types. For example, prostate, ovarian, and bladder cancers all occur in or near regions of normal ^{18}F-FDG distribution. This significantly limits the utility of this approach in detecting tumors in these regions, as the signal from normal localization of ^{18}F-FDG overwhelms the signal localizing in tumor cells.

Oncology imaging

Because of the non-specific nature of ^{18}F-FDG localization, other cellular processes have been targeted for imaging, each representing a presumably more specific pathway in cell proliferation. These include cell wall, nucleic acid, and protein synthesis.

Radiolabeled choline

Choline is an important component of dividing cells, being incorporated into phosphatidylcholine within cell membranes. Carbon-11 choline is rapidly cleared from blood and taken up into dividing cells. Studies with this tracer have been undertaken with a variety of tumor types including brain, prostate (Hara *et al.* 1998; de Jong *et al.* 2003), musculoskeletal system (Yanagawa *et al.* 2003), lung (Khan *et al.* 2003), sinus (Ninomiya *et al.* 2004), bone (Zhang *et al.* 2003), and ovary (Torizuka *et al.* 2003). In comparative studies, ^{11}C-choline shows uptake into tumor in most cases comparable to that seen with ^{18}F-FDG, with considerably less activity observed in the bladder. However, ^{11}C-choline exhibits normal uptake into liver, intestine, and pancreas, which provides a new set of challenges in interpreting tumor uptake in regions that encompass these structures. Both ^{18}F-fluoroethylcholine (Hara *et al.* 2001) and ^{18}F-fluorocholine show distribution similar to ^{11}C-choline, with ^{18}F labeling offering advantages to distribution systems. The prolonged urinary elimination observed with these radiopharmaceuticals further limits their advantages over ^{18}F-FDG (Price *et al.* 2002). Moreover, non-malignant processes that have rapid cell division (i.e. benign tumors) may also exhibit increased uptake of choline.

Radiolabeled thymidine

Thymidine is a well recognized marker of cell proliferation. While some work has been done with ^{11}C-thymidine, most recent research has utilized ^{18}F-thymidine (^{18}F-FLT). This is taken up into cells via a facilitated transport process, where it is phosphorylated by thymidine kinase to the monophosphate. This forms the basis for ^{18}F-FLT to serve as a measure of DNA formation and thus cell proliferation. Imaging with ^{18}F-FLT has been studied in a variety of cancers, including brain (Choi *et al.* 2005), colorectal (Francis *et al.* 2003), pulmonary (Buck *et al.* 2002; Vesselle *et al.* 2002; Yap *et al.* 2006), and lymphoma (Wagner *et al.* 2003). Fluorine-18 FLT shows normal uptake into liver and bone marrow, with renal elimination resulting in kidney and bladder activity (Francis *et al.* 2003). Comparative studies with ^{18}F-FDG have yielded variable results, depending on the tumor type and location, with some studies favoring ^{18}F-FDG, while others have favored ^{18}F-FLT. Unfortunately, many of the published studies have reported only a modest number of patients, making a definitive conclusion about the exact role of ^{18}F-FLT difficult to determine. Currently, efforts are underway to pool research studies and data from ^{18}F-FLT studies to strengthen the evidence for its role in cancer imaging. As with choline, other rapidly dividing, but non-malignant, tissues may be susceptible to false-positive findings with this tracer.

Radiolabeled methionine

Methionine is an essential amino acid that, when labeled, allows for visualization and estimation of amino acid uptake and, by inference, protein formation. It has been extensively used in brain tumors (Jacobs *et al.* 2005), where uptake of ^{18}F-FDG into normal tissue, particularly gray matter, may interfere with identification of tumor (Pirotte *et al.* 2004). Outside of the brain, ^{11}C-methionine shows normal accumulation in the liver, pancreas, intestine, and bone marrow, potentially providing challenges in evaluating and detecting tumors located near or within these organs (Sutinen *et al.* 2000).

Radiolabeled fluorodopa

Fluorodopa (DOPA; 3,4-dihydroxy-5-fluorophenylalanine) labeled with ^{18}F is generally associated with brain imaging; however, it has also been reported in the imaging of neuroendocrine tumors with the capacity to decarboxylate amine precursors, and ^{18}F-DOPA is taken up in carcinoid tumors and pheochromocytoma. This modality may permit visualization of tumors missed by conventional anatomical imaging methods, as well as verifying the endocrine characteristics of the tumor. In carcinoid tumors, the sensitivity of ^{18}F-DOPA exceeds that of ^{18}F-FDG for both the primary tumor and the lymph node metastases of gastrointestinal carcinoid tumors. The relative non-specificity of uptake will need to be better characterized, since false negatives have been reported with undifferentiated carcinoid tumors. Physiological uptake is seen in the duodenum and pancreas, as is non-specific accumulation within the intestine.

Brain imaging

Radiolabeled water

Water labeled with ^{15}O was among the first radiopharmaceuticals used in PET. Using modeling techniques first developed by Kety and Schmidt in the 1940s (Kety & Schmidt 1948), use of $H_2{}^{15}O$ allowed for quantitative measurement (Brooks *et al.* 1986) of blood flow first in the brain and later in other organ systems (Bergmann *et al.* 1984; Bednarczyk *et al.* 1997). The ability to quantitatively measure blood flow with $H_2{}^{15}O$ has a unique place in research. It has several characteristics that make it an excellent tracer for flow measurement, including a high partition coefficient into tissue. While some other diffusible tracers such as ^{15}O-butanol exceed $H_2{}^{15}O$ (Berridge *et al.* 1991) across typical physiological flow rates, it allows for a high rate of validity in measuring cerebral blood flow. While an underestimation of flow is expected at high flow rates, changes in cerebral blood flow with experimental pharmacological vasodilatation are still measurable with $H_2{}^{15}O$ (Bednarczyk *et al.* 2002). Regional cerebral blood flow is usually closely linked to metabolism, allowing for rapid assessment of function. However, this is not true in all conditions as uncoupling of oxidative metabolism from cerebral blood flow has been reported. The short half-life of $H_2{}^{15}O$ led to its early adoption for brain mapping, where serial studies could be performed before, during, and after specific cognitive tasks were presented to a human, verifying expected activities and, in some cases, establishing new and complex relationships between brain regions. Where absolute quantification is not essential (as in brain mapping), $H_2{}^{15}O$ has often been replaced by functional magnetic resonance imaging (fMRI) for assessment of relative change in regional blood flow.

Radiolabeled fluorodopa

In the treatment of Parkinson's disease, levodopa (L-DOPA) is administered as precursor for dopamine. This same process takes place with the administration of labeled levodopa, and ^{18}F-levodopa has been used to study presynaptic nerve terminals of the nigrostriatal dopaminergic system in Parkinson's disease and other movement disorders. This radiopharmaceutical may have a role in the early diagnosis of Parkinson's disease, differentiating it from other movement disorders. Use of ^{18}F-levodopa also permits the follow-up of disease progression and the assessment of medical and surgical therapy strategies. A limitation of ^{18}F-levodopa is that some of its peripheral metabolites cross the blood–brain barrier and degrade the signal-to-noise ratio.

Radiolabeled raclopride

Carbon-11 raclopride is currently the defacto tracer for the imaging of dopamine D_2-receptors *in vivo* in both animals and humans. Initially developed as a clinical antipsychotic agent, raclopride has found a 'second life' as the ^{11}C-labeled form after development of the drug at therapeutic doses was abandoned. Raclopride readily crosses the blood–brain barrier and binds with a high selectivity and affinity to D_2-receptors. A high-affinity ligand with low non-specific binding and good brain uptake, ^{11}C-raclopride provides a reliable tool to study receptor availability. It has been used to study D_2-receptors in ageing, schizophrenia, substance abuse, and in movement disorders including Parkinson's and Huntington's diseases. In spite of widespread use as a research tool, little clinical use has been proposed; however, it has been used to measure the percentage of receptor occupancy following therapeutic doses of antipsychotic agents. Since the extent of receptor occupancy has been shown to correspond with both therapeutic and toxicological thresholds, the possibility exists that this same approach could be employed on an individualized basis, either in patients with refractory disease or in those experiencing apparent dose-related toxicity.

Radiolabeled flumazenil

Flumazenil is a highly specific benzodiazepine receptor antagonist that binds with high affinity to the benzodiazepine recognition site on the gamma-aminobutyric acid ($GABA_A$) receptor. Carbon-11 flumazenil is used to visualize and quantify benzodiazepine receptors in the brain, and it has been used to localize epileptic foci in patients who are candidates for surgery, particularly when MRI and electroencephalography findings are equivocal or contradictory. Carbon-11 flumazenil PET has also been used to provide information in neuropathological conditions known or thought to affect neuronal integrity. It crosses into the brain rapidly, where it binds selectively and reversibly to benzodiazepine receptors. Although several metabolites are formed in the periphery, none is known to cross the blood–brain barrier.

Imaging of opiate receptors

Opiate receptors have long been recognized as targets of narcotic therapy in humans. The understanding of their role in pathophysiology, particularly in addictive disorders, continues to develop. The three radiopharmaceuticals in this section (^{11}C-carfentanil, ^{11}C-diprenorphine, ^{18}F-cyclofoxy) have all been used as probes of the opioid receptors, particularly in the brain. They differ in their characteristics as follows: carfentanil and diprenorphine are both opiate receptor agonists, with carfentanil having a high selectivity for the μ-receptor, while diprenorphine binds non-selectively to the opioid μ-, κ- and δ-receptors; cyclofoxy is an receptor antagonist, selective for the μ- and κ-receptors. The radiopharmaceuticals have been applied to a number of disease states including seizure disorders (Mayberg *et al.* 1991; Prevett *et al.* 1994) and pain (Zubieta *et al.* 2001), and in abuse of cocaine (Zubieta *et al.* 1996), heroin (Zubieta *et al.* 2000), and alcohol (Bencherif *et al.* 2004). While these imaging agents will continue to add to our understanding of the opiate receptor and the endogenous opiates in a variety of conditions, they are also being used to deepen our understanding of drugs that target the opiate receptors in studies that examine the duration of occupancy of opiate receptors by various antagonists (Kim *et al.* 1997). Use of the 'probe' approach may prove important in the targeting of the opioid receptor system in various conditions (Ferrari *et al.* 1998; Kim *et al.* 2001; Krystal *et al.* 2001; Bencherif *et al.* 2005).

Imaging of brain plaques and beta-amyloid

'Pittsburgh Compound B' (PIB; *N*-methyl-2-(4′-methylaminophenyl)-6-hydroxybenzothiazole) is a derivative of histological dye used to stain for beta-amyloid. The ^{11}C-labeled form appears to offer an opportunity for *in vivo* visualization of the deposition of amyloid in the brains of patients with dementia (Mathis *et al.* 2003; Klunk *et al.* 2004; Price *et al.* 2005; Kemppainen *et al.* 2006). This offers substantial potential for both diagnosis of Alzheimer's disease, where deposition of amyloid appears to precede the reductions in ^{18}F-FDG seen with metabolic imaging. This radiopharmaceutical, along with several related compounds (Zhang *et al.* 2005), is expected to add significantly to the understanding of dementing illness and potentially speed the development of drugs for the treatment of dementia. One such compound is ^{18}F-FDDNP (2-(1-(6-[(2-[^{18}F]fluoroethyl) (methyl)amino]-2-naphthyl)ethylidene)malononitrile). This compound exhibits binding to the neurofibrillary tangles that can be observed in the brain later in Alzheimer's disease as well as to beta-amyloid (Shoghi-Jadid *et al.* 2002; Agdeppa *et al.* 2003; Small *et al.* 2006). While not specific for beta-amyloid, it currently has the advantage of being labeled with ^{18}F, potentially allowing for more widespread distribution. Clinical trials of these and other agents are currently ongoing.

Heart imaging

Myocardial metabolism

Long-standing interest in the metabolic pathways of the myocardium has led to the development of numerous substrates labeled with positron-emitting isotopes. Since the normal myocardium preferentially uses fatty acids as a nutritive substrate, labeled fatty acids such as ^{11}C-palmitate were developed. The combination of rapid metabolism to end products that include $^{11}CO_2$ and the preferential utilization of glucose as a substrate by ischemic myocardium have reduced interest in even the research application of this tracer; however, clinical investigation of an ^{18}F-labeled version of the radiopharmaceutical may circumvent limitations of the ^{11}C-labeled form. Acetate labeled with ^{11}C is used to estimate the rate of oxidative metabolism via the tricarboxylic acid cycle by assessing the pharmacokinetics of the clearance of the labeled acetate from the heart. Other metabolic tracers have included $^{15}O_2$ and ^{13}N-labeled amino acids; however, the challenges of administration (a gas in the case of $^{15}O_2$) and metabolite correction (for ^{13}N-amino acids), and the intensive sampling required have limited their use even in myocardial research.

Cardiac perfusion: rubidium-82

While ^{82}Rb is a potassium analog, its use in cardiac imaging provides perfusion rather than viability information. Rubidium-82 is the only generator-produced PET radiopharmaceutical currently in clinical use, allowing for fixed unit cost making it a desirable tracer for use in busy cardiac imaging centers. Use of ^{82}Rb offers two advantages over ^{201}Tl- and ^{99m}Tc-based cardiac imaging agents. The first is that the short half-life offers a short interval between rest and stress imaging sessions, along with a short acquisition interval. The higher energy of the 511 keV emissions allows for better tissue penetration, lessening the possibility of an attenuation artifact possible in patients with significant tissue mass overlying the myocardium, such as in obese patients. With that in mind, the approach to the interpretation of cardiac imaging studies is comparable to that seen with cardiac SPECT tracers (see Chapter 9).

Cardiac perfusion: radiolabeled ammonia

Ammonia labeled with ^{13}N has been used extensively for imaging myocardial perfusion. In centers with easy access to a cyclotron, ^{13}NH$_3$ is well established clinically for the assessment of myocardial perfusion, often in conjunction with ^{18}F-FDG for viability assessment or when photon attenuation is a concern. Outside of centers with easy cyclotron access, the half-life of ^{13}NH$_3$ (approximately 10 minutes) has limited its clinical application. Labeled ammonia has been used to examine therapeutic drug effects ranging from myocardial toxicity seen with chemotherapy to improvements in myocardial flow seen with vasodilators (Bol *et al.* 1993; Gardner *et al.* 1993).

Sympathetic innervation

With SPECT, *meta*-iodobenzylguanidine (mIBG) has been used to image the myocardium; however, fairly extensive mIBG uptake occurs into non-neuronal myocardial tissue, complicating image interpretation. More specific tracers for imaging sympathetic innervation and activity have been sought. Two such tracers are ^{11}C-hydroxyephedrine (Rosenspire *et al.* 1990; Schwaiger *et al.* 1990; Luisi *et al.* 2005) and ^{18}F-fluorocarazolol (Salinas *et al.* 2005). Hydroxyephedrine is a marker of presynaptic norepinephrine uptake that is being used in studies of sudden cardiac death. Beta-blockers such as carazolol have been labeled with ^{11}C and ^{18}F, allowing for visualization of both receptor density and occupancy, although this has not correlated with a patient's clinical state (Spyrou *et al.* 2002; Salinas *et al.* 2005). Research with these tracers is ongoing in dysrhythmia, congestive heart failure, and other cardiovascular conditions. This may result in clinical application in some conditions.

Bone imaging

Fluorine-18

The use of radiofluoride was first reported for bone imaging in humans in 1962, with imaging predating PET scanners. There are USP standards for the production of radiofluoride, and ^{18}F uptake into bone has been shown to reflect both bone perfusion and osteoblastic activity; it is thought that the radiofluoride is incorporated into hydroxyapatite. Currently, radiofluoride is largely used in research into osteoporosis and bone remodeling (Brenner *et al.* 2004; Frost *et al.* 2004), including the assessment of drugs used in the treatment of osteoporosis (Frost *et al.* 2003). However a resurgent interest in clinical use in bone imaging has been suggested. As noted above, radiofluoride is an agent that assesses both bone perfusion and bone remodeling, being incorporated in a distribution similar to that observed with ^{99m}Tc-labeled compounds. Potential advantages for radiofluoride may be found in the higher energy and spatial resolution possible with PET.

Synthesis of radiopharmaceuticals and regulation

Because of the uniquely short half-lives of many positron-emitting isotopes and the lack of 'kits' for labeling, PET radiopharmaceuticals have proven difficult to fit into the existing regulatory and approval mechanisms.

Radioactive Drug Research Committee

In the USA, one mechanism for oversight of investigational radiopharmaceuticals for use in humans (including those radiopharmaceuticals labeled with positron-emitting isotopes) is the Radioactive Drug Research Committees, which operate as local committees of the FDA. They have the ability to supervise clinical research with these agents in specific kinds of study. These studies must be '...intended to obtain basic information regarding the metabolism (including kinetics, distribution, dosimetry, and localization) of a radioactive drug or regarding human physiology, pathophysiology, or biochemistry...' (Food and Drug Administration 2009).

Investigational New Drug Application

For drugs that do not meet the criteria of the Radioactive Drug Research Committee Program for oversight, in investigations that require dosing of more than 30 subjects, or for drugs that are being studied for use as clinical diagnostic agents, an Investigational New Drug Application (IND) must be filed with the FDA. The IND allows for several years of data collection under reviewed study protocols in anticipation of filing a New Drug Application (NDA) if the results of the research support such an outcome.

New Drug Application

The NDA represents the final review and approval by the FDA of a radiopharmaceutical for human use. Currently, two PET radiopharmaceuticals are distributed with FDA approval: ^{82}Rb and ^{18}F-FDG. In the case of ^{18}F-FDG, not all dosages are produced under a NDA.

Summary

Positron emission tomography arguably remains the most versatile and accurate tool for *in vivo* imaging and measurement of multiple molecular processes. PET radiopharmaceuticals, however, are subject to unique synthetic, administrative, and distribution challenges. New drugs need to be evaluated and validated so that their role in understanding physiological, pathophysiological, and pharmacological processes can be accurately interpreted. The challenges and opportunities presented by PET can allow for a nexus of collaboration between physicists, pharmacists, chemists, physicians, and other scientists (including experts in complementary imaging techniques) for further insight into disease and physiology. In addition to application as a research and diagnostic tool, PET continues to mature as a technology for drug development and assessment of clinical pharmacotherapy.

Self-assessment questions

1 What are the three regulatory paths for PET radiopharmaceuticals in the US?
2 What three radiopharmaceuticals can provide information about sympathetic innervation of the heart?
3 Carbon-11 'Pittsburgh Compound B' (PIB) binds to what?
4 Use of ^{11}C-PIB may allow early diagnosis of what disease?
5 Functional magnetic resonance imaging provides comparable information to what parameter measured with ^{15}H$_2$O?
6 What cellular function is imaged by the following radiopharmaceuticals?
   a ^{18}F-FDG
   b ^{11}C-choline
   c ^{18}F-thymidine
   d ^{11}C-methionine.
7 List one or more limitations of ^{18}F-fluorodeoxyglucose (FDG) imaging.
8 What is used in conjunction with a flow tracer to identify 'hibernating' myocardium?
9 In imaging with ^{18}F-FDG, do seizure foci typically appear hyper- or hypometabolic when imaged interictally?
10 What agent used in imaging was initially developed as an antipsychotic agent?
11 What agent is chemically related to fentanyl?

References

Agdeppa E *et al.* (2003). *In vitro* detection of (S)-naproxen and ibuprofen binding to plaques in the Alzheimer's brain using the positron emission tomography molecular imaging probe 2-(1-[6-[(2-[(18)F]fluoroethyl)(methyl)amino]-2-naphthyl]ethylidene)malononitrile. *Neuroscience* 117: 723–730.

Bednarczyk EM *et al.* (1997). Evaluation of the indomethacin nitroglycerin interaction using positron emission tomography. *J Cardiovasc Pharmacol* 30: 732–733.

Bednarczyk EM *et al.* (2002). Brain blood flow in the nitroglycerin (GTN) model of migraine: measurement using positron emission tomography and transcranial Doppler. *Cephalalgia* 22: 749–757.

Bencherif B *et al.* (2004). Mu-opioid receptor binding measured by [¹¹C]carfentanil positron emission tomography is related to craving and mood in alcohol dependence. *Biol Psychiatry* 55: 255–262.

Bencherif B *et al.* (2005). Regional mu-opioid receptor binding in insular cortex is decreased in bulimia nervosa and correlates inversely with fasting behavior. *J Nucl Med* 46: 1349–1351.

Bergmann *et al.* (1984). Quantification of regional myocardial blood flow in vivo with H₂¹⁵O. *Circulation* 70: 724–733.

Berridge M *et al.* (1991). Measurement of human cerebral blood flow with [¹⁵O]butanol and positron emission tomography. *J Cereb Blood Flow Metab* 11: 101–115.

Bol A *et al.* (1993). Direct comparison of ¹³N ammonia and ¹⁵O water estimates of perfusion with quantification of regional myocardial blood flow by microspheres. *Circulation* 87: 512–525.

Brenner W *et al.* (2004). Comparison of different quantitative approaches to ¹⁸F-fluoride PET scans. *J Nucl Med* 45: 1493–1500.

Brooks DJ *et al.* (1986). A comparison between regional cerebral blood flow measurements obtained in human subjects using ¹¹C-methylalbumin microspheres, the C¹⁵O₂ steady-state method, and positron emission tomography. *Acta Neurol Scand* 73: 415–422.

Buck A *et al.* (2002). 3-Deoxy-3-[¹⁸F]fluorothymidine-positron emission tomography for non-invasive assessment of proliferation in pulmonary nodules. *Cancer Res* 62: 3331333–4.

Choi S *et al.* (2005). [¹⁸F]-3′-Deoxy-3′-fluorothymidine PET for the diagnosis and grading of brain tumors. *Eur J Nucl Med Mol Imaging* 32: 653–659.

de Jong I *et al.* (2003). Preoperative staging of pelvic lymph nodes in prostate cancer by ¹¹C-choline PET. *J Nucl Med* 44: 331–335.

Ferrari A *et al.* (1998). Serum time course of naltrexone and 6β-naltrexol levels during long term treatment in drug addicts. *Drug Alcohol Depend* 52: 211–220.

Food and Drug Administration (2009). *Radioactive Drug Research Committee (RDRC) Program.* Washington, DC: Food and Drug Administration; http://www.fda.gov/AboutFDA/CentersOffices/CDER/ucm085831.htm (accessed September 8, 2009).

Francis D *et al.* (2003). Potential impact of [¹⁸F]3′-deoxy-3′-fluorothymidine vs [¹⁸F]fluoro-2-deoxy-D-glucose in positron emission tomography for colorectal cancer. *Eur J Nucl Med Mol Imaging* 30: 988–994.

Frost ML *et al.* (2003). A prospective study of risedronate on regional bone metabolism and blood flow at the lumbar spine measured by ¹⁸F-fluoride positron emission tomography. *J Bone Miner Res* 18: 2215–2222.

Frost ML *et al.* (2004). Dissociation between global markers of bone formation and direct measurement of spinal bone formation in osteoporosis. *J Bone Miner Res* 19: 1797–1804.

Gardner SF *et al.* (1993). High-dose cyclophosphamide-induced myocardial damage during BMT: assessment by positron emission tomography. *Bone Marrow Transplant* 12: 139–144.

Hara T *et al.* (1998). PET imaging of prostate cancer using carbon-11-choline. *J Nucl Med* 39: 990–995.

Hara T *et al.* (2001). Development of ¹⁸F-fluoroethylcholine for cancer imaging with PET: synthesis. biochemistry, and prostate cancer imaging. *J Nucl Med* 43: 187–199.

Jacobs A *et al.* (2005). ¹⁸F-Fluoro-L-thymidine and ¹¹C-methylmethionine as markers of increased transport and proliferation in brain tumors. *J Nucl Med* 46: 1948–1958.

Kemppainen N et al. (2006). Voxel-based analysis of PET amyloid ligand [^{11}C]PIB uptake in Alzheimer disease. Neurology 67: 1575–1580.

Kety SS, Schmidt CF (1948). The nitrous oxide method for the quantitative determination of cerebral blood flow in man: theory, procedure and normal values. J Clin Invest 27: 476–483.

Khan N et al. (2003). A comparative study of ^{11}C-choline PET and [^{18}F]fluorodeoxyglucose PET in the evaluation of lung cancer. Nucl Med Commun 24: 359–366.

Kim S et al. (1997). Longer occupancy of opioid receptors by nalmefene compared to naloxone as measured in vivo by a dual detector system. J Nucl Med 38: 1726–1731.

Kim S et al. (2001). Double-blind naltrexone and placebo comparison study in the treatment of pathological gambling. Biol Psychiatry 49: 914–921.

Klunk W et al. (2004). Imaging brain amyloid in Alzheimer's disease with Pittsburgh Compound-B. Ann Neurol 55: 306–319.

Krystal J et al. (2001). Naltrexone in the treatment of alcohol dependence. N Engl J Med 345: 1734–1739.

Logan J et al. (1996). Distribution volume ratios without blood sampling from graphical analysis of PET data. J Cereb Blood Flow Metab 16: 834–840.

Luisi AJ et al. (2005). Regional ^{11}C-hydroxyephedrine retention in hibernating myocardium: chronic inhomogeneity of sympathetic innervation in the absence of infarction. J Nucl Med 46: 1368–1374.

Mathis C et al. (2003). Synthesis and evaluation of ^{11}C-labeled 6-substituted 2-arylbenzothiazoles as amyloid imaging agents. J Med Chem 46: 2740–2754.

Mayberg HS et al. (1991). Quantification of mu and non-mu opiate receptors in temporal lobe epilepsy using positron emission tomography. Ann Neurol 30: 3–11.

National Institutes of Health (2004–2009). Molecular Imaging and Contrast Agent Database (MICAD). Bethesda, MD: National Library of Medicine; http://micad.nih.gov (accessed September 8, 2009).

Ninomiya H et al. (2004). Diagnosis of tumor in the nasal cavity and paranasal sinuses with [^{11}C] choline PET: comparative study with 2-[^{18}F]fluoro-2-deoxy-D-glucose (FDG) PET. Ann Nucl Med 18: 29–34.

Pirotte B et al. (2004). Comparison of ^{18}F-FDG and ^{11}C-methionine for PET guided stereotactic brain biopsy of gliomas. J Nucl Med 45: 1293–1298.

Prevett M et al. (1994). Opiate receptors in idiopathic generalised epilepsy measured with [^{11}C] diprenorphine and positron emission tomography. Epilepsy Res 19: 71–77.

Price D et al. (2002). Comparison of [^{18}F]fluorocholine and [^{18}F]fluorodeoxyglucose for positron emission tomography of androgen dependent and androgen independent prostate cancer. J Urol 168: 273–2780.

Price J et al. (2005). Kinetic modeling of amyloid binding in humans using PET imaging and Pittsburg compound-B. J Cereb Blood Flow Metab 25: 1528–1547.

Rosenspire KC et al. (1990). Synthesis and preliminary evaluation of carbon-11-meta-hydroxy-ephedrine: a false transmitter agent for heart neuronal imaging. J Nucl Med 31: 1328–1334.

Salinas C et al. (2005). PET imaging of myocardial β-adrenergic receptors with fluorocarazolol. J Cardiovasc Pharm 46: 222–231.

Schwaiger M et al. (1990). Noninvasive evaluation of sympathetic nervous system in human heart by positron emission tomography. Circulation 82: 457–464.

Shoghi-Jadid K et al. (2002). Localization of neurofibrillary tangles and beta-amyloid plaques in the brains of living patients with Alzheimer disease. Am J Geriatr Psychiatry 10: 24–35.

Small G et al. (2006). PET of brain amyloid and tau in mild cognitive impairment. N Engl J Med 355: 2652–2663.

Spyrou N et al. (2002). Myocardial beta-adrenoceptor density one month after acute myocardial infarction predicts left ventricular volumes at six months. J Am Coll Cardiol 40: 1216–1224.

Sutinen E et al. (2000). Nodal staging of lymphoma with whole-body PET: comparison of [^{11}C] methionine and FDG. J Nucl Med 41: 1980–1988.

Theodore WH et al. (1988). Patterns of cerebral glucose metabolism in patients with partial seizures. Neurology 38: 1201–1206.

Torizuka T *et al.* (2003). Imaging of gynecologic tumors: comparison of ^{11}C-choline PET with ^{18}F-FDG PET. *J Nucl Med* 44: 1051–1056.

Vesselle H *et al.* (2002). *In vivo* validation of 3′-deoxy-3′-[^{18}F]fluorothymidine as a proliferation imaging tracer in humans: correlation of [^{18}F]FLT uptake by positron emission tomography with Ki-67 immunohistochemistry and flow cytometry in human lung tumors. *Clin Cancer Res* 8: 3315–3323.

Wagner M *et al.* (2003). 3′-[^{18}F]Fluoro-3′-deoxythymidine ([^{18}F]-FLT) as positron emission tomography tracer for imaging proliferation ina murine B-cell lymphoma model and in human disease. *Cancer Res* 63: 2681–2687.

Yanagawa T *et al.* (2003). Carbon-11 choline positron emission tomography in musculoskeletal tumors: comparison with fluorine-18 fluorodeoxyglucose positron emission tomography. *J Comput Assist Tomogr* 27: 175–182.

Yap C *et al.* (2006). Evaluation of thoracic tumors with ^{18}F-fluorothymidine and ^{18}F-fluorodeoxyglucose positron emission tomography. *Chest* 129: 393–401.

Zhang H *et al.* (2003). ^{11}C-Choline PET for the detection of bone and soft tissue tumours in comparison with FDG PET. *Nucl Med Commun* 24: 273–279.

Zhang W *et al.* (2005). F-18 stilbenes as PET imaging agents for detecting beta-amyloid plaques in the brain. *J Med Chem* 48: 5980–5988.

Zubieta J *et al.* (1996). Increased mu opioid receptor binding detected by PET in cocaine dependent men is associated with increased cocaine craving. *Nat Med* 2: 1225–1229.

Zubieta J *et al.* (2000). Buprenorphine-induced changes in mu-opioid receptor availability in male heroin-dependent volunteers: a preliminary study. *Neuropsychopharmacology* 23: 326–334.

Zubieta J *et al.* (2001). Regional mu opioid receptor regulation of sensory and affective dimensions of pain. *Science* 293: 311–315.

8

Interventional agents used in nuclear medicine

Wendy Galbraith

Learning objectives

- Describe the indication of different interventional agents used in nuclear medicine
- Explain the mechanism of action of the interventional agent that augments the nuclear medicine study
- Evaluate the contraindications and precautions for interventional agents as they apply to use in a patient.

Introduction

Some diagnostic studies are performed with the use of a pharmacological agent, referred to as an interventional agent. In nuclear medicine, these agents will usually augment a function of the body in a short time frame to complement and enhance the sensitivity and specificity of the study. Interventional drugs can be administered before, during, or after the administration of the radiopharmaceutical. This chapter contains information for the interventional agents used most frequently in nuclear medicine. Information on each drug includes its use in nuclear medicine, dose, frequency, route and rate of administration, peak onset or duration, preparation or a description of materials, contraindications, precautions, adverse drug effects, and drug interactions, where applicable. It combines information from primary, secondary, and tertiary sources into one resource that the reader can use as a basis for a nuclear pharmacy practice setting. The chapter is not all-inclusive; rather it covers areas where the pharmacist is frequently called upon to act as a source of information. The chapter finally discusses four of the most common drugs used as part of the *in vitro* preparation of radiopharmaceuticals or the administration of radiopharmaceuticals.

Acetazolamide

Acetazolamide (Diamox) is used as an adjunct in brain imaging to evaluate hemodynamic reserve when identifying ischemic areas from infarct (Loveless 1997). It inhibits carbonic anhydrase, thus reducing the formation of hydrogen and bicarbonate ions from carbon dioxide and water. The result is an increase in carbon dioxide tension in the tissues and a decreased carbon dioxide tension in the pulmonary alveoli. The transient decrease in the rate of carbon dioxide elimination may result in an increase in ventilation and cerebral blood flow to increase oxygenation (American Society of Health-System Pharmacists 1997, p. 2156). Acetazolamide is a non-bacteriostatic sulfonamide that has been used in treating epilepsy, promoting diuresis, decreasing intraocular pressure, and prophylactically to increase respiration for altitude sickness (Acetazolamide package insert 2002; Diamox package insert 2005). When used in cerebral perfusion imaging, acetazolamide increases cerebral blood flow approximately 30 to 40% above baseline in normal patients (Loveless 1997, p. 10). When it is administered intravenously, onset is in two minutes, with peak activity at 15 minutes and a duration of action of four to five hours (American Society of Health-System Pharmacists 1997, p. 2157). Each 500 mg vial containing sterile acetazolamide sodium powder should be reconstituted with at least 5 mL of sterile water for injection prior to use (Acetazolamide package insert 2002). One gram is administered intravenously over two to five minutes before the technetium-labeled perfusion agent is administered 15 to 25 minutes later. Cerebral imaging is carried out 10 to 25 minutes after the perfusion radiopharmaceutical is administered (Loveless 1997, p. 11). Acetazolamide is contraindicated in patients with decreased sodium and/or potassium blood levels (e.g. marked kidney and liver disease or dysfunction, suprarenal gland failure, hyperchloremic acidosis). Since acetazolamide is a sulfonamide, precautions should be observed for patients with sulfa allergies. Adverse reactions occurring most often include paresthesia, particularly a 'tingling' feeling in the extremities, hearing dysfunction or tinnitus, taste alteration, drowsiness, and confusion (Acetazolamide package insert 2002).

Adenosine

Adenosine is used as an adjunct to myocardial perfusion imaging when the stress portion of the study cannot be achieved with exercise alone. Adenosine is a potent peripheral and coronary artery vasodilator. Vasodilatation is mediated by activation of adenosine A_{2A}-receptors on smooth muscle. Adenosine activates all four known adenosine receptor subtypes: A_1, A_{2A}, A_{2B}, and A_3. Activation of the receptors has varying effects: A_{2A} is known to be involved in coronary vasodilatation in stress; A_{2B} is thought to cause the side-effect of flushing/dizziness; A_1 causes slowing of the cardiac atrioventricular node conduction; and A_3 and A_{2B} are thought to be involved in bronchoconstriction (Hinkle 2007, p. 11). Adenosine is rapidly taken up from the vasculature by endothelial cells and metabolized with a biological half-life of less than 10 seconds (Adenoscan package insert 2005). The adult dose is 140 µg/min per kg body weight intravenously over four to six minutes. The perfusion radiopharmaceutical is administered at the half-way point of the adenosine infusion. During the adenosine infusion and for a minimum of five minutes after infusion, the patient's electrocardiogram (ECG) and blood pressure should be monitored (Loveless 1997, p. 3). Adenosine is contraindicated in patients with second- or third-degree atrioventricular block (except in patients with an artificial pacemaker), sinus node disease, bradycardia (except in patients with an artificial pacemaker), known or suspected bronchoconstrictive or bronchospastic lung disease (e.g. asthma) or a known hypersensitivity to adenosine. The most common adverse effects are chest pain, dyspnea, flushing, and headache. Typically, treatment of adverse effects is discontinuance of the infusion as it has a short half-life. The effects of adenosine are inhibited by methylxanthines such as caffeine and theophylline (Adenoscan package insert 2005). Prior to an adenosine study, caffeine products should be withheld for six hours, and theophylline medications should be withheld for 48 hours (Hillard 2008).

Aminophylline

Aminophylline is used to reverse the side-effects of the stress agents dipyridamole, adenosine, and regadenoson (Kowalsky & Falen 2004, p. 524). Aminophylline is a solubilized form of theophylline, which is a xanthine derivative bronchodilator. Its mechanism of action is thought to be twofold: airway smooth muscle relaxation and suppression of the response of the airway to stimuli. Its action in nuclear medicine is thought to be by antagonism of adenosine receptors. To reverse the side-effects of dipyridamole, 100 mg aminophylline is administered by slow intravenous infusion over 60 seconds, or 250 to 500 mg is infused over 20 minutes (Gilbert & Douglas 2001). To reverse the side-effects of adenosine, the adult dose is 100 mg intravenous administered over 60 seconds. The drug is supplied in single-dose 10 and 20 mL vials and in ampules at a concentration of 25 mg/mL. Storage is at room temperature with protection from light. Contraindications include hypersensitivity to theophylline or ethylenediamine. Adverse effects include headache, tremor, and diuresis (Aminophylline package insert 2004).

Atropine

Atropine can be used in myocardial perfusion imaging to increase the heart rate response. It is generally combined with dobutamine stress myocardial perfusion imaging to increase heart rate and oxygen demand (Kowalsky & Falen 2004, p. 523). Atropine is an anticholinergic agent and works by competitively inhibiting the effects of acetylcholine. A usual dose is 0.5 mg administered by intravenous bolus, which may be repeated up to a maximum dosage of 1 mg (Elhendy *et al.* 1998). It is contraindicated in patients with glaucoma, anticholinergic allergies, pyloric stenosis, or prostatic hypertrophy. Adverse effects include tachyarrhythmia, constipation, dry mouth, blurred vision, urine retention, increased intraocular pressure, and respiratory depression (Thomson Micromedex 2009).

Bethanechol

The efficacy of bethanechol for the treatment of gastroesophageal reflux has been directly evaluated with gastroesophageal scintigraphy (Saha *et al.* 1987, p. 122). Bethanechol (Urecholine) is a cholinergic agent that stimulates the parasympathetic nervous system. Bethanechol increases tone, amplitude of contractions, peristaltic activity, and secretions of the gastrointestinal tract. The drug produces contraction of the detrusor muscle of the urinary bladder to enable initiation of micturition and bladder emptying. Initial response to bethanechol when administered subcutaneously is within 5–15 minutes and the duration is up to two hours (Bethanechol package insert 2009). A dose of

2.5–5 mg bethanechol has been administered subcutaneously after ingestion of a solid meal to quantify reflux in comparison to gastric emptying time (Saha *et al.* 1987, p. 123). Bethanechol is contraindicated in asthma; bradycardia; epilepsy; gastrointestinal inflammation or spasms; peritonitis; gastrointestinal or bladder surgery, resection, or obstruction; and hypersensitivity to bethanechol or components (Bethanechol package insert 2009). Adverse effects include abdominal discomfort, flushing, sweating, and a fall in blood pressure. Atropine can be administered for persistent adverse effects. Bethanechol should not be administered intravenously or intramuscularly because of the potential for cholinergic toxicity, including circulatory collapse, severe hypotension, diarrhea, shock, and cardiac arrest (Bethanechol package insert 2009).

Captopril

Captopril is used as an adjunct to renal imaging to diagnose renovascular hypertension (Ziessman *et al.* 2006, p. 231). Captopril is an angiotensin-converting enzyme (ACE) inhibitor. These inhibitors block conversion of angiotensin I to angiotensin II. Patients with renovascular hypertension are relying on the renin–angiotensin I–angiotensin II compensatory mechanism to maintain glomerular filtration perfusion pressure in the affected kidney. Diagnostic administration of an ACE inhibitor prevents compensatory vasoconstriction of the efferent arterioles in the kidney and results in decreased glomerular filtration pressure from the patient's baseline renogram (Kowalsky & Falen 2004, p. 649). When captopril is given orally to fasting patients, its hypotensive effect is apparent within 15 minutes, with maximal effect in 1–1.5 hours and duration of 6–12 hours (US Pharmacopeia 1999, p. 178). The dose for a captopril renogram study is 25–50 mg in adults and 0.5 mg/kg body weight (maximum 25 mg) in children. In renal impairment, the dose should be reduced. For a creatinine clearance of 10–50 mL/min, 75% of the normal dose is administered. For a creatinine clearance of less than 10 mL/min, 50% of the normal dose is used (Thomson Micromedex 2009). The rate of absorption of captopril is improved if the tablets are crushed and given with 240 mL water (8 ounces) on an empty stomach (Kowalsky & Falen 2004, p. 651; Ziessman *et al.* 2006, p. 233). The radiopharmaceutical is administered one hour after the captopril. A diuretic (20–40 mg furosemide intravenous) is often given in conjunction with the radiopharmaceutical to ensure clearance of the collecting system and to improve visual and quantitative interpretation (Ziessman *et al.* 2006, p. 232). Contraindications to captopril are hypersensitivity to any ACE inhibitor, dehydration, high renin levels, and recent dialysis. Blood pressure should be monitored for hypotension, and treatment includes volume expansion with normal saline if the patient continues to be symptomatic (Loveless 1997, p. 6). Concurrent use of an ACE inhibitor decreases the sensitivity by 15% and so captopril should be discontinued three days prior to the study and other longer-acting ACE inhibitors (e.g. oral enalapril, lisinopril, benazepril, ramipril) should be discontinued seven days before the study (Ziessman *et al.* 2006, p. 232). Captopril is available in 25 mg and 50 mg tablets. Captopril solution can be prepared by crushing the tablet and dissolving in as little as 25–100 mL of water and shaking for five minutes. The filler (which does not dissolve) is discarded, and the solution may have a slightly sulfurous odor. Captopril is very unstable when dissolved in water and should be used within one hour of preparation (US Pharmacopeia 1999).

Histamine H$_2$-receptor antagonists

Cimetadine and other histamine H$_2$-receptor antagonists (e.g. ranitidine, famotidine) have been used in the nuclear medicine evaluation of Meckel's diverticulum. Reduction of gastric acid secretion decreases the secretion of pertechnetate from normal stomach gastric mucosa to the small bowel and hence improves the target-to-background ratio, increasing the sensitivity of the study (Saha *et al.* 1987, p. 125; Loveless 1997, p. 9). The oral adult dose of cimetidine is 300 mg four times daily for two days prior to the study. The intravenous adult dose is 300 mg diluted in 100 mL of 5% Dextrose in Water, administered over 20 minutes. The pertechnetate radiopharmaceutical is administered 20 to 60 minutes after cimetidine and followed by imaging. Ranitidine and famotidine have also been used in the evaluation of Meckel's diverticulum: 50 mg ranitidine or 20 mg famotidine produce similar effects on gastric acid secretion to cimetidine (American Society of Health-System Pharmacists 1999, p. 2264; Thomson Micromedex 2009). For children, the oral dose is 20 mg/kg per day for two days prior to the study (Loveless 1997, p. 9; Kowalsky & Falen 2004, p. 623). Intravenous cimetidine is contraindicated for patients known to have hypersensitivity to the product, and adverse effects include mild diarrhea (Loveless 1997, p. 9).

Dipyridamole

Dipyridamole is used as an adjunct to myocardial perfusion imaging when the stress portion of the study cannot be achieved with exercise alone. Dipyridamole is a potent peripheral and coronary artery vasodilator. It inhibits the metabolism of adenosine and consequently indirectly increases endogenous levels of adenosine. The dose for dipyridamole is 0.57 mg/kg body weight up to a maximum dose of 60 mg. It is infused intravenously at 0.142 mg/kg per minute over four minutes (Kowalsky & Falen 2004, p. 522). Plasma dipyridamole concentrations decline in a triexponential fashion following intravenous infusion, with half-lives averaging 3–12 minutes,

33–62 minutes, and 11.6–15 hours. Two minutes after the dipyridamole administration, the serum concentration is at its peak. The cardiac perfusion radiopharmaceutical should be injected at this peak serum concentration, between six and eight minutes from the start of the dipyridamole injection. Dipyridamole is metabolized in the liver and excreted with the bile (Dipyridamole package insert 2004). The biological effects of parenteral dipyridamole last for approximately 30 minutes (Kowalsky & Falen 2004, p. 523). Vital signs, including ECG should be monitored during the intravenous infusion and for 10 to 15 minutes following the infusion. Should severe chest pain or bronchospasm occur, 50–100 mg parenteral aminophylline should be administered over 30 to 60 seconds and this may be repeated within five minutes if symptoms persist (Loveless 1997, p. 4; Dipyridamole package insert 2004). Contraindications include hypersensitivity to dipyridamole, allergy to aminophylline, and severe bronchospastic lung disease. Adverse effects include chest pain, headache, shortness of breath, hypotension, and flushing. Serious adverse effects have been recorded and include four cases of myocardial infarction and six cases of severe bronchospasm (Loveless 1997, p. 4). Since the effects of dipyridamole are the result of an increase in adenosine concentration, the use of methylxanthines will inhibit the vasodilator effects. Caffeine products should be withheld for six hours and theophylline medications should be withheld for 48 hours prior to the test (Hillard 2008). Dipyridamole is supplied at a concentration of 5 mg/mL in vials of 2 mL and 10 mL. Prior to intravenous administration, dipyridamole must be diluted to at least a 1:2 ratio with 0.45% sodium chloride injection, 0.9% sodium chloride injection, or 5% dextrose injection, for a total volume of approximately 20–50 mL. Infusion of undiluted dipyridamole injection may cause local irritation (Dipyridamole package insert 2004).

Dobutamine

Dobutamine is used as an adjunct to myocardial perfusion imaging when the stress portion of the study cannot be achieved with exercise alone and the patient has a contraindications to adenosine or dipyridamole (Kowalsky & Falen 2004, p. 523). Dobutamine is a synthetic catecholamine stimulating β_1-adrenoceptors of the heart, leading to increased coronary output. At the high doses used for pharmacological stress perfusion imaging, both inotropic and chronotropic action of the heart are increased, with resulting increases in myocardial contractility and heart rate. This leads to an increased oxygen demand and increased blood flow in normal coronary arteries, similar to that seen with exercise (Hinkle 2007). The dose of dobutamine needed for myocardial response varies widely from patient to patient, and titration is always necessary (Dobutamine package insert 2007). Dobutamine is given intravenously using a graded infusion beginning at 5–10 µg/kg per minute and increased by 10 µg every three minutes to a maximum of 40 µg/kg per minute. The myocardial perfusion radiopharmaceutical is administered one minute after the last increase in dosage of dobutamine, after which the dobutamine infusion is continued for another two minutes (Hinkle 2007). The onset of action of dobutamine is within one to two minutes, but as long as 10 minutes may be required to obtain the peak infusion rate. The plasma half-life of dobutamine is two minutes. Side-effects frequently occur and often require lowering of the dose rate. Non-cardiac side-effects include nausea, headache, flushing, chills, and dyspnea. Common cardiac side-effects include chest pain, ECG changes, and hypotension. If side-effects persist after stopping the infusion, they can be reversed by administering a short-acting beta-blocker such as metoprolol 0.1 mg/kg or esmolol with a loading dose of 0.5 mg/kg per minute for one minute followed by 0.05 mg/kg per minute for four minutes (Kowalsky & Falen 2004, p. 525; Hinkle 2007). Dobutamine is contraindicated in patients with previous manifestations of hypersensitivity to dobutamine, hypertrophic cardiomyopathy, concurrent use of beta-blockers, or systolic blood pressure greater than 200 mmHg, and diastolic blood pressure greater than 110 mmHg (Loveless 1997, p. 5). Dobutamine is supplied in vials containing 250 mg/20 mL. Dobutamine must be further diluted to at least 50 mL in normal saline or 5% dextrose solution, with a recommendation of 250 mg/250 mL of normal saline for a final concentration of 1000 µg/mL (Dobutamine package insert 2007; Shackett 2009). Calcium-channel blockers and beta-blockers will reduce the effects of dobutamine and should be discontinued 48 hours prior to the study (Hinkle 2007).

Enalaprilat

Enalaprilat is the parenteral dosage form of enalapril and is used as an adjunct in renal imaging to diagnose renovascular hypertension (Ziessman *et al.* 2006, p. 231). Enalapril is an ACE inhibitor. These drugs block conversion of angiotensin I to angiotensin II. Patients with renovascular hypertension are relying on the renin–angiotensin I–angiotensin II compensatory mechanism to maintain glomerular filtration perfusion pressure in the affected kidney. The ACE inhibitor prevents compensatory vasoconstriction of the efferent arterioles in the kidney and results in decreased glomerular filtration pressure from the patient's baseline renogram (Kowalsky & Falen 2004, p. 649). When given intravenously, the peak onset of action of enalaprilat is within 15 minutes and it has a duration of action of up to six hours (US Pharmacopeia 1999, p. 178). The dose for an enalaprilat renogram study is 40 µg/kg, with a maximum of 2.5 mg infused over three to five minutes (Ziessman *et al.* 2006, p. 233). If creatinine clearance is less than 30 mL/min then the dose should be reduced by 50% (Thomson Micromedex 2009). The radiopharmaceutical is administered 15 minutes after enalaprilat. Often a diuretic (e.g. 20–40 mg furosemide intravenous) is given in conjunction with the radiopharmaceutical to ensure clearance of the collecting system and improve visual and quantitative interpretation (Ziessman *et al.* 2006, p. 232). Contraindications to enalaprilat are hypersensitivity to any ACE inhibitor, dehydration, high renin levels, and recent dialysis. Blood pressure should be monitored for hypotension; treatment includes volume expansion with normal saline if the patient continues to be symptomatic (Loveless 1997, p. 6). Concurrent ACE inhibitor use decreases the sensitivity of the test by 15% and should be discontinued three days prior to the study for captopril and seven days for longer-acting ACE inhibitors (e.g. oral enalapril, lisinopril, benazepril, and ramipril) (Ziessman *et al.* 2006, p. 232). Enalaprilat is supplied in a concentration of 1.25 mg/mL as single-dose vials. Enalaprilat injection may be administered undiluted. Caution should be used when administering to neonates because of the benzyl alcohol content (US Pharmacopeia 1999, p. 184).

Furosemide

Furosemide is used with renal imaging in order to differentiate between mechanical obstruction and muscular atony as the cause of upper urinary-tract dilatation (Saha *et al.* 1987, p. 120). Furosemide is a sulfonamide-type loop diuretic that inhibits the reabsorption of electrolytes in the ascending loop of Henle and distal renal tubules. Onset of diuresis is within five minutes of intravenous administration of furosemide, with peak plasma drug concentration occurring at 20 minutes and a duration of action of two hours. Intravenous injection should be given slowly over one to two minutes to reduce adverse effects (American Society of Health-System Pharmacists 1997, p. 2041). The single dose of furosemide used in renal scintigraphy is 40 mg for adults, 1 mg/kg for infants, and 0.5 mg/kg for children aged 1 to 16 years (Kowalsky & Falen 2004, p. 648). For renal failure, the dose may be increased until the desired response is seen, up to a maximum dose of 6 mg/kg (Thomson Micromedex 2009). Furosemide is contraindicated in any condition associated with fluid or electrolyte loss, in patients with anuric renal failure, and in patients allergic to sulfonamides. The potassium depletion associated with furosemide administration may produce cardiotoxic effects. Adverse effects are rare following a single intravenous administration of furosemide. Nausea, vomiting, and dizziness may be observed occasionally (Saha *et al.* 1987, p. 120). Furosemide is supplied in single-use vials with a concentration of 10 mg/mL. Furosemide should be protected from light. Discolored injections or tablets should not be used (American Society of Health-System Pharmacists 1997, p. 2041).

Glucagon

Glucagon has been used as an adjunct to image Meckel's diverticulum when given with pentagastrin. Glucagon has also been utilized in gastrointestinal bleeding studies (Saha *et al.* 1987, pp. 123–125). Exogenous glucagon elicits all the pharmacological responses produced by endogenous glucagon, which is secreted by the alpha-2 cells in the islets of Langerhans in the pancreas. Primarily, glucagon increases blood glucose by stimulating hepatic glycogenolysis. Glucagon also produces relaxation of smooth muscle of the stomach, duodenum, small intestine, and colon, along with inhibiting gastric and pancreatic secretions. Following intravenous administration of glucagon, relaxation of the gastrointestinal smooth muscle occurs within one minute and persists for 9–17 minutes (American Society of Health-System Pharmacists 1997, p. 2445). Glucagon, by decreasing peristalsis, decreases the movement of the radiopharmaceutical (e.g. ^{99m}Tc-labeled RBCs or pertechnetate) that has accumulated at the abnormal site. In Meckel's diverticulum, 50 µg/kg glucagon is administered intravenously one minute after the injection of pertechnetate (Loveless 1997, p. 10). For detection of gastrointestinal bleeding, 0.1–1.0 U glucagon is intravenously administered (Saha *et al.* 1987, p. 123). The most frequent adverse effects of glucagon are nausea and vomiting. Glucagon is supplied in single-dose vials containing 1 U (or 1 mg), which must be reconstituted with 1 mL diluent provided by the manufacturer (American Society of Health-System Pharmacists 1999, p. 246).

Metoclopramide

Metoclopramide (Reglan) has been used in the evaluation of gastric emptying studies. Gastric emptying studies provide a direct method of monitoring the effectiveness of metoclopramide and predicting response to chronic oral therapy (Saha *et al.* 1987, p. 122). Metoclopramide improves gastrointestinal motility by releasing acetylcholine from the myenteric plexus, resulting in contraction of the smooth muscle. In subjects with weak antral and strong duodenal muscle activity, metoclopramide is most effective in promoting gastric emptying; whereas metoclopramide is relatively ineffective in patients with normal gastric emptying (Reglan package insert 2009). A dose of 5–10 mg (20 mg maximum) is administered intravenously over one to two minutes. A rapid injection may result in transient but intense feelings of anxiety and restlessness, followed by drowsiness (Reglan package insert 2009; Shackett 2009). When metoclopramide is administered intravenously, the initial response is seen within one to three minutes, with a duration of action of three hours. Contraindications to metoclopramide are concomitant use of drugs with extrapyramidal adverse effects; gastrointestinal hemorrhage, obstruction (mechanical), or perforation; hypersensitivity to metoclopramide products; pheochromocytoma; and seizure disorders. Metoclopramide is supplied as 5 mg/mL in 2 mL single-dose vials (Reglan package insert 2009).

Morphine sulfate

Morphine sulfate is used as an adjunct in gallbladder imaging in the differentiation of chronic cholecystitis from acute cholecystitis. Morphine sulfate is a Schedule II controlled substance, pure opioid agonist, selective to the opioid μ-receptor, with primary actions in the brain (Thomson Micromedex 2009). It is used in nuclear medicine because it enhances the contraction of the sphincter of Oddi, causing increased intraluminal pressure in the common bile duct and facilitating the flow of tracer into the gallbladder unless the cystic duct is obstructed. If there is no filling after 30 minutes, acute cholecystitis is indicated (Kowalsky & Falen 2004, p. 603). Intravenously administered morphine is readily absorbed, with peak activity at 10 minutes. A terminal half-life of approximately two to four hours after intravenous administration of morphine sulfate has been reported. The dose is 0.04 mg/kg in 10 mL normal saline administered intravenously over three minutes with a maximum dose of 3 mg (Kowalsky & Falen 2004, p. 603). Morphine is contraindicated in patients with hypersensitivity to morphine, morphine salts, or any component of the product; a history of drug abuse; or the presence of pancreatitis (Loveless 1997, p. 8; Thomson Micromedex 2009). At the low dosages administered, no significant adverse effects were reported; however, in the event that morphine effects need to be reversed, 0.1–0.2 mg naloxone can be administered intravenously (Loveless 1997, p. 8).

Pentagastrin

The manufacture and sale of pentagastrin (Peptavlon, Wyeth-Ayerst) was discontinued in the USA in 1998 (Thomson Micromedex 2009). There is currently no USP monograph for this agent and hence its use would require an Investigational New Drug Application. Pentagastrin has been used to increase the localization of sodium pertechnetate in ectopic gastric mucosa when imaging Meckel's diverticulum (Saha *et al.* 1987, pp. 123–125). An alternative to pentagastrin is a histamine H_2-blocker.

Phenobarbital

Phenobarbital is used to differentiate neonatal hepatitis from biliary atresia, a condition present from birth in which the bile ducts inside or outside the liver do not have normal openings. Phenobarbital is a potent inducer of hepatic enzymes and increases bilirubin conjugation and excretion. Phenobarbital administration enhances absorption of the ^{99m}Tc-iminodiacetic acid derivative radiopharmaceuticals and increases canalicular bile flow (Saha *et al.* 1987, p. 125). Phenobarbital pretreatment improves the specificity of the examination from 63 to 94% (Howman *et al.* 1998). Phenobarbital is a long-acting barbiturate and an anticonvulsant. When administered intravenously, onset is within five minutes, and the duration is 10–12 hours. The neonatal dosage for differentiating biliary atresia is 5 mg/kg per day in two divided doses and given over five days (Ziessman *et al.* 2006, p. 181). Intravenously administered phenobarbital should be diluted with at least an equal volume of fluid and administered over three to five minutes, not to exceed 2 mg/kg per minute in infants (Thomson Micromedex 2009). It is suggested that therapeutic levels of phenobarbital should be checked before imaging, with a target therapeutic drug concentration of at least 15 μg/mL for maximal effect (Howman 1998; Ziessman *et al.* 2006, p. 181). Phenobarbital is contraindicated in patients with hypersensitivity to phenobarbital products, porphyria, and respiratory disease (dyspnea or obstruction). Serious adverse effects include agranulocytosis, Stevens–Johnson syndrome, thrombocytopenia, and thrombophlebitis (Thomson Micromedex 2009).

Potassium iodide

Potassium iodide (Saturated Solution of Potassium Iodide [SSKI], Lugol's Solution) is commercially available in several formulations. Potassium iodide is used as a thyroid protectant in diagnostic studies utilizing iodine radiopharmaceuticals and as a protectant from accidental exposure to radioiodine. As a protectant, the adult dosage is 150–300 mg daily for 14 days. The dose for children is 130 mg for those older than one year and 65 mg for infants up to one year. When potassium iodide is administered simultaneously with radiation exposure, the protectant effect is approximately 97%. Potassium iodide administered one and three hours after exposure results in an 85% and 50% protectant effect, respectively. Potassium iodide administered more than six hours after the exposure is thought to have negligible protectant effects (US Pharmacopeia 1999, p. 2355). For adequate blockade of the thyroid gland in diagnostic studies, the dosage is 100–150 mg 24 hours prior to radiopharmaceutical administration and daily for 10 to 14 days following radiopharmaceutical administration (Swanson & Dick 1990, p. 703) Contraindications to potassium iodide are hypersensitivity to iodine or iodide and hyperkalemia. The potassium content is 6 mEq/g potassium iodide (234 mg/g) and it should be used with caution in patients with decreased renal function (American Society of Health-System Pharmacists 1997, p. 2094). Patients receiving potassium-sparing diuretics or ACE inhibitors could develop hyperkalemia; therefore, their serum potassium should be monitored. Adverse effects include gastrointestinal irritation, burning in throat, salivary gland tenderness, and a metallic taste. The oral solution of potassium iodide and the crushed tablets should both be mixed with 240 mL (8 ounces) of water, fruit juice, or milk for ingestion to decrease gastrointestinal adverse effects (US Pharmacopeia 1999, p. 2355). Lugol's solution contains 100 mg/mL of iodide; and SSKI contains 1000 mg/mL; potassium iodide syrup contains 65 mg/mL; and potassium iodide tablets contain 130 mg/tablet (Swanson 1990b, p. 704) Potassium iodide is light sensitive and should be stored in light-resistant containers. Free iodine may be produced by oxidation of potassium iodide, causing the oral solution to turn brownish yellow and these solutions should be discarded (American Society of Health-System Pharmacists 1997, p. 2094).

Potassium perchlorate

Potassium perchlorate is used in nuclear medicine on rare occasions to identify disease states in the thyroid gland where iodide is trapped but not incorporated into organic prodcuts ('organified,' e.g. Hashimoto's thyroid-itis or peroxidase deficiency). The study is termed the 'perchlorate discharge test' (Datz 1993). Perchlorate is a monovalent anion that is trapped by the thyroid and will competitively displace iodide that has not been organified. Lugol's solution or potassium iodide do not have the same discharge effect as the perchlorate ion in the discharge test. Perchlorate competes with iodide for entry through the base membrane, but perchlorate is more highly selected by the thyroid transport system. Perchlorate causes a discharge of stored iodide from the thyroid lumen back to the outer part of the cell. The dumping or discharge initiated by perchlorate has been considered to occur through two mechanisms: stopping the influx of iodide, thus changing the iodide concentration gradient; and increasing the thyroid cell response to thyroid-stimulating hormone (TSH), which increases iodide efflux before it increases the influx (Wolff 1998).

In the perchlorate discharge test, initially, a diagnostic radioiodine dose is given, followed by perchlorate two hours later. Thyroid measurements are taken over the next two hours. A positive test is indicated when the iodide activity in the thyroid falls 10% below baseline levels (Ziessman et al. 2006, p. 99). Onset of blockade action of potassium perchlorate occurs within 30 to 60 minutes after oral administration, with peak plasma concentrations occur-ring within three hours and with a duration of action of six hours (American Society of Health-System Pharmacists 1997, p. 2909). There are no contra-indications or adverse effects to the use of single doses of potassium perchlor-ate in diagnostic imaging procedures with dosages of 1 g or less. The adult dose is 400–1000 mg. A dose of 200 mg has been recommended for children 2 to 12 years of age, and 100 mg may be administered to children under two years of age (Thomson Micromedex 2009). Potassium perchlorate is not manufactured in the USA. If compounded, the preparation must meet the

USP monograph acceptance criteria for potassium perchlorate and all applicable USP compounding procedural chapters.

Regadenoson

Regadenoson (Lexiscan) is a pharmacological stress agent indicated for radionuclide myocardial perfusion imaging in patients unable to undergo adequate exercise stress. Regadenoson is a synthetic adenosine receptor agonist with selective A_{2A}-receptor activity. The coronary vasodilatation effects are similar to those associated with dipyridamole and adenosine. There are four known adenosine receptor subtypes A_1, A_{2A}, A_{2B} and A_3, which mediate varying effects: A_{2A} is known to cause coronary vasodilatation in stress; A_{2B} is thought to cause the side-effect of flushing/dizziness; A_1 causes slowing of the cardiac atrioventricular node conduction; and A_3 and A_{2B} are thought to result in bronchoconstriction (Hinkle 2007, p. 11). Regadenoson has a 10-fold lower affinity for the A_1-receptor and weak, if any, affinity for the A_{2B}- and A_3-receptors (Lexiscan package insert 2009). The selectivity of regadenoson for A_{2A}-receptors should decrease side-effects associated with activation of all adenosine receptors. The peak plasma concentration of regadenoson is within one to four minutes after injection and parallels the onset of the pharmacodynamic response. In healthy volunteers, the regadenoson plasma concentration versus time profile is multiexponential in nature and characterized by a three-compartment model that ranges in biological half-lives from two minutes to two hours. The active half-life of regadenoson is the intermediate phase, with an average half-life of 30 minutes coinciding with loss of the pharmacodynamic effect. The recommended intravenous dose of Lexiscan is 5 mL (0.4 mg regadenoson) administered as a rapid (approximately 10 seconds) injection with a 5 mL saline flush immediately after the injection. The myocardial perfusion radiopharmaceutical is administered 10 to 20 seconds after the saline flush. Regadenoson is contraindicated in patients with second- or third-degree atrioventricular block or sinus node dysfunction unless these patients have an artificial pacemaker. The most common (incidence, 5%) adverse reactions to regadenoson are dyspnea, headache, flushing, chest discomfort, dizziness, angina pectoris, chest pain, and nausea. In clinical studies, 22% of patients had an increase in heart rate to over 100 beats/min within 45 minutes of administration of regadenoson. Aminophylline may be used to attenuate severe and/or persistent adverse reactions to regadenoson (Lexiscan package insert 2009). Since regadenoson's pharmacodynamic effect appears to be similar to that of dipyridamole, 50–100 mg parenteral aminophylline over 30 to 60 seconds should be administered and may be repeated within five minutes if adverse reactions persist (Loveless 1997, p. 4; Dipyridamole package insert 2004; Lexiscan package insert 2009). Studies suggest that the effects of synthetic adenosine agonists such as regadenoson are inhibited by methylxanthines, (e.g. caffeine and theophylline) (Lexiscan package insert 2009). Prior to a regadenoson study, the same measures for adenosine drug interactions should be followed, namely caffeine products should be withheld for six hours and theophylline medications should be withheld for 48 hours (Hillard 2008). Lexiscan is supplied as a single-use vial containing 0.4 mg/ 5mL (0.08 mg/mL) and a single-use prefilled syringe containing 0.4 mg/5 mL (0.08 mg/mL).

Sincalide

Sincalide (Kinevac) is a synthetically prepared C-terminal octapeptide of endogenous cholecystokinin (CCK) (Kinevac package insert 2002). Sincalide is used as an adjunct in gallbladder imaging. Sincalide causes contraction of the gallbladder, relaxation of the sphincter of Oddi, augmentation of pyloric sphincter tone, and enhancement of the motility of the small and large bowel (Loveless 1997, p. 7). Sincalide can be administered before the radiopharmaceutical if the patient has fasted for 24 hours or is on total parenteral nutrition (Kowalsky & Falen 2004, p. 602). The resulting gallbladder contraction clears the gallbladder of its contents, decreasing the pressure in the gallbladder and allowing the radiopharmaceutical to freely flow into the gallbladder if the cystic duct is patent (Loveless 1997, p. 7). Sincalide is also used after radiopharmaceutical administration, when the gallbladder is maximally filled, to quantify gallbladder ejection fraction. Sincalide's onset of action is prompt. When given in a bolus, contraction of the gallbladder becomes maximal in 5 to 15 minutes and returns to baseline size in 60 minutes (Kinevac package insert 2009).

The dose of 0.02 μg/kg is administered intravenously over two to three minutes or infused over 30 minutes when diluted in 50 mL normal saline. The longer administration time is reported to provide more reliable gallbladder contraction, with less variability and fewer adverse effects (Kowalsky & Falen 2004, p. 603; Ziessman *et al.* 2006, p. 549). The preparation is contraindicated in patients hypersensitive to sincalide and in patients with intestinal obstruction. Adverse effects include nausea and abdominal or stomach pain in 20% of patients. The incidence of other adverse reactions, including vomiting, flushing, sweating, rash, hypotension, hypertension, shortness of breath, urge to defecate, headache, diarrhea, sneezing, and numbness was less than 1%; dizziness was reported in approximately 2% of patients. These manifestations are usually lessened by slower injection rate (Kinevac package insert 2002). Sincalide should not be given after morphine sulfate since morphine counteracts the action of sincalide (Loveless 1997, p. 8). Sincalide is supplied in single-dose vials containing 5 μg. The contents are reconstituted with 5 mL sterile Water for Injection for a concentration of 1 μg/mL (Kinevac package insert 2002).

Thyroid-stimulating hormone

Nuclear medicine uses TSH (thyrotropin) to mimic the endogenous hormone from the pituitary gland that stimulates all thyroid enzymatic processes. Thyrogen (thyrotropin alfa) is recombinant human TSH, often referred to as rhTSH. Thyrogen has replaced purified thyrotropin because of the transient hypotension adverse effects that appear to be part of an allergic reaction to the bovine purified thyrotropin product (American Society of Health-System Pharmacists 1997, p. 1901). TSH stimulates the thyroid gland to secrete the thyroid hormones: thyroxine (T_4) and triiodothyronine (T_3). The production of TSH is inhibited by somatostatin, produced by the hypothalamus. Thyroid hormones also inhibit TSH production and secretion, in a regulatory negative feedback loop. TSH was used to differentiate primary hypothyroidism from secondary hypothyroidism, but it is no longer necessary now that measurement of TSH concentrations is readily available. Thyrogen is currently used in nuclear medicine to improve sensitivity for detecting residual or metastatic thyroid tissue in patients with thyroid carcinoma. The traditional procedure for performing a follow-up whole-body radioiodine scan required the withdrawal of thyroid medications (over two to six weeks) to allow endogenous TSH levels to increase to above 40 mU/mL in order to stimulate residual thyroid tissue. However, most patients became clinically hypothyroid during this period and were exposed to the potential risk of increased tumor growth associated with elevated serum TSH levels. Administration of Thyrogen has been shown to increase plasma TSH to over 200 mU/mL (Meier 1994). After a single intramuscular injection of Thyrogen, the peak serum concentration is reached between 3 and 24 hours after injection (median of 10 hours). An intramuscular dose of 0.9 mg is administered every 24 hours for two days and TSH and thyroglobulin are monitored 72 hours after the last injection. The ^{131}I-labeled sodium iodide therapy or diagnostic whole-body dose is administered orally 24 hours after the last injection, with imaging performed 72 hours after the last injection (Thyrogen package insert 2004). Thyrogen is contraindicated in patients who have experienced hypersensitivity reactions to bovine TSH. Because of the potential rise in serum thyroid hormone levels, caution should be exercised in patients with a known history of heart disease and with significant thyroid tissue. The most common adverse effects include nausea (10.5%) and residual headache (7.3%). Thyrogen is supplied as a single-dose vial containing 1.1 mg (4–12 IU/mg) thyrotropin alfa lyophilized product, intended for intramuscular administration after reconstitution with 1.2 mL sterile Water for Injection to obtain a concentration of 0.9 mg/mL. The package insert states that clinical trials have demonstrated that even when Thyrogen-stimulated thyroglobulin testing is performed in combination with radioiodine imaging, there remains a meaningful risk of missing a diagnosis of thyroid cancer or of underestimating the extent of disease. Therefore, thyroid hormone withdrawal testing of thyroglobulin with radioiodine imaging remains the standard diagnostic modality to assess the presence, location, and extent of thyroid cancer (Thyrogen package insert 2004).

Miscellaneous agents used with *in vitro* preparations

Anticoagulant Citrate Dextrose Solution

Anticoagulant Citrate Dextrose Solution USP differs from Bracco's Anticoagulant Citrate Dextrose Solution Modified Formula in the ratio of ingredients. Anticoagulant Citrate Dextrose (ACD) is an anticoagulant primarily used in the *in vitro* radiolabeling of red blood cells (RBC) with ^{51}Cr for intravenous administration (A-C-D package insert 1994). Some radiopharmaceuticals suggest ACD as an anticoagulant in their preparation; however, ACD is not employed widely for this purpose (Ceretec package insert 2006). Each reaction vial contains 80 mg citric acid, 224 mg anhydrous sodium citrate, and 120 mg anhydrous dextrose in a sterile, non-pyrogenic aqueous 10 mL solution; the pH is 4.5–5.5. *In vitro*, citrate ions combine with ionic calcium in blood; the resulting lack of ionic calcium prevents coagulation. The A-C-D Solution Modified is supplied in 75 mL vials containing 10 mL of solution. The procedure calls for 30–50 mL of whole blood to be added to the vial (A-C-D package insert 1994). As ACD is toxic to cells, its uses for blood collection should not exceed 0.15 mL/mL blood. Excess incubation of ACD and blood has been shown to decrease the RBC labeling efficiency (Swanson 1990, p. 619).

Ascorbic acid

Ascorbic acid is used in the *in vitro* process to prepare ^{51}Cr-labeled RBC for RBC mass and plasma volume calculations and as an antioxidant to stabilize ^{99m}Tc-hydroxymethylene diphosphonate (HDP). Ascorbic acid, 50–100 mg, is used to reduce the unbound hexavalent state of the chromate ion to the trivalent state (chromic ion) with the purpose of terminating the RBC labeling process. The trivalent chromic ion is not ncorporated into the RBC and will be renally excreted when the final preparation is administered to the patient (Swanson 1990, p. 617). Ascorbic acid is also used as an antioxidant to protect ^{99m}Tc-labeled diphosphonates from the effects of oxidation and, therefore, to increase both the *in vitro* and *in vivo* stability of the complex. Ascorbic acid (0.5–2 mg) is added to ^{99m}Tc-HDP preparations to extend the shelf-life beyond the package insert expiration of eight hours (Chilton *et al.* 1990). The ascorbic acid must be added at the end of the preparation process to avoid a ^{99m}Tc-labeled ascorbic acid complex, which will distribute to and be eliminated from the kidneys. Ascorbic acid 500 mg/mL is supplied as vials and ampules from various manufacturers. It is recommended that ampules of ascorbic acid be stored under refrigeration. A color change may occur during storage but this does not decrease therapeutic activity (Thomson Micromedex 2009).

Heparin

Heparin is an anticoagulant used in nuclear medicine for procedures requiring collection of whole blood or in a regular process to maintain a patient's intravenous access site. Fatal medication errors have occurred with the use of heparin, so careful attention to the various strengths of heparin is imperative. Fatal hemorrhages have occurred in children through medication errors in which 1 mL heparin vials were confused with 1 mL 'catheter lock flush' vials. All heparin sodium injection vials should be carefully examined to confirm the correct vial choice prior to administration of the drug (Thomson Micromedex 2009). Heparin acts as a catalyst that markedly accelerates the rate at which antithrombin III neutralizes thrombin and activated coagulation factor X. Antithrombin III generally neutralizes these coagulation factors slowly, but the presence of heparin allows this neutralization to occur almost instantaneously; it addition it can also neutralize factors IX, XI, XII, and plasmin. The antidote for heparin is protamine sulfate (American Society of Health-System Pharmacists 1997, p. 1085). When heparin is used as an *in vitro* anticoagulant for blood samples, the ratio is 7–15 U heparin to 1 mL of whole blood. The process of leukocyte separation and labeling requires up to 50 mL of whole blood. When choosing a heparin concentration to coat the collection syringe, both the number of units and volume must be considered. Usually, a minimum of 1000 U heparin (1 mL of 1000 U/mL solution) is used for coating the collection syringe. Heparin 'catheter lock flush' solution is used to maintain patency of indwelling peripheral or central access sites. The dose for maintaining patency in these situations should be the lowest concentration of heparin that has been shown to be effective, 10 U/mL. Heparin is contraindicated in patients who are hypersensitive to the drug or have uncontrollable bleeding. It must be used with caution as there is an increased risk of bleeding with the concurrent administration of some drugs (American Society of Health-System Pharmacists 1997).

Hetastarch

Heatastarch (HES; hydroxyethyl starch) is a synthetic polymer that is classified as a plasma volume expander (Thomson Micromedex 2009). The colloidal properties of 6% hetastarch solution resemble those of human albumin. When added to whole blood, hetastarch increases the erythrocyte sedimentation rate. Hetastarch is used in nuclear medicine as an adjunct to the *in vitro* process to increase the yield of granulocytes. The addition of 6% hetastarch to whole blood is usually in the ratio of 1:8. Kowalsky & Falen explain a labeling procedure where 10 mL of 6% hetastarch is added to approximately 43 mL whole blood, mixed well, and the red cells settle to the bottom in approximately 45 minutes (Kowalsky & Falen 2004, p. 302). When used for isolating leukocytes, the hetastarch is nearly completely removed in the process before reinjection into the patient. Precautions to be aware of include allergic or sensitivity reactions and interference of hetastarch with platelet function. Hetastarch is supplied at 6% hetastarch in 0.9% sodium chloride and is commonly referred to by its trade name, Hespan (American Society of Health-System Pharmacists 1997, p. 1995).

Summary

Diagnostic nuclear medicine procedures can include the use of a non-radioactive agent known as an interventional drug. It is important for these drugs to be used properly in order to enhance the effectiveness of the study. Even though these drugs will only be administered once, attention to the dose and contraindications for these drugs is imperative for their safe use in the nuclear medicine department.

Self-assessment questions

1 An order is received for a hepatobiliary assessment with a 'EF' procedure. What interventional agent would be appropriate for this indication?
2 Describe the mechanism of action of phenobarbital as the interventional agent to rule out biliary atresia.
3 A patient arrives for a cardiac stress test using the pharmacological stress agent regadenoson. The patient has taken the following medications the morning of the study: Trandate (labetalol) 200 mg, Lotensin HCT 10/12.5 (benazepril and hydrochlorothiazide combination), and Fiorinal (aspirin, butalbital, and caffeine). What would be the most appropriate recommendation for this patient?

References

A-C-D package insert (1994). *A-C-D Solution Modified.* Princeton, NJ: Bracco Diagnostics.

Acetazolamide package insert (2002). *Acetazolamide for Injection USP.* Bedford, OH: Bedford Laboratories.

Adenoscan package insert (2005). *Adenoscan Adenosine Injection.* Deerfield, IL: Astellas Pharma US.

American Society of Health-System Pharmacists (1997). *American Hospital Formulary Service Drug Information*. Bethesda, MD: American Society of Health-System Pharmacists.

Aminophylline package insert (2004). *Aminophylline Dyhydrate Injection*. Lake Forest, IL: Hospira.

Bethanechol package insert (2009). *Urecholine*. Irvine, CA: Teva Pharmaceuticals.

Ceretec package insert (2006). *Ceretec for the Preparation of Technetium Tc99m Exametazine Injection*. Arlington Heights, IL: GE Healthcare, Medi-Physics.

Chilton HM *et al.* (1990). Radiopharmaceuticals for bone and bone marrow imaging. In: Swanson DP *et al.* eds. *Pharmaceuticals in Medical Imaging*. New York: Macmillan, p. 542.

Datz FL (1993). *Handbook of Nuclear Medicine*, 2nd edn. St. Louis, MO: Mosby-Year Book, pp. 2, 7.

Diamox package insert (2005). *Diamox Sequels: Acetaxolamide Capsules, Extended Release*. Pamona, NY: Duramed Pharmaceuticals.

Dipyridamole package insert (2004). *Dipyridamole for Injection*. Bedford, OH: Bedford Laboratories.

Dobutamine package insert (2007). *Dobutamine Injection USP*. Bedford, OH: Bedford Laboratories.

Elhendy A *et al.* (1998). Safety of dobutamine–atropine stress myocardial perfusion scintigraphy. *J Nucl Med* 39: 1662–1666.

Gilbert GM, Douglas NA (2001). Pharmacologic interventions in nuclear medicine assessment of cardiac perfusion. *J Pharm Pharmaceut Sci* 4: 255–262.

Hillard N (2008). *Drug Radiopharmaceutical Interactions Handout*. The Nuclear Pharmacy; http://nuclearpharmacy.uams.edu/resources/Interactions.htm (accessed May 12, 2009).

Hinkle GH (2007). Interventional agents in stress myocaridal perfusion imaging. In: Norenberg J, ed. *Continuing Education for Nuclear Pharmacists and Nuclear Medicine Professionals*, Vol. 13(2). Albuquerque, NM: University of New Mexico.

Howman GR *et al.* (1998). Hepatobiliary scintigraphy in infancy. *J Nucl Med* 39: 311–319.

Kinevac package insert (2002). *Sincalide*. Princeton, NJ: Bracco Diagnostics.

Kowalsky R, Falen S (2004). *Radiopharmaceuticals in Nuclear Pharmacy and Nuclear Medicine*, 2nd edn. Washington, DC: American Pharmacists Association.

Lexiscan package insert (2009). *Lexiscan (Regadenoson) Injection Solution for Intravenous Use*. Deerfield, IL: Astellas Pharma US.

Loveless VS (1997). Drugs used as interventional agents in nuclear medicine. In: Hladik WB III, ed. *Correspondence Continuing Education Courses for Nuclear Pharmacists and Nuclear Medicine Professionals*, Vol. 7(2). Albuquerque, NM: University of New Mexico.

Meier CA (1994). Diagnostic use of recombinant human thyrotropin in patients with thyroid carcinoma. *J Clin Endocrin Metab* 78: 188–196.

Reglan package insert (2009) *Metoclopramide*. Deerfield, IL: Baxter Healthcare.

Saha GB *et al.* (1987). Interventional studies in nuclear medicine. In: Hladik III WB *et al.* eds. *Essentials of Nuclear Medicine Science*. Baltimore, MD: Williams & Wilkins.

Shackett P (2009). *Nuclear Medicine Technology: Procedures and Quick Reference*, 2nd edn. Philadelphia, PA: Lippincott, Williams & Wilkins.

Swanson DP (1990). Radiopharmaceuticals for hematological applications. In: Swanson DP *et al.* eds. *Pharmaceuticals in Medical Imaging*. New York: Macmillan.

Swanson DP, Dick TJ, (1990). Drugs for the mitigation of internal radiocontamination. In: Swanson DP *et al.* eds. *Pharmaceuticals in Medical Imaging*. New York: Macmillan.

Thomson Micromedex (2009) *DRUGDEX-EV*. Greenwood Village, CO: Thomson Micromedex; http://www.micromedex.com/products/drugdex/ (accessed 19 May 2009).

Thyrogen package insert (2004). *Thyrogen (Thyrotropin Alfa for Injection)*. Cambridge, MA: Genzyme.

US Pharmacopeia (1999). Dispensing Information, Vol. I: Drug Information for the Health Care Professional, 19th edn. Englewood, CO: Micromedex.

Wolff J (1998). Perchlorate and the thyroid gland. *Pharm Rev* 50: 89–105.

Ziessman HA *et al.* (2006). *Nuclear Medicine: The Requisites In Radiology*. Philadelphia, PA: Elsevier Mosby.

9

Clinical applications of radiopharmaceuticals in the nuclear medicine department

Vesper Grantham and Jan M. Winn

Learning objectives

- Counsel and educate patients and healthcare providers on nuclear medicine procedures and radiopharmaceuticals based on knowledge of procedure indications, patient preparation, and radiopharmaceutical and pharmaceutical dosages
- Optimize diagnostic imaging and therapy results using clinical information
- Assess the appropriateness of the nuclear medicine examination requested.

Introduction

Nuclear pharmacists and nuclear medicine technologists benefit from a strong working relationship and understanding of each other's roles in nuclear medicine imaging. A nuclear pharmacist who is highly knowledgeable in clinical aspects of nuclear medicine and what occurs to the patient after the radiopharmaceutical is shipped to the department and administered is a valuable resource for patients, nuclear medicine technologists, and other healthcare providers. He or she can assist in analyzing altered biodistributions, investigating new radiopharmaceuticals and/or problem solving unique clinical situations. A strong working relationship between the pharmacist and technologist improves overall patient care.

Overview of instrumentation and imaging devices

Both nuclear pharmacists and nuclear medicine technologists utilize common radiation detection equipment, including the dose calibrator, Geiger–Mueller (GM) survey meter, and well counter. These instruments are used for similar applications although more directly related to patient procedures in the nuclear medicine department.

Instrumentation that nuclear pharmacists may not be familiar with includes the imaging and counting devices, which will be briefly discussed. There are two main types of imaging cameras utilized in nuclear medicine, the gamma scintillation camera (Figure 9.1) and the PET camera (Figure 9.2). The gamma scintillation camera produces images based on the absorption of single-photon emissions from the patient after the patient has been given the radiopharmaceutical. Scintillation cameras can have single, dual, or triple detector heads. To produce images, these cameras utilize different collimators, which are based primarily on the energy of the radionuclide being imaged (low, medium, and high).

There are a variety of image acquisitions that the gamma camera can procure, including static, whole-body, dynamic, gated, and SPECT (single photon emission computed tomography). The acquisition method used for a particular patient study is dependent on the physiological information the technologist needs to collect. Static imaging involves simply imaging the patient for a given period of time, usually 5–10 minutes. The image produced is a representation of the patient's physiology for that period of time. Whole-body

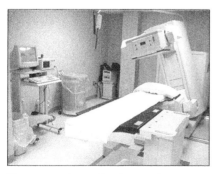

Figure 9.1   A typical nuclear medicine gamma camera in a department.

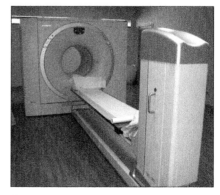

Figure 9.2   A typical positron emission tomography (PET) camera.

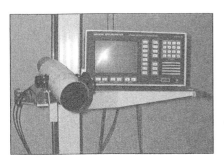

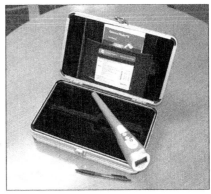

Figure 9.3 An uptake probe used for counting radioiodine during thyroid uptake studies.

Figure 9.4 A surgical probe used for radioactivity localization.

imaging is simply the imaging of a patient's entire body from head to toe. The camera can move slowly over the patient's body to acquire the image. Dynamic imaging involves segmental imaging of a patient's physiology over time, images of two seconds in duration for a total of one minute for example. The dynamic acquisition is sometimes referred to as a flow, when the technologist is imaging the dose as it is transported through the vascular system to the area of uptake. Gating is a unique type of imaging, utilizing the patient's physiological triggers to acquire and organize the image data. Finally, SPECT allows for the production of tomographic (transverse, sagittal, and coronal) images and requires the camera detector head to rotate around the patient.

The PET camera (Figure 9.2) creates images based on the annihilation reaction of the electrons and positrons from the PET radiopharmaceutical. One of the key benefits of PET imaging is the ability to create attenuation-corrected images from a transmission/computed tomography (CT) scan. Following the CT scan, the emission of the photons in opposite directions is acquired by the circular array of crystals in the PET camera to form the patient's image.

In addition to the imaging devices, technologists may use the scintillation uptake probe or intraoperative gamma probe for other counting. The uptake probe (Figure 9.3) is a scintillation counter used for counting radioiodine during thyroid uptake calculations. The intraoperative probe (Figure 9.4) is a very small probe used to localize radioactive sources during surgery.

Procedures

Cardiology

Nuclear cardiology is a specialized area of nuclear medicine that may be performed in a general nuclear medicine department or in a separate department within cardiology services. There are three main procedures performed

Table 9.1 Cardiology procedures

Procedure	Radiopharmaceutical	Adult dosage range	Route administration	Clinical applications
Myocardial perfusion	^{99m}Tc-sestamibi, ^{99m}Tc-tetrofosmin	Rest: 8–30 mCi (296–1110 MBq); Stress: 20–30 mCi (740–1110 MBq)	IV	Detect and evaluate coronary artery disease
	^{201}Tl-thallous chloride	Rest: 2–5 mCi (74–185 MBq); Stress: 3–5 mCi (111–185 MBq)	IV	
PET myocardial perfusion	^{82}Rb-rubidium chloride	Rest: 30–60 mCi (1110–2220 MBq); Stress: 30–60 mCi (1110–2220 MBq)	IV	Detect and evaluate coronary artery disease
Cardiac viability	^{201}Tl-thallous chloride	3–5 mCi (111–185 MBq)	IV	Assess viable ischemic myocardium
PET cardiac viability	^{18}F-FDG	10–15 mCi (370–555 MBq)	IV	Assess viable ischemic myocardium
Gated blood pool	^{99m}Tc-labeled red blood cells	20–30 mCi (740–1110 MBq)	IV	Evaluation of left ventricular function, ejection fraction, wall motion

IV, intravenous; see text for other abbreviations.

in nuclear cardiology: myocardial perfusion, myocardial viability, and gated blood pool studies. There are several radiopharmaceutical options for each of these procedures, which even vary in the type of acquisition (SPECT or PET). The procedures and radiopharmaceuticals are summarized in table 9.1.

Nuclear cardiologists often read the nuclear cardiology studies. A technologist who is specifically certified in nuclear cardiology has credentials as an NCT or Nuclear Cardiology Technologist.

Myocardial perfusion

One of the most common nuclear cardiology procedures is the myocardial perfusion study. This cardiac test assesses the radiopharmaceutical distribution to the myocardium at rest and stress as a way of indirectly assessing coronary artery patency. A patient may undergo treadmill or chemical stress depending on the patient's physiological and mental state. After the dose is administered intravenously to the patient, the patient is imaged using a SPECT acquisition. Imaging technology allows the technologist to 'gate' the

SPECT images by connecting the patient to a three-lead ECG monitor while the imaging data are collected. The technologist reconstructs the SPECT data with the ability to produce a left ventricular ejection fraction and other quantitative data.

For a normal perfusion study, the left ventricular myocardial wall should demonstrate homogeneous uptake throughout the myocardium in all cardiac walls (anterior, posterior, lateral, septal, and apical). Any areas of decreased radiopharmaceutical uptake indicate a lack of vascular blood flow to the area of the myocardium, which indirectly indicates coronary vessel blockage. Figure 9.5 demonstrates a myocardial perfusion study, showing both a normal situation and decreased dose uptake to the inferior wall.

The PET myocardial perfusion study is performed in a similar manner to the SPECT study but at a much faster pace because of the short half-life of the PET radiopharmaceutical. A basic protocol for a PET perfusion study involves the following: rest transmission scan, injection of ^{82}Rb; rest images for 5–10 minutes, chemical stress, injection of ^{82}Rb, stress imaging and stress transmission scan (Di Carli 2004). Images are reconstructed and interpretation is very similar to a SPECT myocardial perfusion study.

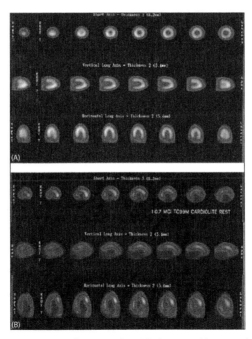

Figure 9.5 Resting myocardial perfusion studies. (A) The normal heart, with homogeneous radiopharmaceutical uptake throughout the myocardium on short, vertical long, and horizontal long slices. (B) An abnormal heart with an inferior wall defect. Decreased blood flow is shown by the decreased dose uptake.

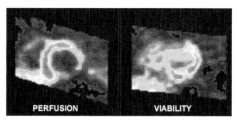

Figure 9.6 Myocardial perfusion and PET viability study. The compared study images demonstrate the 'mismatch' presentation correlating with viable myocardial tissue.

Myocardial viability

Myocardial viability assessment is a useful procedure to differentiate between chronic/silent ischemia, stunned myocardium, hibernating myocardium, and infarcted myocardium. Assessing the specific physiological status of the myocardium helps to determine the reversibility of the defect with revascularization. Use of ^{201}Tl delayed imaging and PET metabolic imaging with ^{18}F-fluorodeoxyglucose (FDG) in viability studies are summarized in table 9.1.

To perform a viability study, the radiopharmaceutical is injected, and imaging starts at the appropriate time depending on the radiopharmaceutical. A 24 hour delayed/redistribution SPECT scan is often performed with ^{201}Tl while a 45 minute delay is needed for ^{18}F-FDG PET imaging.

A viability study should not be performed without an abnormal myocardial perfusion study. These two studies (perfusion and viability) must be compared for interpretation. With both viability studies, if the perfusion defect demonstrates dose distribution or 'fills-in,' the myocardial tissue can be successfully revascularized. This results in a mismatch abnormality on the perfusion and viability studies (Figure 9.6). If the perfusion defect does not demonstrate dose distribution on the viability study, the myocardial tissue is infarcted and cannot be successfully revascularized.

Gated cardiac blood pool

A gated cardiac blood pool study is one procedure that is known by more names than any other procedure performed in nuclear medicine. The study can be referred to as a nuclear ventriculogram (NVG) or multigated acquisition (MUGA). Regardless of the name, the procedure involves imaging the blood within the left ventricle to provide a quantitative assessment of the left ventricular ejection fraction, systolic and diastolic blood volumes, cardiac output, stroke volume, and cardiac wall motion (Figure 9.7).

The study involves labeling the patient's red blood cells (RBC) and injecting the radiolabeled cells back into the patient intravenously. The patient is imaged with a gating acquisition for approximately 20 minutes and the technologist processes the images. A normal left ventricular ejection fraction should be approximately 50–80% (Shackett 2009, p. 74).

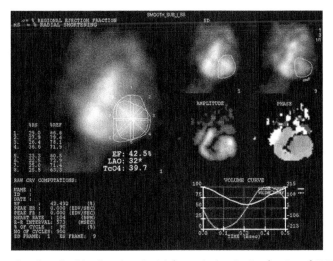

Figure 9.7 Gated cardiac blood pool study. A left ventricular ejection fraction of 42.5% is considered abnormal.

Central nervous system

Nuclear medicine can image three different aspects of the central nervous system including cerebral spinal fluid physiology, blood flow assessment to the brain, and metabolic brain imaging using PET. Table 9.2 identifies common central nervous system studies and the radiopharmaceuticals available to perform them.

Table 9.2 Central nervous system procedures

Procedure	Radiopharmaceutical	Adult dosage range	Route of administration	Clinical applications
Cisternogram	^{111}In-DTPA	500 µCi (18.5 MBq)	Intrathecal	Evaluate CSF physiology
CSF shunt patency	^{99m}Tc-DTPA	1–3 mCi (37–111 MBq)	Shunt reservoir	Assess shunt function
Brain perfusion SPECT	^{99m}Tc-HMPAO	10–20 mCi (370–740 MBq)	IV	Evaluation of brain death, cerebral ischemia, seizure foci
	^{99m}Tc-ECD	10–20 mCi (370–740 MBq)	IV	
Brain metabolism PET	^{18}F-FDG	10–20 mCi (370–740 MBq)	IV	Evaluation of epilepsy, movement disorders, cerebrovascular disease, dementia

CSF, cerebrospinal fluid; IV, intravenous; see text for other abbreviations.

Cisternogram

To perform a cisternogram, the radiopharmaceutical is injected into the intrathecal space of the lumbar spine where it dilutes with the patient's CSF. It then travels through the CSF space around the spine and up to the brain, where it is absorbed into the bloodstream and then excreted from the body. Because this physiological process occurs slowly, imaging does not begin for at least six hours and possibly not until 24 hours after radiopharmaceutical injection. Imaging sessions occur over two to three days to ensure adequate documentation of the physiological transit of the CSF.

The images taken for this procedure include anterior, right lateral, and left lateral views of the head for approximately five minutes each. A vertex view, which is an image of the top of the head, may also be acquired. For consistency, the same images are repeated at each imaging session.

This procedure is performed to detect the presence of normal pressure hydrocephalus, which may slow CSF transit time and cause delay in CSF absorption into the bloodstream. This condition is also associated with CSF reflux into the cerebral ventricles (Figure 9.8B). A normal scan will demonstrate significant clearance of the radiopharmaceutical from the CSF

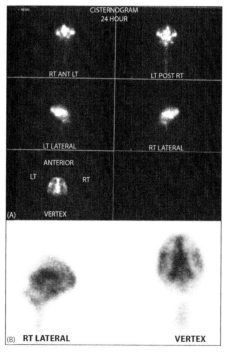

Figure 9.8 Cisternography. (A) In a normal situation, there is no radiopharmaceutical accumulation in the cerebral ventricles. It accumulates diffusely in the basal cisterns and over the convexities of the brain. (B) In the abnormal image, the radiopharmaceutical is seen in the cerebral ventricles at 24 hours. RT, right; LT, left; ANT, anterior; POST, posterior.

space within 24–48 hours and no visualization of the cerebral ventricles (Figure 9.8A).

Cerebrospinal fluid shunt patency

Patients diagnosed with forms of hydrocephalus are frequently treated by placement of a shunt system comprising a tube that begins in one of the lateral cerebral ventricles and empties into the peritoneal cavity. A reservoir device under the skin behind the patient's ear allows flow of CSF out of the ventricles when the pressure reaches a predetermined value. The shunt provides a pathway for excess CSF to leave the ventricular system and be excreted. The shunts are effective but may become blocked by objects floating in the CSF or by a kink in the tubing, resulting in a return of patient symptoms as a result of a build-up of CSF in the ventricles.

To determine if the return of symptoms indicates a malfunctioning shunt, a CSF shunt patency study can be performed in the nuclear medicine department. A dose of ^{99m}Tc-DTPA in a small volume is injected under sterile conditions into the shunt reservoir. A lateral image of the head on the side of the reservoir and an anterior view of the patient's chest and abdomen are taken at 5, 10, and 20 minutes after radiopharmaceutical injection. If the shunt is operating normally the radiopharmaceutical will flow down the tubing and empty into the peritoneal space (Figure 9.9A). If the radiopharmaceutical traverses part of the tubing then stops, it is an indication that the tubing is blocked at the point where the dose stops (Figure 9.9B). Another sign of a malfunctioning shunt is failure to visualize the peritoneal cavity.

Brain perfusion with SPECT scanning

In the mid 1980s, nuclear brain imaging was limited to assessing the blood flow to the head in a single plane. With modern radiopharmaceuticals and SPECT imaging, nuclear medicine now assesses radiopharmaceutical perfusion of the brain in three dimensions, providing greater image detail and more information to physicians.

Common clinical indications for the performance of a perfusion brain study include confirmation of brain death, localization of the origin of seizure foci, and assessment of cerebral ischemia. The imaging protocol used in the nuclear medicine department varies based on the specific indication for the scan.

If the scan is ordered for confirmation of brain death, initial flow of radiopharmaceutical through the major cerebral vessels with dynamic imaging of the head at the time of radiopharmaceutical injection may be performed along with delayed images after the radiopharmaceutical has perfused into the brain. If the procedure has been ordered to assess seizure foci, it is critical to inject the radiopharmaceutical within 30 to 60 seconds of the onset of a seizure, followed by imaging two hours later. For all other indications, the primary diagnostic images are acquired approximately two hours after

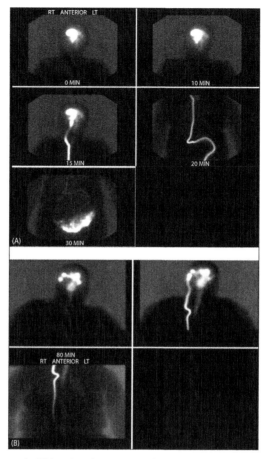

Figure 9.9 Shunt study. (A) Imaging demonstrates the catheter end and the accumulation of the radiopharmaceutical in the peritoneum. This indicates the shunt is not malfunctioning or blocked. (B) Here, neither the entire shunt catheter nor dose accumulation in the peritoneum is visualized. This indicates a possible blockage or malfunction of the shunt catheter.

injection. For all indications except brain death, delayed SPECT images are acquired so the perfusion pattern can be assessed in three dimensions through the entire volume of the brain.

On a normal brain perfusion scan, there should be homogeneous distribution of the radiopharmaceutical throughout the gray matter (Figure 9.10A). The cerebral ventricular structures do not contain radiopharmaceutical and will present as areas lacking perfusion. If a patient is brain dead, there will be no perfusion of the brain (Figure 9.10B). In the presence of cerebral ischemia there will be reduced or absent perfusion in the area experiencing ischemia (Figure 9.10C). Since seizure foci are hypermetabolic, they present as focal areas of radiopharmaceutical uptake greater than the surrounding tissue.

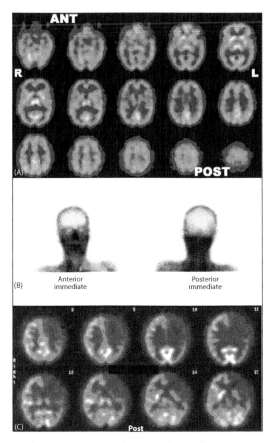

Figure 9.10 Brain perfusion. (A) In a normal brain perfusion, there is homogeneous dose accumulation throughout the brain. (B) In brain death, there is lack of blood flow in the brain. (C) A baseline cerebral perfusion study demonstrates decreased radiopharmaceutical distribution which is associated with lack of cerebral vascular blood flow.

Brain metabolism with PET scan

Though the actual scan time for PET imaging of brain metabolism is less than 30 minutes, the preparation time is significant. An intravenous line must first be started in the patient. The patient then relaxes for several minutes in a quiet, dimly lit room prior to radiopharmaceutical injection. The injection is then made through the intravenous line to avoid stimulating pain receptors in the brain and altering radiopharmaceutical distribution. The patient remains in the quiet setting for another hour before scanning begins. These environmental precautions ensure normal distribution of the radiopharmaceutical throughout the gray matter without additional accumulation in pain receptor centers or the visual or auditory cortex.

On a normal PET brain scan, there should be homogeneous distribution of the radiopharmaceutical throughout the gray matter. The cerebral ventricular structures do not contain radiopharmaceutical and will present as areas lacking perfusion. Seizure foci are hypermetabolic and present as focal areas of radiopharmaceutical uptake greater than the surrounding tissue. In the presence of cerebral ischemia, there will be reduced perfusion in the area experiencing ischemia. In patients with Alzheimer's dementia, there is decreased perfusion bilaterally in the temporoparietal regions.

Endocrine disorders

A variety of diagnostic and therapeutic nuclear medicine procedures are available to assess and treat endocrine disorders. Table 9.3 identifies common endocrine procedures with basic details for each.

Thyroid scan

Patient preparation for all thyroid procedures is critical. Medications given to patients with thyroid conditions, along with some vitamins, foods, and iodinated contrast media may alter radiopharmaceutical uptake, which is why extensive lists of such compounds indicating when they must be discontinued are available in many nuclear medicine resources (Ziessman *et al.* 2006, p. 77). If an oral radiopharmaceutical is to be administered, the patient should not consume food or drink for at least two hours before and after

Table 9.3 Endocrine procedures

Procedure	Radiopharmaceutical	Adult dosage range	Route of administration	Clinical applications
Thyroid scan	^{99m}Tc-pertechnetate	3–10 mCi (111–370 MBq)	IV	Assess palpable thyroid nodules
	^{123}I-sodium iodide	100–500 µCi (3.7–18.5 MBq)	Oral	
Thyroid uptake	^{123}I-sodium iodide	10–20 µCi (0.4–0.7 MBq)	Oral	Differentiate Grave's disease from thyroiditis
	^{131}I-sodium iodide	5 µCi (0.2 MBq)	Oral	
Parathyroid scan	^{99m}Tc-sestamibi	20–25 mCi (740–925 MBq)	IV	Localize parathyroid adenomas
Adrenal medulla scan	^{123}I-MIBG	3–10 mCi (81–370 MBq)	IV (slowly)	Localization of pheochromocytomas, neuroblastomas, and their metastases
	^{131}I-MIBG	500 µCi–1 mCi (18.5–37 MBq)	IV (slowly)	

IV, intravenous; see text for other abbreviations.

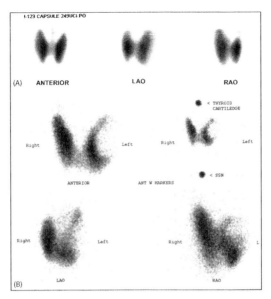

Figure 9.11 Thyroid scans. (A) Typical images in a normal thyroid scan: anterior (top left), left anterior oblique (top middle) and right anterior oblique (top right). (B) A cold nodule can be seen in the left superior lobe.

radiopharmaceutical administration to ensure that the radiopharmaceutical does not bind to food.

Imaging begins approximately 30 minutes after intravenous administration of ^{99m}Tc-pertechnetate or 24 hours after oral administration of radioiodine. The scan consists of a set of three images, each taken for 10 minutes. The images include anterior, right anterior oblique, and left anterior oblique angles of the thyroid.

Under normal circumstances, there is homogeneous distribution of the radiopharmaceutical throughout a thyroid gland of normal size (Figure 9.11A). Hyperthyroidism may cause intense uptake of the radiopharmaceutical, while thyroid nodules may demonstrate more or less radioactivity than the surrounding gland depending upon whether the nodules are functional or not. Figure 9.11B demonstrates a cold nodule appearance on a thyroid scan.

Thyroid uptake

All thyroid uptake procedures are performed approximately 24 hours after oral administration of either isotope of radioiodine. If paired with a thyroid scan using ^{123}I, a single radiopharmaceutical dose may be administered to perform both procedures. Patient preparation for a thyroid uptake procedure is the same as for a thyroid scan.

Thyroid uptake is most commonly assessed with an uptake probe, though a protocol exists for using a gamma camera. Counts are collected over the patient's lower thigh to determine background activity and over the anterior neck for the thyroid. A mathematical equation is used to compute the percentage of the administered radiopharmaceutical that localizes in the thyroid. A normal 24 hour thyroid uptake ranges from 10 to 30%. Below 10% suggests hypothyroidism and above 30% indicates hyperthyroidism.

Parathyroid scan

Since the late 1980s, the parathyroid scan has evolved from using a technically challenging dual radiopharmaceutical protocol to one using a single radiopharmaceutical with early and delayed imaging. The procedure, which requires no patient preparation, is performed to detect the presence of parathyroid adenomas and to guide their surgical extraction. The patient is injected with ^{99m}Tc-sestamibi and then anterior static images of the neck are acquired immediately and approximately two hours after injection. A focal area of increased radiopharmaceutical uptake present on both early and late images is indicative of a parathyroid adenoma (Figure 9.12).

With the development of intraoperative radiation detection probes, radiation accumulation in an adenoma is used to guide its surgical removal. Probe guidance benefits patients by reducing surgical time and scar size.

Adrenal medulla scan

Protocols and radiopharmaceuticals exist for scanning both the adrenal cortex and the adrenal medulla. Nuclear medicine imaging of the adrenal cortex, primarily used in diagnosing Addison's disease or Cushing's disease, has been replaced with CT and MRI (Ziessman *et al.* 2006, p. 105). Medullary imaging is performed infrequently but serves a role in the management of patients with pheochromocytoma or neuroblastoma.

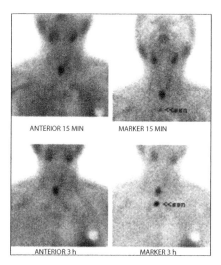

Figure 9.12 Parathyroid study showing an adenoma in the midline of the neck, which could be visualized at 15 minutes.

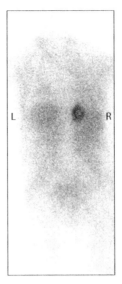

Figure 9.13 A pheochromocytoma is visualized on the patient's right side 18 hours after administering the radiopharmaceutical.

The procedure uses [131]I- or ^{123}I-labeled *meta*-iodobenzylguanidine (mIBG). Based on radiation dosimetry and the fact that many of these procedures are performed on children, ^{123}I-mIBG is preferred. Regardless of the iodine isotope used, the thyroid is blocked by pretreatment with a saturated solution of potassium iodide. Many medications affect adrenergic tissue uptake of mIBG and must be discontinued at an appropriate time prior to the procedure (Ziessman *et al.* 2006, p. 110). The radiopharmaceutical is injected slowly to minimize the potential for adverse reaction. Whole-body imaging may begin as early as four hours after injection with ^{123}I but optimal images are acquired at 24 hours because of the reduced background activity at this point. SPECT imaging is possible and frequently helpful when using ^{123}I-mIBG.

The spleen, liver, heart, and salivary glands routinely take up the radiopharmaceutical. Focal areas of increased mIBG uptake may confirm the presence of the primary tumor and metastases (Figure 9.13).

Gastrointestinal disorders

There are numerous quantitative and qualitative nuclear medicine procedures that assess the gastrointestinal system (table 9.4).

Gastric emptying

Quantitative assessment of gastric motility is accomplished by observing a radiolabeled meal being emptied from the patient's digestive system. Prior to

Table 9.4 Gastrointestinal procedures

Procedure	Radiopharmaceutical	Adult dosage range	Route of administration	Clinical applications
Gastric emptying	^{99m}Tc-sulfur colloid	100 µCi–1 mCi (3.7–37 MBq)	Oral	Assess gastric emptying rate
Liver/spleen	^{99m}Tc-sulfur colloid	2–7 mCi (74–259 MBq)	IV	Detect and evaluate diffuse hepatic parenchymal diseases; evaluation when CT contrast is contraindicated
Hepatobiliary	^{99m}Tc-mebrofenin, ^{99m}Tc-disofenin	3–15 mCi (111–555 MBq)	IV	Evaluate cholecystitis, biliary atresia, bile leaks
Hemangioma	^{99m}Tc-labeled red blood cells	20–30 mCi (740–1110 MBq)	IV	Detect and localize hepatic hemangiomas
Hepatic pump	^{99m}Tc-MAA	1–6 mCi (37–222 MBq)	Pump catheter	Assess position and patency of hepatic arterial perfusion pump
Gastrointestinal bleed	^{99m}Tc-labeled red blood cells	20–30 mCi (740–1110 MBq)	IV	Detection and localization
Meckel's diverticulum	^{99m}Tc-pertechnetate	10–15 mCi (370–555 MBq)	IV	Detection and localization
Denver/LeVeen shunt	^{99m}Tc-MAA	1.5–5 mCi (55.5–187 MBq)	IP	Evaluation of shunt patency
	^{99m}Tc-sulfur colloid	3 mCi (111 MBq)		

IV, intravenous; IP, intraperitoneal; see text for other abbreviations.

the procedure, patients are asked not to eat or drink for six to eight hours and may be asked to stop taking any drugs affecting gastric motility. A ^{99m}Tc-sulfur colloid labeled meal (chicken liver, eggs, or oatmeal) is ingested by the patient over 10–15 minutes so imaging can begin before gastric emptying takes place. The patient is imaged for approximately 90 minutes with a dynamic or static acquisition. The radiolabeled contents are observed moving from the stomach to the small intestines.

Following imaging, the technologist will process the image data to determine the percentage gastric emptying rate. A normal solid emptying rate is

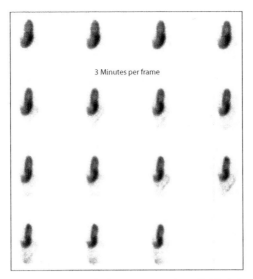

3 Minutes per frame

Figure 9.14   Solid gastric emptying study demonstrating the radiolabeled stomach contents and intestines. Quantitative results would also be presented but are not seen here.

approximately 50% of the contents emptied at 90 minutes, but this varies depending on the normal criteria for the department's patients (Shackett 2009, p. 112).

Qualitatively, images will demonstrate the stomach and small intestines. The radioactivity should slowly decrease in the stomach throughout the study. A patient can have a slower than normal emptying rate or a faster than normal emptying rate depending on the pathology (Figure 9.14).

Gastrointestinal bleeding

Gastrointestinal bleed localization can take place with CT angiography and with imaging using radiolabeled RBC. The patients' RBC are labeled and reinjected. A 60 minute dynamic acquisition of the patient's abdomen is used to detect and localize the bleeding site. The nuclear medicine study is best at assessing bleeds in the lower gastrointestinal tract.

Normally, the heart, liver, and other major vascular structures are visualized. A gastrointestinal bleed is identified as a focal accumulation of radioactivity that increases in intensity and/or size over time and progresses through the bowel (Figure 9.15).

Meckel's diverticulum

Diverticuli composed of gastric mucosa may be detected with ^{99m}Tc-pertechetate imaging. The radiopharmaceutical is administered to the patient and then dynamic imaging is performed for 30–60 minutes. A positive study will demonstrate focally increased radiopharmaceutical uptake in the right lower

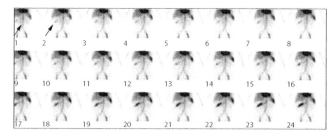

Figure 9.15 Gastrointestinal bleed study. The gastrointestinal bleed is indicated by the arrow.

quadrant that appears at the same time as the radiopharmaceutical appears in the stomach.

Liver and spleen imaging

Liver/spleen imaging began in the 1950s and has changed little since its inception except for the advent of SPECT imaging. The number of liver/spleen procedures has steadily decreased since CT became readily available. Nuclear medicine is unique in that it is the only modality that can image both organs in their entirity rather than cross-sectionally (CT, MRI, sonography). This can provide a better overall picture of both organs and their functional relationship.

Fifteen minutes after the administration of the radiopharmaceutical, a SPECT procedure is performed. The images are processed and transverse, sagittal, and coronal images are produced. A normal liver and spleen demonstrate homogeneous dose distribution throughout both and no bone marrow visualization. The liver and spleen can be quite variable in shape. Diffuse hepatic diseases such as cirrhosis and hepatitis produce non-homogeneous uptake throughout the liver. Focal diseases (liver metastases, cysts, and abscesses) will appear as localized focal decreased areas of uptake.

Hepatobiliary assessment

One of the most frequently performed studies is of the hepatobiliary system to evaluate cholecystitis. The study can also be used to diagnosis biliary atresia, biliary obstruction, and postsurgical bile leaks. The patient should fast for at least two to five hours but not for longer than 12 hours. Patients should also not be taking pain medications that contain opium or morphine derivatives for two to six hours (Christian and Waterstram-Rich 2007). All of these can cause inaccurate results if the gallbladder ejection fraction is calculated.

The patient is given the radiopharmaceutical and imaged dynamically for approximately 60 minutes or until the liver, gallbladder, and small intestines are visualized. The patient is then given an interventional agent, cholecystokinin, to stimulate gallbladder contraction. The patient is again imaged dynamically for approximately 30 minutes to determine the gallbladder

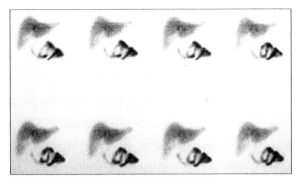

Figure 9.16 Hepatobiliary study, showing visualization of liver and small intestines. Lack of gallbladder visualization at one hour and delayed imaging is suggestive of acute cholecytitis.

ejection fraction. The gallbladder ejection fraction is calculated by drawing regions of interest around the gallbladder and processing the data.

A normal gallbladder ejection fraction is approximately 35% or greater. A value of less than 35% indicates impaired gallbladder contraction suggestive of chronic cholecystitis, cystic duct syndrome, sphincter of Oddi spasm, or gallbladder dyskinesia (Shackett 2009, p. 130). Failure of the gallbladder to visualize is indicative of acute cholecystitis (Figure 9.16) and cholecystokinin would not be administered in these circumstances.

Hemangioma

Hepatic hemangiomas are benign vascular tumors that are often incidentally found on CT or other anatomical imaging techniques. Prior to a biopsy to determine if the tumor is cancerous, physicians will often want to determine if the tumor is a vascular hemangioma to prevent excessive bleeding and/or rupture. The nuclear medicine hemangioma study plays a significant role in this process. The patient's RBC are labeled and reinjected. A SPECT study is performed one to two hours after the radiolabeled RBC are administered. Areas of increased radiopharmaceutical accumulation that correlate with the anatomical tumor site are determined to be hemangiomas (Figure 9.17) because of the blood supply to the area, while decreased or normal areas of uptake require further investigation with biopsy.

Hepatic pump

Patients who have been diagnosed with cancerous liver lesions may receive a hepatic arterial infusion pump so that the chemotherapy can be delivered directly to the cancerous sites. This is necessary because liver tumors receive a majority of their blood supply via the hepatic artery, whereas normal liver tissue receives the majority of its blood supply from the portal vein. Any intravenous treatments will be less effective as a result of this blood supply issue.

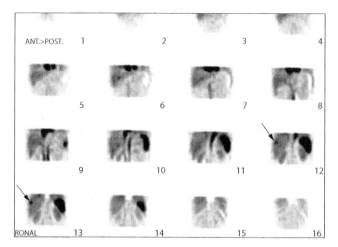

Figure 9.17 A hemangioma can be seen on coronal SPECT views. Normal vasculature is also seen, including the heart, spleen, liver, aorta, and other vascular structures.

Nuclear medicine can assist in confirming the placement and patency of the hepatic pump. A small volume of ^{99m}Tc-labeled macroaggregated albumin (MAA) is injected intraarterially through the hepatic pump catheter by the physician. If the catheter is placed correctly, the radiopharmaceutical uptake will appear non-homogeneous because of the level of radioactivity in the liver lesions versus the minimal localization in the normal liver tissue. If the catheter is not placed correctly and is shunting to the venous system, then the lungs will visualize. If there is extrahepatic perfusion, then the stomach, spleen, and bowel will visualize.

LeVeen/Denver shunt

A LeVeen/Denver shunt assists in draining excess ascites fluid from the peritoneal cavity into the vascular system, usually the right jugular vein. After the fluid is dispersed into the vascular system it is filtered and excreted by the kidneys. To evaluate the patency of this peritoneovenous shunt, the radiopharmaceutical (^{99m}Tc-MAA or ^{99m}Tc-sulfur colloid) is administered intraperitoneally by the physician. The abdomen is imaged with static images every five minutes for 20–30 minutes. After the injection, the radiopharmaceutical distributes compartmentally into the peritoneal cavity and is diluted into the ascites. The 'radioactive ascites' is taken up by the shunt, demonstrating the shunt tubing running from the abdomen to the neck. If the shunt is patent, the lungs or liver will be visualized depending on the radiopharmaceutical injected. Non-patent shunts present persistent abdominal activity and absent or partially absent tubing. In addition, the liver or liver/spleen is not visualized.

Table 9.5 Genitourinary procedures

Procedure	Radiopharmaceutical	Adult dosage range	Route of administration	Clinical applications
Renal function studies	^{99m}Tc-DTPA, ^{99m}Tc-MAG-3	3–20 mCi (111–740 MBq)	IV (bolus)	Evaluate renal function
Cystogram	^{99m}Tc-pertechnetate, ^{99m}Tc-sulfur colloid, ^{99m}Tc-MAG-3	Direct: 0.5–1 mCi (18.5–37 MBq); indirect: 3–10 mCi (111–370 MBq)	Via bladder catheter (direct), IV (indirect)	Evaluate and detect vesicoureteral reflux

IV, intravenous; see text for other abbreviations.

Genitourinary imaging

Nuclear genitourinary imaging encompasses several different procedures; this chapter focuses on the two most commonly performed procedures: renal function studies and cystography (table 9.5).

Renal function

There are two physiological renal processes that can be evaluated with nuclear medicine, glomerular filtration with ^{99m}Tc-DTPA or tubular secretion with ^{99m}Tc-MAG-3. The latter has many advantages for imaging the renal system and is more commonly used (Ziessman *et al.* 2006, p. 219). Both procedures are very similar when imaging. Patients should be well hydrated prior to the study so the radiopharmaceutical excretion and washout will not be delayed. Patients are also asked to empty their bladder prior to beginning the study. Patients may or may not be asked to stay off their medications depending on the physician's preference. Either radiopharmaceutical is injected intravenously while a dynamic flow image is acquired, documenting the blood flow to the kidneys. A one hour dynamic image follows to document the physiological uptake and excretion of the radiopharmaceutical from the kidney. Frequently, a diuretic may be administered half way into the study to differentiate dilation of the renal collecting system from obstruction.

Following the imaging, the technologist processes the images for quantitative data. The physician analyzes the images based on kidney visualization, quantitative graphs, and quantitative values (Figure 9.18). A normal glomerular filtration rate in a healthy young adult is 125 mL/min, while a normal effective renal plasma flow that reflects tubular secretion is 500–600 mL/min. These values decrease normally with ageing (Shackett 2009, p. 252).

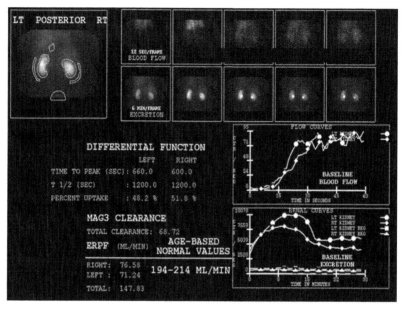

Figure 9.18 Functional renal study using ^{99m}Tc-MAG-3. The patient has decreased tubular secretion associated with a low effective renal plasma flow. The acquired data are compared with the institution's normal age-based values.

Cystography

Nuclear medicine offers an alternative to the radiographic cystogram to assess bladder filling and determine if vesicoureteral reflux is present. This procedure is typically performed in children. The patient must be catheterized and a saline intravenous bag is connected to the catheter to fill the bladder. The radiopharmaceutical is diluted in the saline so the bladder can be seen on the camera along with any other structures that fill with the 'radioactive urine.'

A series of dynamic images are acquired as the bladder is filling. A predicted maximum bladder volume is calculated based on the patient's age and weight to ensure the bladder is not overfilled. The study may be terminated if the patient becomes too uncomfortable, leaks around the catheter, demonstrates bilateral vesicoureteral reflux, or if the maximum volume is reached. The fluid is drained from the bladder or the patient is asked to empty their bladder at the conclusion of the study.

A normal cystogram demonstrates radiopharmaceutical accumulation into the bladder with no radioactivity in either ureter (Figure 9.19A). An abnormal cystogram may demonstrate unilateral or bilateral radiopharmaceutical reflux from the bladder up through the ureter(s) (Figure 9.19B). In severe vesicoureteral reflux, radioactivity may be seen in the kidneys.

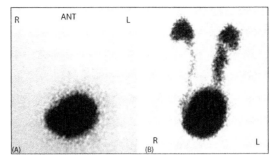

Figure 9.19 Cystography. (A) Radiopharmaceutical accumulation seen in the bladder on a normal cystogram. (B) Bilateral reflux is demonstrated by retrograde movement of the radiopharmaceutical from the bladder, through the ureters, and into the kidneys.

Infection imaging

Several radiopharmaceuticals are available for the detection of occult infection, though each is not suitable for every clinical indication. Because of this, patient history is important in determining which radiopharmaceutical is appropriate. Table 9.6 gives an overview of infection imaging procedures.

Gallium imaging

Gallium-67 citrate scanning has been used for detection of infection for several decades. Though it has shortcomings affecting image quality that are addressed with the newer labeled leukocyte agents, gallium still has a role in specific clinical situations such as immunocompromised patients.

The gallium scan requires no preparation of the patient or the radiopharmaceutical. Imaging does not begin until approximately 24 hours after injection to permit normal excretion of the radiopharmaceutical and clearance

Table 9.6 Infection procedures				
Procedure	**Radiopharmaceutical**	**Adult dosage range**	**Route of administration**	**Clinical applications**
Gallium scan	^{67}Ga-citrate	5–10 mCi (185–370 MBq)	IV	Detection of chronic infection located outside the abdomen, especially in immunocompromised patients
Leukocyte scan	^{111}In-oxine	500 µCi (18.5 MBq)	IV	Detection of acute infection in any location
	^{99m}Tc-HMPAO	10–25 mCi (370–925 MBq)	IV	

IV, intravenous; see text for other abbreviations.

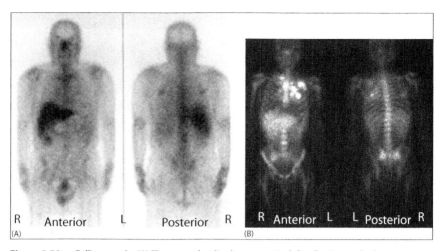

Figure 9.20 Gallium study. (A) The normal radiopharmaceutical distribution to the bone marrow, liver, spleen, salivary and lachrymal glands, external genitalia, bladder, and kidneys. (B) Increased radiopharmaceutical uptake in the mediastinal region at 72 hours, indicating an area of infection.

from the soft tissue. Because of its long half-life, imaging with gallium can continue up to 76 hours after initial injection if needed. A whole-body scan is most commonly performed, though static images of specific areas may also be taken.

Gallium normally localizes in the skeleton, marrow, liver, spleen, salivary and lachrymal glands, external genitalia, bladder, and kidneys (Figure 9.20A). The renal excretory route is active for the first 24–48 hours. Around 48 hours after injection, radiopharmaceutical excretion changes from the kidneys to the gastrointestinal tract, making it visible on later images. An area of infection will present as a focal area of increased radiopharmaceutical uptake that does not move over sequential imaging sessions (Figure 9.20B).

Leukocyte imaging

Two radiopharmaceutical options exist for the labeling of leukocytes: ^{99m}Tc-HMPAO and ^{111}In-oxine. The ^{99m}Tc-labeled option is preferred because it provides less radiation exposure to patients and a larger dose can be given, which improves image quality.

Whichever radiopharmaceutical is utilized, approximately 60 mL of blood must be withdrawn from the patient for radiolabeling. Transportation and labeling time result in a two to three hour delay before the labeled radiopharmaceutical is ready for injection into the patient. Imaging with ^{99m}Tc-labeled leukocytes can begin one to two hours after radiopharmaceutical injection, while imaging with ^{111}In-labeled leukocytes does not begin until approximately 24 hours after injection. A whole-body scan is performed if the location of the infection is unknown or multiple areas of infection are

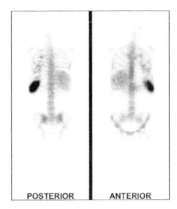

Figure 9.21   Abnormal ^{111}In-labeled leukocytes demonstrating pulmonary infiltrates.

suspected. Static images of a specific area can be taken if the location of interest is known.

For both agents, the spleen shows normal radiopharmaceutical uptake, although it is more intense with the ^{111}In-labeled dose. Liver and bone marrow also visualize with both agents. A lack of care in the radiolabeling process can damage the leukocytes, resulting in lung uptake of the radiopharmaceutical. Any unbound technetium will be excreted through the genitourinary tract, resulting in early visualization of the kidneys and bladder. A scan indicating infection will demonstrate a focal area of increased radiopharmaceutical accumulation (Figure 9.21).

Lymphatic clinical procedures

There are two methods to assess physiological lymphatic flow (table 9.7). The sentinel node study maps the location of the first lymph node(s) draining a lesion site. This approach is primarily used for patients with breast cancer and melanoma, but it can be used in many types of malignancy. The lymphangiogram images the lymphatic flow in extremities to demonstrate blockages in flow.

Sentinel node imaging

The sentinel node study is an important presurgical assessment in the management of cancer patients to minimize the number of lymph nodes removed during surgery. This limits chronic problems such as lymphedema and improves the patient's quality of life. The theory is that if the sentinel node (the first node to which a malignancy drains) can be identified, removed, and analyzed during surgery then the lymphatic excision need go no further if the first draining node is identified as not cancerous. If the node is cancerous, then a wider lymphatic removal process must occur since the cancer has obviously entered the lymphatics and is at a more severe stage.

Table 9.7 Lymphatic procedures

Procedure	Radiopharmaceutical	Adult dosage range	Route of administration	Clinical applications
Sentinel node study	^{99m}Tc-sulfur colloid (filtered and unfiltered)	0.2–7.0 mCi (7.4–259 MBq)	Variable depending on indication and physician (intradermal; intraglandular; periareolar)	Evaluation of lymphatic flow patterns and staging of cancers
Lymphangiogram	^{99m}Tc-sulfur colloid (filtered)	200 μCi–7 mCi (7.4–259 MBq)	Intradermal in the web between fingers or toes	Evaluation of lymphatic drainage for blockage; chronic lymphedema or swollen extremity; primary and secondary lymphedema

This procedure involves multiple injections around the lesion of interest. The administration technique is dependent on the type of malignancy and the physician's preference. The radiopharmaceutical will migrate through the lymphatics draining the cancerous area and be taken up in the first draining node(s). After the radiopharmaceutical is administered and allowed to migrate, the patient is taken to the surgical suite and the surgeon locates the sentinel node with an interoperative probe.

The sentinel node study is not interpreted as positive or negative. The study is performed to locate the first draining lymph node(s) for easier localization and removal during surgery (Figure 9.22). The nuclear physician or

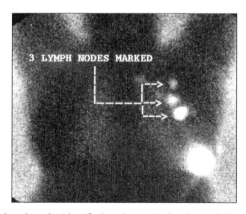

Figure 9.22 Three lymph nodes identified on the sentinel node study. The larger area inferior to the three nodes is the injection site.

radiologist indicates for the report when and how many nodes were detected after radiopharmaceutical injection.

In some instances, no nodes will be visualized, which causes a dilemma. This presentation may occur if the injection is performed at the wrong depth or if the lymphatics are so congested with malignancy that the radiopharmaceutical cannot migrate.

Lymphangiography

The routine lymphangiogram is performed to assess lymphatic flow in an affected extremity and the contralateral extremity for comparison purposes. The ^{99m}Tc-sulfur colloid may be filtered or unfiltered. It is injected into the webs of the fingers or toes and is then drained into the lymphatic system to be cleared by the body. The nuclear medicine technologist typically performs the injections, which occur in two web spaces on each extremity. Imaging begins immediately and may be a series of static images or a dynamic acquisition that demonstrates radiopharmaceutical flow through the extremity. Most frequently, a whole-body scan that includes the entire length of both extremities is utilized.

A normal lymphangiogram study (Figure 9.23A) demonstrates the lymphatic flow through the deep channels to the pelvic lymph nodes and dose accumulation in the liver. An abnormal study will demonstrate the level of lymphatic blockage and severity. Lymphatic blockage is evidenced by radiopharmaceutical flow that progresses to a point in the patient's extremity and then goes no further. The presence of extensive collateral lymphatic channels

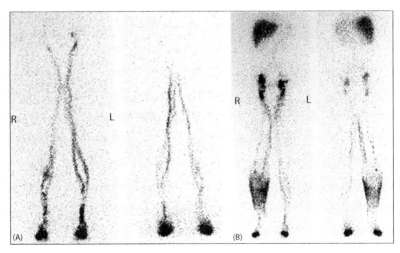

Figure 9.23 Lymphangiography. (A) In the normal situation, radiopharmaceutical accumulation can be seen in the inguinal nodes and liver. This is typically seen in both early (as here) and delayed imaging. (B) Blockage in the right lower extremity is identified by the radiopharmaceutical moving from the deep lymphatic channels to the superficial channels, producing the appearance of 'radioactive skin.' Normal dose accumulation in the liver and pelvic lymph nodes is seen.

and/or the identification of dermal backflow, which occurs when the injected dose cannot be pulled into the lymphatics and so causes a large area of radioactive skin, indicates abnormality in the lymphatic system (Figure 9.23B).

Non-imaging procedures

Nuclear medicine procedures that do not involve imaging are fairly rare in nuclear medicine departments because of the sensitivity and specificity of many blood chemistry tests. Two primary procedures fall in the non-imaging category, including the test for *Helicobacter pylori* and studies of RBC mass and plasma volume (table 9.8). These procedures assess the patient's physiology by counting samples such as urine, RBCs, plasma, and breath instead of imaging.

Helicobacter pylori test

The *H. pylori* test is a procedure that detects the presence of gastric urease as an aid in the diagnosis of *H. pylori* infection as this bacterial species is commonly found in patients suffering from gastric or duodenal ulcers. Its eradication is an essential part of treatment of ulcers.

Patients should not eat or drink for six hours prior to the test, should not have taken any antibiotics or bismuth for one month prior to the test, or any proton pump inhibitors for two weeks prior to the test (Shackett 2009, p. 48). Patients swallow a capsule of ^{14}C-labeled urea with water without handling or chewing the capsule, which could alter the results. After ten minutes, a sample of the patient's breath is collected in a mylar balloon supplied by the manufacturing company. The breath sample is typically sent back to the

Table 9.8 Non-imaging procedures

Procedure	Radiopharmaceutical	Adult dosage range	Route of administration	Clinical applications
Helicobacter pylori breath test	^{14}C-urea	1 µCi (0.037 MBq)	Oral	Detect gastric urease to aid in diagnosis of *H. pylori*
Red cell mass	^{51}Cr-labeled red blood cells	10–30 µCi (0.37–1.11 MBq)	IV	Evaluate polycythemia vera, anemia, trauma, blood loss replacement therapy
Plasma volume	^{123}I-serum albumin	10 µCi (0.37 MBq)	IV	

IV, intravenous; see text for other abbreviations.

manufacturing company for counting in a liquid scintillation counter or it may be processed in the department.

Patients who do not have *H. pylori* in the stomach will excrete the ^{14}C in their urine, while patients with the bacteria will excrete the radioactivity in their breath as a result of hydrolysis of the urea to carbon dioxide and ammonia by the bacterial urease. The ^{14}C-labeled carbon dioxide enters the patient's bloodstream and is transported to the lungs to be exhaled. Patient samples with high amounts of radioactivity are considered as positive for *H. pylori*, while samples with low amounts of radioactivity are considered normal.

Red cell mass and plasma volume

Procedures to measure the RBC mass and plasma volume are indicated in patients suspected of having polycythemia vera, or overproduction of RBCs. The study is really two separate procedures that are performed simultaneously. The red cell mass study utilizes ^{51}Cr-labeled RBC, while the plasma volume utilizes ^{125}I-human serum albumin. The technologist follows the procedure protocol and administers the two radiopharmaceuticals intravenously and waits a period of time before drawing a sample of the patient's blood. The RBC and plasma samples are counted in a well counter after several complex separation and dilution techniques, and the results are calculated. These results are compared with a departmental chart of normal values. The plasma volume range is 30–45 mL/kg for males and females, while the RBC volume ranges are 25–35 mL/kg for males and 20–30 mL/kg for females (Shackett 2009, p. 241). Currently, there is also an option to use an automated total blood volume system that performs the complex steps of this protocol automatically (Manzone *et al.* 2007).

Oncology

Nuclear medicine offers a variety of procedures for the localization and assessment of suspected and proven cancers. In most instances, the nuclear medicine procedure is not considered the gold standard for initial diagnosis but is utilized to detect metastatic spread after initial diagnosis and tumor recurrence after surgery or therapy. Table 9.9 lists the oncological imaging procedures that will be reviewed.

Somatostatin receptor imaging

There is a category of malignant tumors, known as neuroendocrine tumors, which secrete hormones and have somatostatin receptors on their cell membranes. Specific malignancies in this category include carcinoid tumors, gastrinomas, pheochromocytomas, and insulinomas.

Table 9.9 Oncological imaging procedures

Procedure	Radiopharmaceutical	Adult dosage range	Route of administration	Clinical applications
Somatostatin receptor imaging	^{111}In-pentetreotide	6 mCi (222 MBq)	IV	Detect primary and metastatic neuroendocrine tumors, neuroblastoma
Prostate cancer	^{111}In-capromab pendetide	5 mCi (185 MBq)	IV	Detection and localization
Scintimammography	^{99m}Tc-sestamibi	25 mCi (925 MBq)	IV	Detection and localization in primary breast carcinoma and axillary metastases
PET imaging	^{18}F-FDG	10–20 mCi (370–740 MBq)	IV	Detection and localization of primary and metastatic cancers including head and neck, lymphoma, lung, colorectal

IV, intravenous; see text for other abbreviations.

Indium-111 pentetreotide is a radiolabeled synthetic form of somatostatin. The radiopharmaceutical will accumulate in neuroendocrine tumors or their metastases, producing abnormally increased uptake on the images.

Imaging using ^{111}In-pentetreotide typically occurs at 4 and 24 hours after radiopharmaceutical injection to permit adequate time for radiopharmaceutical accumulation in areas of abnormality. Since spread of the primary tumor is always a consideration, whole-body imaging is typically performed from the anterior and posterior. At the 24 hour imaging session, SPECT images of the primary tumor location may be performed for added diagnostic information.

Images from this procedure will demonstrate normal uptake of the radiopharmaceutical in the pituitary, thyroid, liver, spleen, kidneys, and bladder (Figure 9.24A). Normal bowel clearance of the radiopharmaceutical will be visualized on the 24 hour images. Generalized lung uptake of the radiopharmaceutical may be present in patients who have recently completed radiation therapy owing to residual inflammation. Recent surgical and colostomy sites may also accumulate this radiopharmaceutical. Figure 9.24B shows abnormal uptake with dose accumulation in the liver.

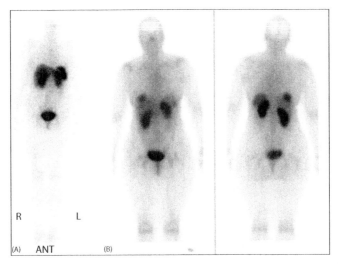

Figure 9.24   Indium-111 pentetreotide study. (A) In the normal situation, there is typical uptake in the liver, spleen, kidneys, and bladder. (B) Here there is a focal area of abnormal radiopharmaceutical accumulation in the dome of the liver at four hours.

Prostate cancer imaging

Indium-111 capromab pendetide is a monoclonal antibody radiopharmaceutical used to detect tumor recurrence in the prostate fossa and disease spread into pelvic lymph nodes in patients with diagnosed prostate cancer. Scan results aid in staging and determining the effective treatment management.

The dose is injected into the patient slowly over five minutes to reduce the probability of an adverse reaction. An initial set of SPECT and planar images is acquired at 30 minutes after injection to produce a vascular map of the pelvic area. This map aids the interpreting physician in differentiating normal vascular areas from abnormal areas of radiopharmaceutical accumulation on later images. The delayed images to demonstrate radiopharmaceutical localization may be acquired at 48, 72, 96, and 120 hours after radiopharmaceutical injection. A hemi-body scan from head to mid-femur and a SPECT acquisition of the pelvis are the typical images acquired at each session.

Normal areas of radiopharmaceutical activity include the blood pool, bone marrow, liver, and spleen. Focal areas of increased uptake in the prostate fossa indicate tumor recurrence while uptake in any lymph nodes indicates metastatic spread of the disease (Figure 9.25).

Scintimammography

Scintimammography is considered a second-line diagnostic tool, after mammography, to evaluate patients with breast lesions detected by palpation or mammogram. Images are taken of the breasts to assess primary tumors and

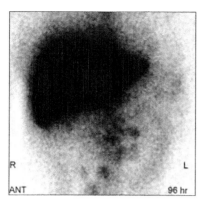

Figure 9.25 Indium-111 capromab pendetide scan demonstrates radiopharmaceutical accumulation in the abdominal and pelvic lymph nodes.

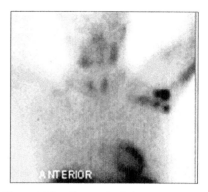

Figure 9.26 Abnormal scintimammogram with left axillary uptake of the radiopharmaceutical.

axillary images are acquired to assess lymph nodes for metastatic spread. Clinical use of this procedure is increasing with the recent development of dedicated breast imaging cameras, which are smaller and easier to position than traditional gamma cameras.

For a scintimammogram, the radiopharmaceutical must be injected in the arm contralateral to the side of the breast lesion. If the patient has lesions in both breasts, then the dose is injected through a vein in the top of the foot (Shackett 2009, p. 270). This injection technique is used to reduce the probability that dose infiltration will result in axillary pooling, which may obscure uptake in lymph nodes on the side of interest.

Imaging begins 5 to 10 minutes after radiopharmaceutical injection. A lateral static view of each breast is acquired along with an anterior view of the chest with the patient's arms overhead to expose the axillary area.

The heart will demonstrate increased uptake of the radiopharmaceutical since the radiopharmaceutical is also used for cardiac imaging. Focal areas of increased uptake in the breast are indicative of primary tumor. Focal areas of increased uptake in the axilla indicate the presence of metastatic lesions (Figure 9.26).

Glucose metabolism imaging

Imaging cancerous tissue with radioactive glucose is ideal since most cancerous cells metabolize glucose at a rate approximately five times higher than surrounding normal cells. It should be noted that not all cancers demonstrate this higher glucose metabolism rate, which is why a thorough cancer history is needed to determine if PET imaging is appropriate.

Patient preparation for the scan includes no food or drinks other than water for approximately six to eight hours prior to radiopharmaceutical injection. This preparation places the body in a glucose-starved state so that uptake of the ^{18}F-FDG is maximized. As low insulin levels reduce muscle uptake of the radiopharmaceutical, an adequate insulin level is ensured by checking the patient's blood sugar prior to injection of ^{18}F-FDG. Optimal serum glucose level is below 1.5 g/L, though adequate images can be obtained in patients as long as the serum glucose level is below 2.0 g/L (Mettler & Guiberteau 2006).

After the radiopharmaceutical is injected through an intravenous catheter, the patient relaxes in a room for 60 to 90 minutes before scanning begins. The duration of the wait depends upon the patient's type of cancer. During the waiting period, the patient should not undergo any physical exercise and should be kept warm to avoid abnormal distribution of the radiopharmaceutical to the muscles through shivering.

After the radiopharmaceutical has localized, the patient is placed supine on the PET imaging bed. On state-of-the-art PET/CT hybrid cameras, the entire scanning session lasts 20 minutes or less. These two imaging methods are complementary to one another in that the PET scan provides metabolic information while the CT scan provides anatomical information. Images created by fusing the PET and CT data provide optimal information for diagnostic assessment.

Normal areas of ^{18}F-FDG accumulation include the brain, myocardium, liver, bone marrow, kidneys, and bladder (Mettler & Guiberteau 2006) (Figure 9.27A). Many other anatomical structures may also demonstrate uptake of radioactivity based on patient age, medications, and surgical sites. Abnormalities present as focal areas of increased radiopharmaceutical uptake, particularly in the lymph nodes and at the site of the primary tumor (Figure 9.27B).

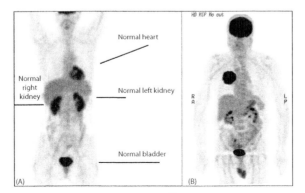

Figure 9.27 Positron emission tomography using ^{18}F-fluorodeoxyglucose to assess excessive glucose metabolism in tumors. (A) Normal areas of uptake are noted, excluding the brain. (B) Here there is abnormal increased uptake in the right lung region.

Respiratory function

Ventilation and perfusion lung imaging for the detection of pulmonary emboli have been performed for decades in nuclear medicine departments. Since the end of the 1990s, there has been a reduction in the number of scans ordered as CT has gained prominence in the detection of pulmonary emboli. Table 9.10 identifies the radiopharmaceuticals available for both the ventilation and perfusion portions of the scan.

The ventilation scan is typically performed first using ^{133}Xe gas or ^{99m}Tc-DTPA aerosol. Both radiopharmaceuticals are inhaled by the patient through a special breathing apparatus and require a high level of patient cooperation. When using ^{133}Xe gas, the dynamic ventilation images are acquired as the patient inhales the radiopharmaceutical since it does not remain in the respiratory system. Since ^{99m}Tc-DTPA is administered as an aerosol, it adheres to the airway, permitting multiple images to be taken after the patient has completed inhalation of the radiopharmaceutical.

After the ventilation imaging is completed, the patient is administered ^{99m}Tc-MAA intravenously. The syringe is agitated prior to injection to suspend the particles throughout the volume and the dose is injected with the patient lying supine. Failure to do these things may result in an abnormal distribution of the dose within the lungs, making image interpretation difficult. Six to eight static images of the lungs from various angles are then acquired.

The diagnosis of pulmonary embolism is most accurately made using ventilation and perfusion images along with chest radiographs taken within 24 hours of the nuclear medicine procedure. In general terms, a pulmonary embolism results in reduced blood flow to the affected lung segment on the perfusion scan, while causing no visual changes on the ventilation scan or the radiograph. In patients with chronic obstructive pulmonary disease, the

Table 9.10 Respiratory procedures

Procedure	Radiopharmaceutical	Adult dosage range	Route of administration	Clinical applications
Perfusion scan	^{99m}Tc-MAA	4 mCi (148 MBq)	IV	Diagnosis pulmonary embolism by ventilation–perfusion mismatch
Ventilation scan	^{133}Xe gas	4–20 mCi (185–740 MBq)	Inhalation	Diagnosis pulmonary embolism by ventilation–perfusion mismatch
	^{99m}Tc-DTPA aerosol	25–35 mCi (900–1300 MBq)	Inhalation	

IV, intravenous; see text for other abbreviations.

ventilation scan typically shows mottled radiopharmaceutical distribution throughout the lungs with retention and slower than normal clearing of ^{133}Xe from the lungs.

Skeletal clinical procedures

Nuclear skeletal imaging is one of the most commonly performed nuclear medicine procedures and is used predominantly to image skeletal metastases. The general imaging protocol (bone scan or three-phase scan) is determined based on the patient's indication and history. Three primary diagnostic nuclear medicine procedures assess the skeletal system (table 9.11).

Whole-body bone scan

Prior to administering the radiopharmaceutical or performing the scan, it is important for the nuclear medicine technologist to do a full assessment of the patient's history. The nuclear medicine technologist interviews the patient to assess the relevant history, including cancer, trauma, and pain. A nuclear medicine physician or radiologist requires the history to interpret the physiological skeletal images accurately.

Patient preparation for the nuclear bone scan primarily takes place between dose administration and imaging. After injection of the radiopharmaceutical, patients are asked to follow several instructions to increase the quality of the image and decrease their radiation exposure. Patients are instructed to drink liquids to promote hydration, which encourages soft tissue clearance of the

Table 9.11 Skeletal procedures

Procedure	Radiopharmaceutical	Adult dosage range	Route of administration	Clinical applications
Whole body bone scan	^{99m}Tc-MDP, ^{99m}Tc-HDP	20–30 mCi (740–1110 MBq)	IV	Detection and staging of bone metastases; evaluation of benign and primary malignant bone lesions; assessment of bone viability
Three-phase bone scan	^{99m}Tc-MDP, ^{99m}Tc-HDP	20–30 mCi (740–1110 MBq)	IV (bolus injection)	Differentiate osteomyelitis from cellulitis; evaluation of prosthesis for loosening or infection
PET bone scan	^{18}F-sodium fluoride	10–20 mCi (370–740 MBq)	IV	Detect benign and malignant bone disease

IV, intravenous; see text for other abbreviations.

radiopharmaceutical and subsequent excretion. Radiopharmaceutical elimination from the soft tissue increases the count ratio of target (bone) to background (soft tissue), resulting in more resolved images. Two to three hours after administration of the bone imaging agent, patients are imaged. The time delay allows sufficient uptake of the phosphorus compound in the bone matrix and further elimination of the radiopharmaceutical from the soft tissue. Immediately prior to imaging, patients are asked to use the restroom to empty their bladder. This decreases the likelihood for increased uptake in the bladder, which could mask any abnormalities in the pelvis.

The whole-body bone scan images from head to toe utilizing a dual head camera to scan both the anterior and posterior sides. The camera slowly moves over the patient who is lying supine on the imaging table. Following the whole-body scan, the technologist may follow up with static bone images of more specific areas of the skeleton or areas that may have overlapped during the whole-body scan (e.g. scapula and ribs). SPECT imaging may also be used to further evaluate vertebral lesions.

A normal bone scan demonstrates symmetrical radiopharmaceutical uptake on both the right and left sides of the patient (Figure 9.28A). Any areas demonstrating increased or decreased radiopharmaceutical uptake are evaluated by the radiologist as abnormalities or artifacts. Most skeletal abnormalities demonstrate as increased radiopharmaceutical uptake; hence the importance of the patient's medical history for interpretation.

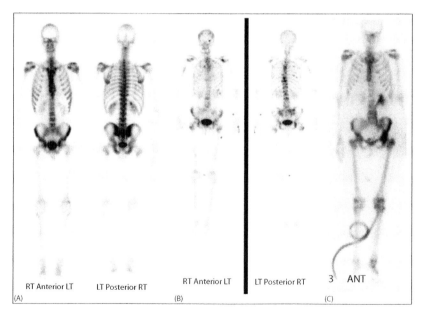

RT Anterior LT   LT Posterior RT   RT Anterior LT   LT Posterior RT   3   ANT
(A)   (B)   (C)

Figure 9.28 Whole-body bone scans. (A) The normal image. (B) The occurrence of bone metastases. (C) Bone scan demonstrating attenuation artifact, catheter, and renal dose retention in the left kidney.

Abnormalities that result in increased uptake include metastatic bone lesions, trauma such as fractures, Paget's disease, and degenerative joint disease (Figure 9.28B). Common artifacts that attenuate the photons to create focal decreased areas of uptake include pacemakers, prostheses, and implants (Figure 9.28C).

Three-phase bone scan

Most commonly, the three-phase study is used to differentiate osteomyelitis from cellulitis. The technologist positions the camera over the anatomical area of the suspected abnormality. Once the positioning is accurate, the technologist injects the radiopharmaceutical and begins imaging immediately to obtain the flow of the radiopharmaceutical to the area of interest. The dynamic acquisition consists of brief sequential images taken one after the other. This dynamic acquisition usually continues for one to two minutes. This acquisition is followed by static images of the area and then more imaging after a delay of two to three hours to allow the dose to incorporate.

The three phases are necessary for an accurate interpretation of the study as infection of the bone or soft tissue. A study that is positive for osteomyelitis will demonstrate increased uptake in all three phases (dynamic, immediate statics, and delayed statics) (Figure 9.29), whereas a study that is negative for osteo-myelitis will not demonstrate increased uptake on the delayed static images.

Bone scan for physiological information

Patient preparation is similar for a PET bone scan to that for general gamma bone imaging. After obtaining a complete history, the patient is injected with approximately 370 MBq (10 mCi) of ^{18}F-sodium fluoride. A delay time of 60 minutes is recommended before imaging for the PET radiopharmaceutical. Often this involves the patient waiting in a lead-shielded waiting room resting in a recliner and watching television.

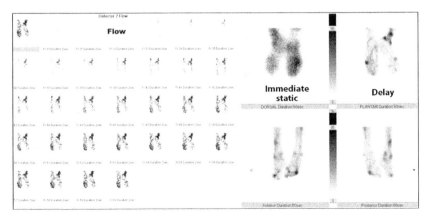

Figure 9.29 Positive three phase bone scan with increased activity in the left foot during flow, immediate static and delayed imaging.

The patient is scanned in the PET/CT scanner for approximately 15–30 minutes. The patient lies supine as the scanner acquires the CT image of the patient for attenuation correction and anatomical localization. The PET procedure immediately follows the CT. The PET scan involves imaging the patient for several bed positions. The result is a three-dimensional image of the patient's entire skeleton with both anatomical (CT) and physiological (PET) information. Interpretation of the PET/CT scan is similar in assessment of increased and decreased radiopharmaceutical uptake.

Radionuclide therapy procedures

Nuclear medicine offers several therapeutic procedures utilizing unsealed radiation sources. The procedures and the pathological conditions they treat are outlined in table 9.12.

Table 9.12 Therapeutic procedures

Procedure	Radiopharmaceutical	Adult dosage range	Route of administration	Clinical applications
Thyroid therapy	^{131}I-sodium iodide	Variable	Oral	Treatment hyperthyroidism and some thyroid cancers
Bone pain palliation	^{89}Sr-strontium chloride	4 mCi (148 MBq)	IV (slow rate)	Reduce pain in patients with bone metastases
	^{153}Sm-lexidronam	1 mCi/kg (37 MBq/kg)	IV (slow rate)	
Polycythemia vera	^{32}P-sodium phosphate	3–5 mCi (111–185 MBq)	IV	Reduce overabundance of red blood cells
Non-Hodgkin's lymphoma	^{111}In-ibritumomab tiuxetan	5 mCi (185 MBq)	IV	Biodistribution infusion
	^{90}Y-ibritumomab tiuxetan	0.4 mCi/kg (platelets $> 150 \times 10^9$/L) or 0.3 mCi/kg (platelets 100×10^9 to 150×10^9/L)	IV	Therapeutic infusion
	^{131}I-tositumomab	5 mCi (185 MBq)	IV	Dosimetric infusion
		30–200 mCi (1110–7400 MBq)	IV	Therapeutic infusion

IV, intravenous; see text for other abbreviations.

Thyroid therapy

Thyroid therapy procedures are performed using ^{131}I-sodium iodide in liquid or capsule form. Of all the radiopharmaceuticals used to assess the thyroid, the radiation dosimetry of ^{131}I makes it the only suitable radiopharmaceutical for effectively destroying overactive thyroid tissue and well-differentiated thyroid cancers.

Patient preparation for thyroid therapy is the same as for a thyroid uptake procedure. In patients with primary hyperthyroidism, a therapeutic dosage may be computed using gland size and the radioiodine uptake value, with doses commonly ranging from 185 to 1110 MBq (5–30 mCi). Multiple treatments may be administered over time to keep the condition under control.

In patients with well-differentiated thyroid cancer, the initial radioiodine treatment follows surgical resection and is intended to ablate any remaining cancerous tissue in the thyroid bed along with any metastases. The dose of radioiodide may be as high as 300 mCi for an ablation or treatment of thyroid cancer metastases. Additional therapy procedures may be performed later if recurrence of cancer is noted.

Bone pain palliation

Approximately 50% of patients with breast or prostate cancer develop skeletal metastases (Robinson *et al.* 1992). For many, these metastases cause intractable pain and a loss in ambulatory capacity. Two radiopharmaceuticals, ^{89}Sr-strontium chloride and ^{153}Sm-lexidronam, are currently used to reduce skeletal pain in these patients and improve quality of life.

For both radiopharmaceuticals, the patient must have confirmed bone metastases. The radiopharmaceutical is administered through a secure intravenous line to ensure it is not injected outside the circulatory system. Since both radiopharmaceuticals are high-energy beta emitters, the patient does not have to be hospitalized after injection since they pose little hazard to those around them. Pain relief generally occurs within 7 to 10 days after therapy and may last for a variable period of time. Retreatment may occur at intervals of 10 weeks. Complete blood count should be monitored periodically after treatment since this therapy results in bone marrow suppression, which may require medical attention.

Polycythemia vera treatment

Polycythemia vera is a condition in which the bone marrow makes an excessive quantity of RBC, causing the blood to thicken and placing the patient at increased risk for blood clots and resulting tissue infarction.

Phosphorus-32 sodium phosphate is injected through an established intravenous line to avoid infiltration into the soft tissue. It localizes in the bone matrix and irradiates the nearby bone marrow, resulting in reduced blood counts. The patient's blood count may require monitoring since all blood components will be reduced, not just the RBC.

Reduced RBC counts are typically seen within 10 to 12 weeks after therapy. Retreatment can occur in three months if no response is noted, with the second dose 25% greater than the initial. Treatment can be repeated up to three times but retreatment doses should never exceed 7 mCi.

Non-Hodgkin's lymphoma treatment

Two radioimmunotherapy treatments are available for patients with non-Hodgkin's lymphoma (NHL): ^{90}Y-ibritumomab tiuxetan and ^{131}I-tositumomab. Both radiopharmaceuticals provide tumor-targeted therapy directed toward the CD20 antigen found on normal and malignant B cell lymphocytes. The treatment is radiological since a beta-emitting radionuclide is used to cause cell destruction, yet it is also immunological in nature since it creates an immune response that damages tumor cells. It should be noted that at the present time use of these radiopharmaceuticals is limited to patients who have failed to respond to traditional therapies or whose cancer has returned after traditional therapy.

Yttrium-90 ibritumomab tiuxetan is used in patients meeting specific criteria relative to platelet count and percentage of bone marrow demonstrating disease. The amount of radioactivity administered is also determined based on platelet count in an attempt to reduce drastic blood count reduction. Because of the extent of bone marrow suppression that follows this therapy, patients must be screened carefully to ensure that their bone marrow can withstand the treatment.

The patient is pretreated with non-radioactive rituximab to saturate normal CD20 binding sites and to protect the critical organ, which is the spleen. Within four hours of the conclusion of the rituximab infusion, the patient is given ^{111}In-ibritumomab tiuxetan intravenously. The ^{111}In label permits imaging with a gamma camera 48–72 hours after administration to document biodistribution and determine if the patient can proceed with the radiotherapy. If the biodistribution is acceptable, then the patient is given rituximab followed by ^{90}Y-ibritumomab tiuxetan approximately seven days after the biodistribution is documented. Blood count is monitored closely after therapy.

Iodine-131 tositumomab is the other radioimmunotherapy agent available for the treatment of NHL. It is similar to ^{90}Y-ibritumomab in that blood count assessment before and after therapy is important. With this radiopharmaceutical, thyroid protection is necessary since the radiopharmaceutical may contain free ^{131}I.

The treatment protocol is similar to that with ^{90}Y-ibritumomab tiuxetan yet more complex. Pretreatment with a supersaturated sodium iodide solution begins 24 hours prior to the procedure and continues until 14 days after the final therapy infusion. On the first day, an infusion of the non-radioactive immunological agent is administered to bind normal CD20 sites. Next a small dose of ^{131}I-tositumomab is administered intravenously so biodistribution can be imaged and quantified over the next 24 to 72 hours. The biodistribution quantification will determine if the patient is a candidate for therapy and how much radioactivity should be administered.

If the patient is a candidate for therapy, then non-radioactive tositumomab is administered intravenously followed by the ^{131}I-tositumomab. This therapeutic infusion may occur as soon as seven days or as late as 14 days after biodistribution documentation.

In patients studied to date, both radiopharmaceuticals demonstrate higher response and efficacy rates than the non-radioactive immunotherapy treatment.

Summary

Nuclear pharmacists benefit from knowledge of how radiopharmaceuticals are utilized in the nuclear medicine department and applied to patient care. This knowledge will enhance a pharmacist's ability to effectively communicate with nuclear medicine technologists, to problem solve, and to critically think about clinical situations.

Self-assessment questions

1 What nuclear medicine procedure or procedures utilize the following radiopharmaceuticals?
   a ^{99m}Tc sulfur colloid
   b ^{111}In-pentetreotide
   c ^{89}Sr-chloride
   d ^{99m}Tc-sestamibi
   e ^{99m}Tc-DTPA
   f ^{99m}Tc-MDP
   g ^{99m}Tc-mebrofenin.
2 What nuclear medicine procedure or procedure combination is used to assess each of the following conditions?
   a pulmonary embolism
   b myocardial infarction
   c breast cancer
   d gall stones
   e neuroblastoma
   f Alzheimer's dementia
   g osteomyelitis.

---

3 Provide at least one example of a nuclear medicine procedure for each of the following image acquisition methods:

 a dynamic

 b static

 c gated

 d SPECT

 e PET.

4 Name a radiopharmaceutical commonly administered by the following routes:

 a oral

 b intravenous

 c intrathecal.

References

Christian PE, Waterstram-Rich KM (2007) *Nuclear Medicine and PET, Technology and Techniques*, 6th edn. New York: Elsevier Mosby, p. 541.

Di Carli MF (2004). Advances in positron emission tomography. *J Nucl Cardiol* 11: 719–732.

Manzone TA *et al.* (2007). Blood volume analysis: a new technique and new clinical interest reinvigorate a classic study. *J Nucl Med Technol* 35: 55–63.

Mettler FA, Guiberteau MJ (2006). *Essentials of Nuclear Medicine Imaging*, 5th edn. Philadelphia, PA: Saunders Elsevier.

Robinson RG *et al.* (1992). Radionuclide therapy of intractable bone pain: emphasis on strontium-89. *Semin Nucl Med* 22: 28–32.

Shackett P (2009). *Nuclear Medicine Technology: Procedures and Quick Reference*, 2nd edn. Philadelphia, PA: Lippincott, Williams & Wilkins.

Ziessman HA *et al.* (2006) *Nuclear Medicine: The Requisites*, 3rd edn. Philadelphia, PA: Mosby Elsevier.

Chapter 1

1	b	7	b
2	d	8	d
3	c	9	a
4	e	10	e
5	a	11	c
6	c		

Chapter 2

1   Neutrons, protons, and electrons.

2   The major components of the nucleus: protons and neutrons.

3   Isotopes differ in number of neutrons and atomic number. Isobars differ in number of neutron and protons. Isomers differ in excitation; one is in an excited, metastable state. Isotones differ in number of protons and in atomic number. Ions differ in net electrical charge owing to excess or deficiency in electrons.

4   Gravitational, electromagnetic (coulombic), strong interaction (strong nuclear), and weak interaction (weak nuclear).

5   Strong interaction (strong nuclear) is most important, then weak interaction (weak nuclear), electromagnetic (coulombic), and finally gravitational.

6   (a) 263.3 MeV; (b) 8.23 MeV/nucleon. These are calculated as follows. For ^{32}P, $A = 32$ and $Z = 15$ (15 protons). Since $A = Z + N$, there are 17 neutrons. Finding the mass units for these using the standards at the beginning of the chapter (proton $= 1.00728$ AMU, neutron $= 1.00867$ AMU): $15(1.00728) + 17(1.00867) = 32.2566$ AMU. The unit difference is $32.2566 - 31.9739 = 0.2826$ AMU. Since 1 AMU $= 931.5$ MeV, 0.2826 AMU $\times 931.5$ MeV/AMU $= 263.3$ MeV (answer a). Then 263.3 MeV/31 nucleons $= 8.23$ MeV/nucleon (answer b).

7   As the ratio increases in relative neutron abundance, beta emission tends to dominate. As the ratio increases in relative

proton abundance, positron emission and electron capture tend to dominate.

8 Alpha decay is by

$$^A_Z X_N \rightarrow ^{A-4}_{Z-2} Y_{N-2} + ^4_2 He^{2+}.$$

Beta decay is by

neutron → positron + antineutrino.

Positron decay is by

positron → neutron + neutrino.

9 Alpha decay.

10 Gamma, beta, positron, rarely alpha decay.

11 Excitation and ionization.

12 Beta emission.

13 (a) Beta and other; (b) positron and other; (c) gamma.

14 The half-life equals $0.693/\lambda$, where λ is the decay constant. So $\lambda = 0.693/14.262$, which is $0.04859/day$ ($0.04859 \, day^{-1}$).

15 Half-life equals $0.693/\lambda$, where λ is the decay constant. So half-life is $0.693/0.0825$, which is $8.400 \, h$.

16 $550 \, \mu Ci = 0.55 \, mCi$ and $1 \, mCi = 37 \, MBq$. So $0.55/1 \times 37 = 20.35 \, MBq$.

17 $37 \, MBq = 1 \, mCi$. So $132 \, MBq$ is equal to $132/37 \times 1$, which is $3.6 \, mCi$.

18 $1 \, MBq = 1 \times 10^6 \, dps$. So $5.15 \times 10^7 \, dps$ ($51.5 \times 10^6 \, dps$) is equal to $51.5 \, MBq$.

19 $1 \, MBq = 1 \times 10^6 \, dps$ and $37 \, MBq = 1 \, mCi$. So $13.25 \, mCi = 37 \times 13.25 \, MBq = 490 \, MBq$. This is equal to $490 \times 10^6 \, dps$ (or $4.90 \times 10^8 \, dps$).

20 Radioactivity decay is given by the equation $A_t = A_0 e^{-\lambda t}$. The decay constant λ is given by $0.693/half$-life; so for a half-life of $6.02 \, h$, λ is 0.1155.

    a   At 10 am, $A_t = 19 \, mCi$ ($703 \, MBq$). Time zero is $8{:}00 \, am$ (A_0) and $t = 2 \, h$.

$$19 = A_0 e^{-(0.1155)(2)} = A_0 e^{-0.2310}.$$
$$A_0 = 19/e^{-0.2310} = 23.9 \, mCi \, (885 \, MBq).$$ This is the radioactivity at $8{:}00 \, am$.

    b   From 10:00 am to 5:00 pm is $7 \, h$. So $A_0 = 19 \, mCi$, $t = 7$, and $A_t = 19 e^{-(0.1155)(7)} = 19 e^{-0.8085} = 8.47 \, mCi \, (313 \, MBq)$. This is the radioactivity at $5{:}00 \, pm$.

21 $\ln N/N_0 = -\lambda t$, where N is quantity at time t, N_0 is quantity at time 0, and λ is the decay constant.

    a $\ln(187.5/750) = -1.3863 = -\lambda t$
$$\lambda = 1.3863/16 = 0.0866/day \, (0.0866 \, day^{-1}).$$

    b   The half-life is given by $0.693/\lambda$, which is $0.693/0.0866$ or 8.0 days.

22 The decay constant λ for ^{99m}Tc is given by 0.693/6.02, which is 0.1151/h.

$$6.02\,h = 2.17 \times 10^4\,s. \text{ So}$$
$$\lambda = 0.693/(2.17 \times 10^4\,s) = 3.19 \times 10^{-5}/s.$$

a $A = 8\,mCi$

$$A = 8 \times (37 \times 10^6\,dps) = 2.96 \times 10^8\,dps.$$
$$N = A/\lambda = (96 \times 10^8\,dps)/(3.19 \times 10^{-5}/s) = 9.28 \times 10^{12}\,atoms.$$

b   1 mol ^{99m}Tc $= 6.02 \times 10^{23}$ atoms. Therefore, the mass of ^{99m}Tc in 8 mCi (296 MBq) is $(9.28 \times 10^{12}$ atoms$)(99\,g/mol)/$ $(6.02 \times 10^{23}\,g/mol)$. This is 1.53×10^{-9}g or 1.53 ng.

23 Roentgen measures exposure to gamma and X-rays, and only in air. Rad (radiation absorbed dose) is the absorbed dose from either particulate or electromagnetic radiation. Rem (roentgen equivalent man) quantifies equivalent or effective dose, relating absorbed dose to the effective biological damage. A quality factor is used. Gray (Gy) is the deposition of one joule of energy per kilogram of a material by any type of radiation. 1 Gy = 100 rads. Sievert is the absorbed dose (Gy) multiplied by a quality factor 1 Sv = 100 Rem.

24 Alpha is the most damaging as it is very massive and it carries a 2+ charge, allowing many ionizations to occur.

25 Gamma radiation has the longest range. It is uncharged and electro-magnetic so it does not interact with matter as much as particles do.

Chapter 3

1	True	6	a
2	c	7	False
3	True	8	d
4	c	9	a
5	d	10	a

Chapter 4

1	d	5	d
2	a	6	False
3	False	7	f
4	True		

Chapter 5

1	a	6	False
2	d	7	d
3	b	8	True
4	d	9	a
5	a	10	c

Chapter 6

1   Technetium-99m-labeled red blood cells would be appropriate for blood
     pool imaging. Iodine-125-labeled human serum albumin is confined to
     the plasma but has primary gamma energy of 30 keV and is not suitable
     for imaging. Pyrophosphate vials for the stannous ion could be used
     either with the *in vivo* method or the modified *in vivo* method.
     UltratagRBC could be used for the *in vitro* labeling process. The reason
     for the blood pool imaging procedure is not given. If the reason is possible
     gastrointestinal bleeding, then the *in vitro* method has a higher labeling
     efficiency and should be prepared. If the reason is for evaluation of right
     and left ventricular function, than the pyrophosphate stannous ion
     in vivo method would be more efficient.
2   During the first hour following injection of ^{99m}Tc-exametazime-labeled
     white blood cells, activity is seen in the lungs, liver, spleen, blood pool,
     bone marrow, and the bladder. Bowel activity is routinely visualized by
     three to four hours and increases with time. Because of this normal bowel
     and renal clearance of ^{99m}Tc-exametazime, imaging of the abdomen
     should be performed between one and two hours after administration in
     order to avoid this background hepatobiliary and urinary clearance.
3   When preparing the kit, special attention must be paid to removal of
     nitrogen gas from vial with a vented needle and to avoid the addition of a
     concentration of technetium of greater than 30 mCi/mL. An unknown
     complex forms in compounding if the proper venting does not take place
     when adding the technetium to the kit. The unknown complex has been
     shown to have the same biodistribution and elimination as
     ^{99m}Tc-tetrofosmin but has no retention in the cardiac tissues.

Chapter 7

1   Radioactive Drug Research Committee, Investigational New Drug
     Application and, New Drug Application RDRC, IND, NDA.
2   Hydroxyephedrine, fluorocarazolol, and *meta*-iodobenzylguanidine
     (mIBG).
3   Beta-amyloid.
4   Alzheimer's disease.
5   Relative blood flow.
6   a   glucose uptake (metabolism)
     b   cell membrane synthesis
     c   nucleic acid synthesis
     d   amino acid metabolism (protein synthesis).
7   Non-specific uptake (also impaired glucose uptake such as might occur
     in diabetes).

8   Fluorine-18 fluorodeoxyglucose.
9   Hypometabolic.
10 Raclopride (used in imaging as ^{11}C-raclopride).
11 Carfentanil.

Chapter 8

1   Hepatobiliary imaging is synonymous with gallbladder imaging.
    Sincalide is used as an adjunct in gallbladder imaging. Sincalide causes
    contraction of the gallbladder, relaxation of the sphincter of Oddi,
    augmentation of pyloric sphincter tone, and enhancement of the motility
    of the small and large bowel. Sincalide is used after the
    radiopharmaceutical is administered and after the gallbladder is filled, as
    seen on the image. Regions of activity in the gallbladder are compared
    with the regions of activity after the sincalide has been administered and
    the gallbladder has contracted. The percent difference quantifies the
    gallbladder ejection fraction (EF).
2   Phenobarbital is used to differentiate neonatal hepatitis from biliary
    atresia. Phenobarbital causes elevation of drug-metabolizing enzymes
    (the phenobarbital inducer effect). The increase is seen in the CYP-
    dependent monooxygenase enxymes, of which one function is the
    metabolism of fatty acids. The increase in enzymes causes an increase in
    the absorption of bile and of calicular bile flow. The ^{99m}Tc-labeled
    iminodiacetic acid derivatives mimic the bile pharmacokinetics and
    hence are taken up and excreted in patients with patent bile ducts. In
    prolonged elevation of serum conjugated bilirubin, the clearance from
    the liver to the bile duct is sometimes difficult to see because of the
    slow clearance rate. The administration of phenobarbital ensures the
    best possible excretion of hepatobiliary agents and visualization of the
    biliary tree.
3   Labetalol is a non-selective beta-blocker and a selective alpha-1 blocker.
    Patients taking beta-blockers or calcium-channel blockers may not be
    able to exercise adequately during the stress portion of the study. A
    pharmacological test is in order for this patient. There are no
    contraindications or precautions with the angiotensin-converting enzyme
    inhibitors (benazepril) or thiazide diuretics (hydrochlorothiazide).
    Fiorinal contains 40 mg caffeine. Regadenoson effects are inhibited by
    methylxanthines such as caffeine and theophylline. Prior to a
    regadenoson study, the same measures for adenosine drug interactions
    should be followed, namely caffeine products should be withheld for
    six hours. The best course would be to reschedule the patient for the
    next day. The other pharmacological stress agents would be
    contraindicated in this patient. The actions of both adenosine and

dipyridamole are inhibited by methylxanthines, and dobutamine would not be appropriate because the labetalol would antagonize dobutamine's mechanism of action.

Chapter 9

1. a Gastric emptying, liver/spleen scan, Denver/LeVeen shunt assessment, cystogram, sentinel node study, lymphangiogram.
   b Somatostatin receptor imaging.
   c Bone pain palliation.
   d Myocardial perfusion, parathyroid scan, scintimammography.
   e CSF shunt patency, functional renal scan, ventilation lung scan (if aerosolized).
   f Whole body and three-phase bone scans.
   g Hepatobiliary scan.
2. a Ventilation and perfusion lung scans.
   b Myocardial perfusion scan, PET myocardial perfusion scan, cardiac viability scan, PET cardiac viability scan.
   c Scintimammography, sentinel node scan, bone pain palliation, PET imaging.
   d Hepatobiliary scan.
   e Adrenal medulla scan or somatostatin receptor imaging.
   f Brain metabolism PET scan.
   g Bone scan.
3. a Brain perfusion, gastric emptying, hepatobiliary assessment, gastrointestinal bleed, Meckel's diverticulum, functional renal studies, cystogram, lymphangiogram, lung ventilation with ^{133}Xe, three-phase bone scan.
   b Cisternogram, gastric emptying, LeVeen/Denver shunt, thyroid scan, parathyroid scan, adrenal medulla scan, sentinel node scan, scintimammography, perfusion scan, ventilation scan.
   c Gated cardiac blood pool.
   d Myocardial perfusion, cardiac viability, brain perfusion, liver/spleen scan, hemangioma, ^{111}In-capromab pendetide prostate cancer scan.
   e PET myocardial perfusion, PET myocardial viability, brain metabolism PET, ^{18}F-FDG PET scan, PET bone scan with ^{18}F-sodium fluoride.
4. a ^{123}I-sodium iodide, ^{131}I-sodium iodide, ^{99m}Tc-sulfur colloid for gastric emptying, ^{14}C-urea.
   b Many: refer to the Route of administration column on each procedure table in this chapter.
   c ^{111}In-DTPA.

Index